MW00791562

Training Manual for Health Care Central Service Technicians

American Society for Healthcare Central Service Professionals of the American Hospital Association

Training Manual for Health Care Central Service Technicians

Fifth Edition

JOSSEY-BASS
A Wiley Imprint
www.josseybass.com

Copyright © 2006 by John Wiley & Sons, Inc. All rights reserved.

Published by Jossey-Bass
A Wiley Imprint
989 Market Street, San Francisco, CA 94103-1741 www.josseybass.com

No part of this publication may be reproduced, stored in a retrieval system, or transmitted in any form or by any means, electronic, mechanical, photocopying, recording, scanning, or otherwise, except as permitted under Section 107 or 108 of the 1976 United States Copyright Act, without either the prior written permission of the publisher, or authorization through payment of the appropriate per-copy fee to the Copyright Clearance Center, Inc., 222 Rosewood Drive, Danvers, MA 01923, 978-750-8400, fax 978-646-8600, or on the Web at www.copyright.com. Requests to the publisher for permission should be addressed to the Permissions Department, John Wiley & Sons, Inc., 111 River Street, Hoboken, NJ 07030, 201-748-6011, fax 201-748-6008, or online at http://www.wiley.com/go/permissions.

Limit of Liability/Disclaimer of Warranty: While the publisher and author have used their best efforts in preparing this book, they make no representations or warranties with respect to the accuracy or completeness of the contents of this book and specifically disclaim any implied warranties of merchantability or fitness for a particular purpose. No warranty may be created or extended by sales representatives or written sales materials. The advice and strategies contained herein may not be suitable for your situation. You should consult with a professional where appropriate. Neither the publisher nor author shall be liable for any loss of profit or any other commercial damages, including but not limited to special, incidental, consequential, or other damages.

Jossey-Bass books and products are available through most bookstores. To contact Jossey-Bass directly call our Customer Care Department within the U.S. at 800-956-7739, outside the U.S. at 317-572-3986, or fax 317-572-4002.

Jossey-Bass also publishes its books in a variety of electronic formats. Some content that appears in print may not be available in electronic books.

Library of Congress Cataloging-in-Publication Data

Training manual for health care central service technicians / American Society
for Healthcare Central Service Professionals (ASHCSP). — 5th ed.
p. ; cm. — (Jossey-Bass/AHA Press series)
Includes bibliographical references.
ISBN-13: 978-0-7879-8244-7 (alk. paper)
ISBN-10: 0-7879-8244-X (alk. paper)
1. Hospitals—Central service department. 2. Hospitals—Staff.
I. American Society for Healthcare Central Service Professionals. II. Series.
[DNLM: 1. Central Supply, Hospital—manpower. 2. Personnel,
Hospital—education. WX 165 T768 2006]
RA975.5.C4T735 2006
362.11068'3—dc22 2005029308

Printed in the United States of America

FIFTH EDITION

PB Printing 10 9 8 7 6 5 4 3 2

Contents

Foreword to the Fifth Edition

THE FIFTH EDITION of the American Society for Healthcare Central Service Professionals' *Training Manual for Health Care Central Service Technicians* provides a broad base of necessary information for the training or self-education of entry-level staff in the central service/sterile processing profession. This manual also serves as a comprehensive resource for experienced service/sterile processing staff and other health care workers involved in the safe handling of materials and instruments. The fifth edition is an effective tool for preparing for a national certification test, whether as a technician, supervisor, or manager. The text is equally valuable whether used as a foundation for developing continuing education programs or for creating tests to measure staff competency.

The *Training Manual for Health Care Central Service Technicians* is produced independently and non-commercially by the American Society for Healthcare Central Service Professionals to support members' and health care staff's professional competency.

The first edition was published in 1985, and this edition follows three intervening editions. Much credit continues to be due to those members who created the document that has served as a foundation and guide for the editions that followed, and to those volunteers who have worked to ensure that subsequent versions of the manual have reflected the most current technology, practices, and regulations.

This edition was developed in 2004 through the combined efforts of the Education and Publication Committee members, each of whom is a leader in the central service/sterile processing community. Throughout the year these volunteers generously committed much of their personal time and energy to producing this comprehensive resource. Boundless gratitude is due this group for documenting, double-checking, and sharing their knowledge.

Special recognition goes to the 2004 Education and Publication Committee:

Pamela Caudell, RN, CNOR, CSPDS

Ernesto Gonzalez

Paul Hess, RN, BSN, CRCST

Jean Hodge, RN, CSPDT, FCSP

Nyla Japp, RN, PhD, ACSP

Mike Murphy, ACSP, CSPDT

Patricia Hooker-Nothum

Claudia Pence

Corrine Reamer

Penny Sabrosky

Robin Sandrick

Tamela Sharp

Toni M. Smith

Alice Marie Stewart

Raymond Taurasi

Carol Wicki

David Wise, CSPDT

Martha Young

Additional thanks to the individuals who served as fifth edition fact checkers, proofreaders, and editors:

Jean Hodge, RN, CSPDT, FCSP
Michael Murphy, ACSP

Dorothea Conroy, RN, BS, ACSP, CSPDM
Education and Publications Committee Chair

Foreword to the Fourth Edition

THE FOURTH EDITION of the *Training Manual for Central Service Technicians* was developed in 2001 by a national committee of leaders in the central service and sterile processing profession (CS/SPD). The committee wishes to note, however, that the book reflects the wisdom and practical knowledge of leaders who have contributed over the last sixteen years as well. Originally developed in 1985, the *Training Manual for Central Service Technicians* has proven to be a valuable resource for central service managers, educators, and technicians. It is a concise, applicable tool that can be used for orientation, training, and instructional programs in health care facilities and in institutions for learning. Designed to help both those who are taking a formal class and those who are studying on their own, the fourth edition of the manual provides students with current regulations, techniques, and trends in the central service/sterile processing profession.

CS/SPD is a dynamic field: information and technology are constantly changing. Regular updates on regulations and procedural innovations are crucial for keeping those working in this field abreast of changes and for building and maintaining an efficient, safe work environment. While this text can be used as a guide, each individual central service manager develops the policies and procedures appropriate for his or her facility, given its particular resources and complex needs.

The *Training Manual for Central Service Technicians,* Fourth Edition, is an independent, non-commercial effort. Any reference to manufacturers or their products should not be construed as an endorsement by ASHCSP or the American Hospital Association.

ASHCSP is grateful for the considerable amount of time and effort given by all who participated in the development and review of this publication and for the contributions of those who worked on previous editions. The central service personnel and other health care professionals who have contributed to this book represent a diversity of experience and expertise that ensures a comprehensive approach to the subject matter.

Special thanks and recognition go to the following:

The 2001 ASHCSP Fourth Edition Training Manual Review Committee: Nancy Chobin, RN, CSPDM; Dorothea Conroy, RN, ACSP; Jean Hodge, RN, CSPDT, FCSP; Sue McManus, RN; Michael Murphy, ACSP; and Linda Petty, RN, CNOR

Patti Costello, Executive Director

Catherine Futrell, Committee Liaison

And to the following individuals who helped complete this publication:

Cathy Bickerstaff, RN, CSPDM; Randy Corn; Clare Daly; Rose Seavey, RN, CNOR, ACSP; Frank Sizemore, ACSP; and Francis Vincent

ASHCSP would also like to recognize the individuals and organizations that contributed to the first three editions:

Paula Adams

Betty L. Andersen

Betty Baker

G. Edward Becker

Sara Beddow

Harley D. Berlant

Judith Borland, RN

Veronica Brundage

Walter E. Bruso, RN

Mary Virginia Bunting, RN

Terry Burnett

Nancy Chobin, RN

Jerry L. Cleveland

Mary Linda Cole

Randall L. Corn

Carol Freudenstein

Ernesto Gonzales

Jean Haywood

Caryl Hebert, RN

G. Sue Henderson, RN

Jean Hodge, RN, CSPDT, FCSP
Cynthia A. Hunstiger, RN
Nyla Japp, RN, PhD., ACSP
Miriam Kalmbach, RN
Rose Lohmann
Carol Meosching
Cindy Molko
Reny E. Moses
Marimargaret Reichert, RN
Carol Reilly
Mary Eleanor Reilly, RN
Glenn A. Runnels, RN
Janet K. Schultz, RN
Al Schutta
Catherine A. Sisk
Frank Sizemore
Sally Smith
Terri Stoner
Donna Swenson
Jo Taylor, RN
Therese Taylor
Harriet Thorsfeldt, RN
Joseph B. VanDerwerken
Judith A. Veale
Ursula Carda Webb
Guinevere Wilson
Eva M. Zazo, RN
The Central Service/Central Supply staff of Shriner's Hospital for Crippled Children in Chicago
Evanston Hospital in Evanston, Illinois

Michael C. Murphy, ACSP
Publications Committee Chairman

Foreword to the Third Edition

CENTRAL SERVICE EMPLOYEES are responsible for many tasks within the department, depending on its size and the services provided by the health care facility. Services that are not provided today may, in fact, be implemented in the near future due to redesign and right-sizing. ASHCSP, in its effort to keep central service technicians aware of their present and future responsibilities, felt it necessary to update the second edition of the *Training Manual for Central Service Technicians.* The third edition of this manual does just that. Filled with new and innovative information, the revised 1997 edition will be an effective tool for years to come.

The *Training Manual for Central Service Technicians* is an introductory text developed to acquaint entry-level aides and technicians with the scope of the central service profession and with the scientific principles that underlie their daily work. The American Society for Healthcare Central Service Professionals (ASHCSP) intends this manual to serve as a powerful tool for today's central service technician. With revised and updated chapters on anatomy and physiology, microbiology and infection control, decontamination, instrumentation, sterilization, storage, distribution, and inventory control, this manual provides students with the knowledge needed to become efficient, safe, and informed in their work.

Designed to help both those who are taking a formal class or for those who have decided to study on their own, the third edition of the *Training Manual for Central Service Technicians* provides students with current trends, regulations, and techniques.

It is important, however, that users do not restrict learning to the information contained in the manual. It is imperative, in this era of change, that all members of the health care profession keep abreast of changes and developments in their field. Use this manual as a primary resource but remember to supplement studies with other sources when available.

In today's health care environment, knowledgeable employees are essential for the safe and effective delivery of patient care.

Thanks and recognition are due to all those involved in this third edition of the *Training Manual for Central Service Technicians.* Because of these individuals' hard work and often time-consuming effort, central service technicians of the present and of the future are better equipped to deal with their fast-paced and everchanging profession.

Special thanks, for their review and contributions to the third edition of the *Training Manual for Central Service Technicians,* are due the following:

Jean Hodge, RN
Material Services Education Coordinator/Infection Control Practitioner
Meriter Hospital
Madison, WI

Nancy Chobin, RN
Medical Center Educational Services
Saint Barnabus Medical Center
Livingston, NJ

Nyla Japp
Director of Infection Control Services
St. Catherine Hospital
Garden City, KS

Miriam Kalmbach, RN
Director, Central Services
Scott and White Hospital
Temple, TX

Eleanor Reilly, RN
Director, Central Services
The Cleveland Clinic Hospital
Cleveland, OH

Frank Sizemore
Manager, Central Service
North Carolina Baptist Hospital, Inc.
Winston-Salem, NC

Sally Smith
Director, Patient Care Services
Deckerville Community Hospital
Deckerville, MI

Without their help, this revised 1997 edition would not have been possible.

Dennis Moore
1996 ASHCSP President

Foreword to the Second Edition

HEALTH CARE IS in an unprecedented state of upheaval and change. Managed care, national health coverage, reengineering or "right-sizing," CQI, and functional work teams are some of the forces having an impact on health care. Add new sterilant alternatives, off-site processing, changing regulations, and an increase in reusable items—it's easy to see how central service/SPD departments feel pressured! However, one constant is the need to provide a good, strong knowledge base and continuing education for staff. The *Training Manual for Central Service Technicians* provides the basics necessary for such a program.

In creating the second edition of this book, the intent of the Research and Development Committee of the American Society for Healthcare Central Service Personnel was to

- Retain the original work whenever possible
- Revise when necessary due to changing regulations, written recommended practices, or established standards
- Enhance the usability for technicians by

  In the chapter on anatomy and physiology, adding representative CS supplies and equipment for each organ system

  Reorganizing material in Chapters Four, Five, Six, and Seven

  Adding a primer on roots of medical terminology

Special thanks and recognition are due the following:

Research and Development Committee

Caryl Hebert, R.N.
Director, SPD
St. Frances Cabrini Hospital
Alexandria, LA

Donna Swenson
Manager, Central Supply
Evanston Hospital
Evanston, IL

PRIMARY REVIEW GROUP

Nancy Chobin, R.N.
Assistant Director, Materials Management
St. Barnabas Hospital
Livingston, NJ

Marimargaret Reichert, R.N.
Olmsted Falls, OH

Mary Eleanor Reilly, R.N.
Director, Central Service
Cleveland Clinic Hospital
Cleveland, OH

Additional thanks to

G. Edward Becker
Microsystems, Inc.
Milwaukee, WI

Reny Moses
Director, Supply Processing and Distribution
Mid-Maine Medical Center
Waterville, ME

Al Schutta
Director, Central Service/Materials Management
HealthEast St. Joseph's Hospital
St. Paul, MN

Ernesto Gonzales
Director, Central Service/Materials Management
HealthEast St. John's Hospital
Maplewood, MN

Eva M. Zazo, R.N.
Coordinator, Central Service
St. Luke's Hospital
Saginaw, MI

Rose Lohmann
Minneapolis, MN

Cindy Molko
Supervisor, Central Service
St. Mary's Hospital
Rochester, MN

Photography Services Division
Audio/Visual Department
Evanston Hospital
Evanston, IL

Also, the Staffs of the Central Services and Central Supply Departments of

Shriner's Hospital for Crippled Children
Chicago, IL

Evanston Hospital
Evanston, IL

Without their help, this first complete revision would not have been possible.

October 1993

Catherine A. Sisk
Chairman, Research and Development Committee
Children's Hospital and Medical Center, Seattle

Foreword to the First Edition

TRAINING MANUAL FOR CENTRAL SERVICE TECHNICIANS is an introductory text developed to acquaint entry-level aides and technicians with the scope of the central service profession and with the scientific principles that underlie their daily work. The American Society for Hospital Central Service Personnel (ASHCSP) intends the manual to serve as the core of the ASHCSP technician training program, the development of which was undertaken at the long-standing request of the society membership. The other two elements of the program materials, to be available in 1987, are a student workbook and an instructor's guide. The manual is also intended to serve as a concise, practical resource tool that can be used by central service managers and educators in their own orientation, training, and instructional programs. To provide additional information on ethylene oxide for a more comprehensive training program, *Ethylene Oxide Use in Hospitals: A Manual for Health Care Personnel* (AHA catalog no. 031826) is recommended.

The manual is not intended to define criteria for optimum performance of central service responsibilities. This purpose is served by the ASHCSP *Recommended Practices for Central Service.* The manual does not spell out detailed methodologies and procedures for specific central service functions. It remains the task of each central service manager to develop policies and procedures that are best suited to the resources and complex needs of his or her institution.

This manual is a committee effort that brings into one book practical information from all parts of the country. The central service personnel and other health care professionals who contributed to this book represent a diversity of experience and interest that ensures a well-rounded effort. However, participation by these individuals and their institutions or agencies in the development of this manual does not constitute endorsement by the individuals, institutions, or agencies. This manual is published with the understanding that neither the committee nor the committee members assume responsibility for any inadvertent misinformation, omissions, or results due to the use of this manual. In addition, any reference to manufacturers or their products cannot be construed as an endorsement by ASHCSP or the American Hospital Association.

The society is grateful for the time and effort contributed by those who participated in the development and review of this manual. In particular, special thanks and recognition are due the following:

Jerry L. Cleveland (director, central service, St. Luke's Hospital, Cedar Rapids, IA): 1985 ASHCSP president and principal project director

Randall L. Corn (director, supply, processing, and distribution, St. Joseph's Hospital, Tucson, AZ), 1986 ASHCSP president: gathered the original resource materials, principal contributor to initial drafts of the manual

G. Sue Henderson, R.N. (assistant manager, central service, Wesley Medical Center, Wichita, KS), 1984 ASHCSP president: facilitated progress on the project as president, principal reviewer of the final text

Cynthia A. Hunstiger, R.N. (director, central service, Saint Mary's Hospital of Rochester, MN), 1985 ASHCSP board of directors: principal reviewer of the final text

Marimargaret Reichert, R.N. (director, central service, Robinson Memorial Hospital, Ravenna, OH): illustrator (see Illustration Credits), principal reviewer of the final text

Glenn A. Runnells, R.N. (specialist, O.R. Aseptic Practice, Superior Surgical Mfg. Co., Inc., Seminole, FL): principal reviewer of the final text

Janet K. Schultz, R.N. (manager for OR systems, American V. Mueller, Chicago, IL): contributed Chapter Five, principal reviewer, technical editor for the final text

Therese Taylor (central sterile reprocessing supervisor, Robinson Memorial Hospital, Ravenna, OH): illustrator (see Illustration Credits)

Harriet Thorsfeldt, R.N. (director, materials management, Holladay Park Medical Center, Portland, OR), 1985 chair, ASHCSP Research and Development Committee: supervised the project, principal reviewer of the final text

Judith A. Veale (JV Biomedical Consultants, Rehoboth, MA); edited the original contributions, coordinated the final development and revision of the text

The society also wishes to gratefully acknowledge the resource material, suggestions, and helpful criticisms contributed by the following project participants:

Paula Adams (director, materials management, Huron Valley Hospital, Detroit, MI)

Betty L. Andersen (central service supervisor, Queen of the Valley Hospital, Napa, CA)

Betty Baker (retired manager, central processing and distribution, Lansing General Hospital, Lansing, MI)

Sara Beddow (supervisor, central supply, Memorial Hospital, Colorado Springs, CO)

Harley D. Berlant (assistant director, materials management, St. Sinai Medical Center, Miami Beach, FL)

Judith Borland, R.N. (manager, central service, Smyrna Hospital, Smyrna, GA)

Veronica Brundage (clinical specialist, GeriCare, Passaic, NJ)

Walter E. Bruso, R.N. (health occupation supervisor, Clover Park Vocational Technical, Tacoma, WA)

Mary Virginia Bunting, R.N. (director, supply, processing, and distribution, St. Francis Medical Center, Trenton, NJ)

Terry Burnett (Herman Miller Company, San Francisco, CA)

Mary Linda Cole (central service consultant, Criticare of Oregon, Portland, OR)

Carol Freudenstein (orientation and continuing education supervisor, central service, Saint Mary's Hospital of Rochester, Rochester, MN)

Jean Haywood (chief, supply, processing and distribution, U.S. Veterans Administration Medical Center, Tucson, AZ)

Carol Moesching (manager, central service, Community Hospital of San Gabriel, San Gabriel, CA)

Reny E. Moses (director, supply processing, and distribution, Mid-Maine Medical Center, Waterville, ME); member, 1985 ASHCSP board of directors

Carol Reilly (director, central service, Long Island Jewish Hospital, Hillside Division, New Hyde Park, NY)

Terri Stoner (manager, central sterilizing, University of Iowa Hospitals and Clinics, Iowa City, IA)

Jo Taylor, R.N. (director, central supply, St. Luke's Regional Medical Center, Boise, ID); member, 1985 ASHCSP board of directors

Joseph B. VanDerwerken (director, central service, Glens Falls Hospital, Glens Falls, NY); member, 1985 ASHCSP board of directors

Ursula Carda Webb (director, materials management, Bannock Regional Medical Center, Pocatello, ID)

Guinevere Wilson (manager, central service, Cook County Hospital, Chicago, IL); member, 1985 ASHCSP board of directors

The project was guided by Clarence Daly, executive director, ASHCSP, under the supervision of Edward Bertz, director, Personal Membership. Editorial and production support was provided by Christie Enman and Karen Bennett, AHA Division of Marketing Services.

The society very much appreciates the cooperation of the American Sterilizer Company, American V. Mueller, Ethicon, Inc., and the Association for the Advancement of Medical Instrumentation, in contributing illustrations for the text (see Illustration Credits), and of AMMA, Inc., in contributing Appendix A, Central Service Terminology.

October 1985

Jerry L. Cleveland
President, American Society for Hospital Central Service Personnel

Illustration Credits

Except as noted below, all photographs and line drawings were contributed by Marimargaret Reichert, R.N., and Theresa Taylor, Robinson Memorial Hospital, Ravenna, OH. Figures 2.1 through 2.10 were reprinted, with the permission of the publisher, from *The Human Body*, copyright 1986 by Ethicon, Inc., Somerville, NJ. Figure 4.6 was provided courtesy of the American Sterilizer Company, Erie, PA. Figures 5.4 and 5.5 were reprinted, with the permission of the publisher, from *Care and Handling of Surgical Instruments,* copyright 1980 by American Hospital Supply Corporation, Evanston, IL. Figures 6.4, 6.6, 7.3, and 7.7 were reprinted, with the permission of the publisher, from *Good Hospital Practice: Steam Sterilization and Sterility Assurance*, copyright 1980 by the Association for the Advancement of Medical Instrumentation, Arlington, VA. The photographs at the beginning of each chapter were provided courtesy of St. Luke's Hospital, Cedar Rapids, IA. The cover photograph is reprinted, with permission, from the *Journal of Hospital Supply, Processing, and Distribution,* September 1983.

Training Manual for Health Care Central Service Technicians

Chapter 1

Introduction to Central Service

EDUCATIONAL OBJECTIVES

At the completion of this assignment, the student will be able to

- Describe the historical development of the central service department (CSD) within health care
- Describe the organizational structure and objectives of the CSD
- List the five major functional areas of a typical CSD
- Describe the basic functions of each CSD area
- Define the ethical responsibilities of the central service technician
- List the categories of hazards associated with work in the CSD
- List the means of preventing safety hazards
- Describe proper attire to be worn in the CSD (how it varies within the department) and the importance of personal cleanliness
- State the purpose and outline of the continuous quality improvement process
- List agencies involved with the development of standards and their application to the CSD
- Define and give reasons for work flow, people flow, and airflow patterns
- Demonstrate an understanding of the purpose of a procedure manual and be able to differentiate between policies and procedures
- Describe the relationship between CSD functions and written policies and procedures
- Describe the four types of communication
- List basic rules for telephone communications
- Define medical terminology

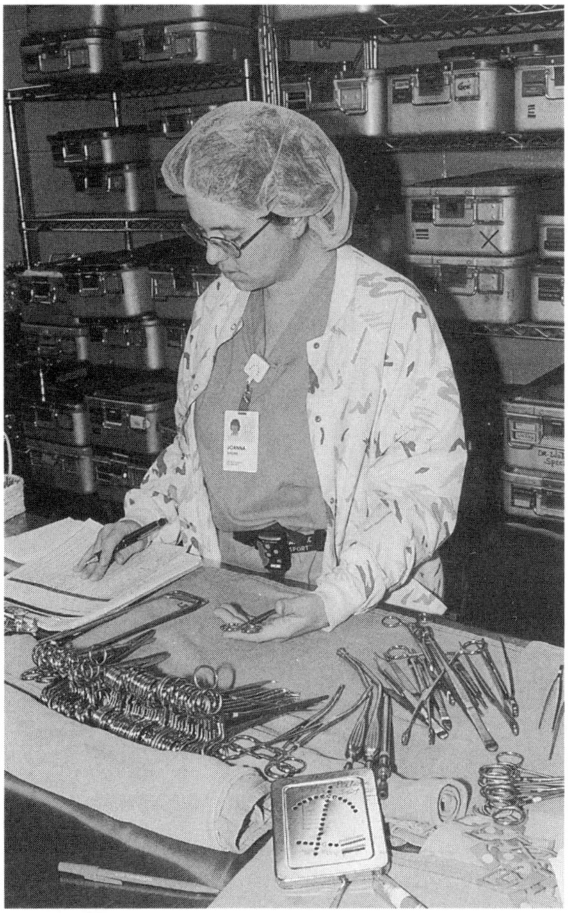

THE CENTRAL SERVICE DEPARTMENT (CSD) is the department within a health care facility in which medical/surgical supplies and equipment, both sterile and nonsterile, are cleaned, prepared, processed, sterilized, stored, and issued for patient care.

Until the 1940s, medical/surgical supplies were, for the most part, processed and maintained in the departments and patient care areas in which they were to be used. Under this system, there was considerable duplication of effort and equipment, and it was difficult to maintain consistently high standards of sterilization technique and product quality throughout the health care facility. Sterilization processing was "everybody's business but no one's responsibility" (Perkins, 1983).

As the number and variety of surgical procedures grew and the types of medical devices, equipment, and supplies proliferated, it became apparent that centralized processing was needed for efficiency, economy, and patient safety. The work of scientists W. B. Underwood and John J. Perkins was instrumental in encouraging health care facilities to establish a separate and distinct department, the central service department, with specialized expertise and direct responsibility for providing clean and sterile medical/surgical supplies and equipment to patient care areas.

This chapter provides an overview of the organizational structure, objectives, and functions of the CSD and an introduction to the responsibilities of CSD technicians.

Organizational Structure

The health care field of sterile processing and distribution has commonly been known as either *central service* or *central supply,* although neither of these names accurately reflects the functions or duties of the people who work in this field. A number of other names are also used to refer to the department that performs these functions. Among these names are central processing, central sterile, supply processing and distribution, and sterile processing and distribution. Whatever the department is called, the functions performed by the staff include the following: (1) cleaning, decontamination, processing (inspection, assembling, and packaging), and sterilization of reusable patient care supplies and equipment, and (2) distribution of these supplies and equipment to the units that use them.

Other logistical services may also be part of the CSD, such as mailroom, linen, and patient transport. Regardless of how the department is structured, any or all of these functions may be included in the services provided. Some of these functions may be performed by other departments.

Not only are the functions performed by the central service department different from one health care facility to another, but the organizational reporting structure varies also. For example, in many facilities the CSD reports to materials management, in others it reports to surgery, and in still others, to fiscal services, nursing, pharmacy, infection control, or administration. Some facilities have the cleaning, decontamination, processing, and sterilization functions report to one department and distribution to another department.

Every health care facility is organized into divisions and departments, each with a defined scope of activities and an organizational structure of its own. Managers are placed in charge of each of the departments, and their authority relationships are defined. Figure 1.1 shows one type of organizational structure for a health care facility. Figure 1.2 shows an example of an organizational structure for a large CSD.

Objectives and Functions

In general, central service provides the health care facility with services in the areas of supply processing and distribution. The distribution area is responsible for the delivery of supplies to designated customers. The decontamination processing areas are responsible for the cleaning, decontamination, inspection, assembly, packaging, and sterilization of all reusable patient care equipment and supplies. Sterile and nonsterile items must be separated and placed in defined and separate storage areas. This will help avoid confusion as to the items' sterile status.

The objectives of central service include the following:

- Provide inventoried supplies and equipment to customer areas
- Promote better patient care by providing prompt, accurate service
- Provide supplies of sterile linen packs, basins, instruments, trays, and other sterile items
- Maintain an accurate record of the effectiveness of the cleaning, disinfecting, and sterilizing processes
- Strive for uniformity and simplicity in the trays and sets that the department provides

- Maintain an adequate inventory of supplies and equipment
- Monitor and enforce controls necessary to prevent cross-infection according to infection control policies
- Establish and maintain sterile processing and distribution standards
- Operate efficiently to reduce overhead expense
- Stay abreast of developments in the field and to implement changes as needed to stay current with new regulations and recommended practices
- Review current practice for possible improvements in quality or services provided
- Provide consulting services to other departments in all areas of sterile processing and distribution, including in-service education programs, review of policies and procedures, and implementation of new processes

Other objectives may be included depending on the scope of the services provided by the individual department.

Major Areas in Central Service

The CSD is usually divided into five major areas: decontamination, processing (inspection, assembly, and packaging), sterilizing, sterile storage, and distribution.

Decontamination is the area where reusable patient care equipment and supplies are cleaned and rendered safe to handle. This can be done manually or with mechanical equipment depending on the item being decontaminated and the resources of the department. Whether manual or mechanical means are used, chemical detergents and disinfectants will be utilized as part of the process.

Processing is the area where decontaminated or clean supplies, instruments, and trays are prepared for additional processing, storage, or distribution. There may be a linen room where packs of reusable linen are folded, assembled, and packaged. This is normally separate from the processing areas because of the large amount of lint that is generated. Lint can act as a vehicle for the movement of microorganisms, and can invade a patient wound and cause the body to attack it as a foreign object. Both of these possibilities can cause an infection to develop. For this reason the amount of lint (and other dust) must be minimized in the processing area. In addition to a linen room, many CSDs have an assembly area for house trays as well as single packaged items. Larger central service departments process operating room instruments through their CSD. Many CSDs also process reusable RT and anesthesia equipment. Clinics and other hospitals sometimes share processing services with one CSD to centralize processing and reduce costs.

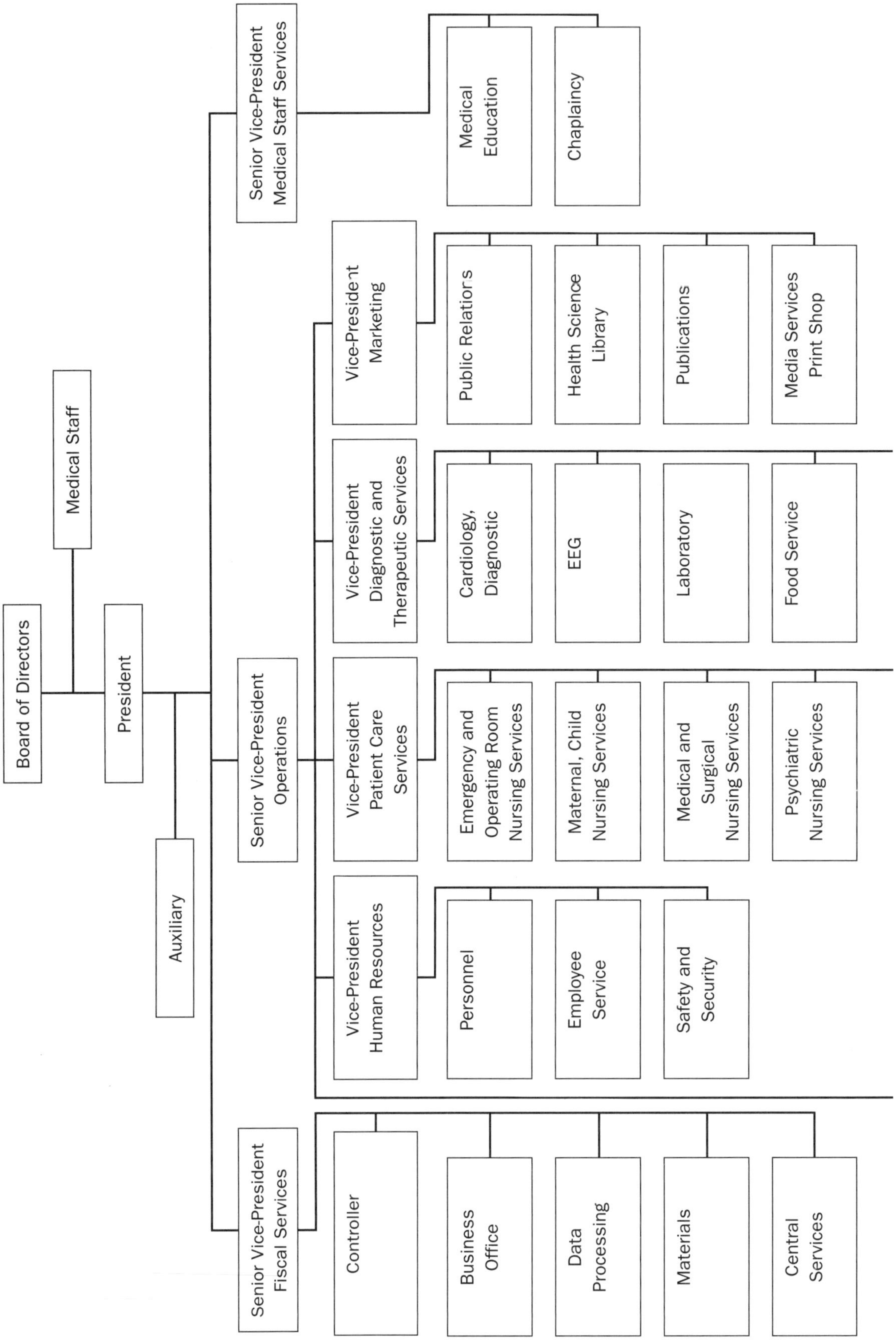
Board of Directors
Medical Staff
President
Auxiliary
Senior Vice-President Fiscal Services
Senior Vice-President Operations
Senior Vice-President Medical Staff Services
Controller
Business Office
Data Processing
Materials
Central Services
Vice-President Human Resources
Vice-President Patient Care Services
Vice-President Diagnostic and Therapeutic Services
Vice-President Marketing
Personnel
Employee Service
Safety and Security
Emergency and Operating Room Nursing Services
Maternal, Child Nursing Services
Medical and Surgical Nursing Services
Psychiatric Nursing Services
Cardiology, Diagnostic
EEG
Laboratory
Food Service
Public Relations
Health Science Library
Publications
Media Services Print Shop
Medical Education
Chaplaincy

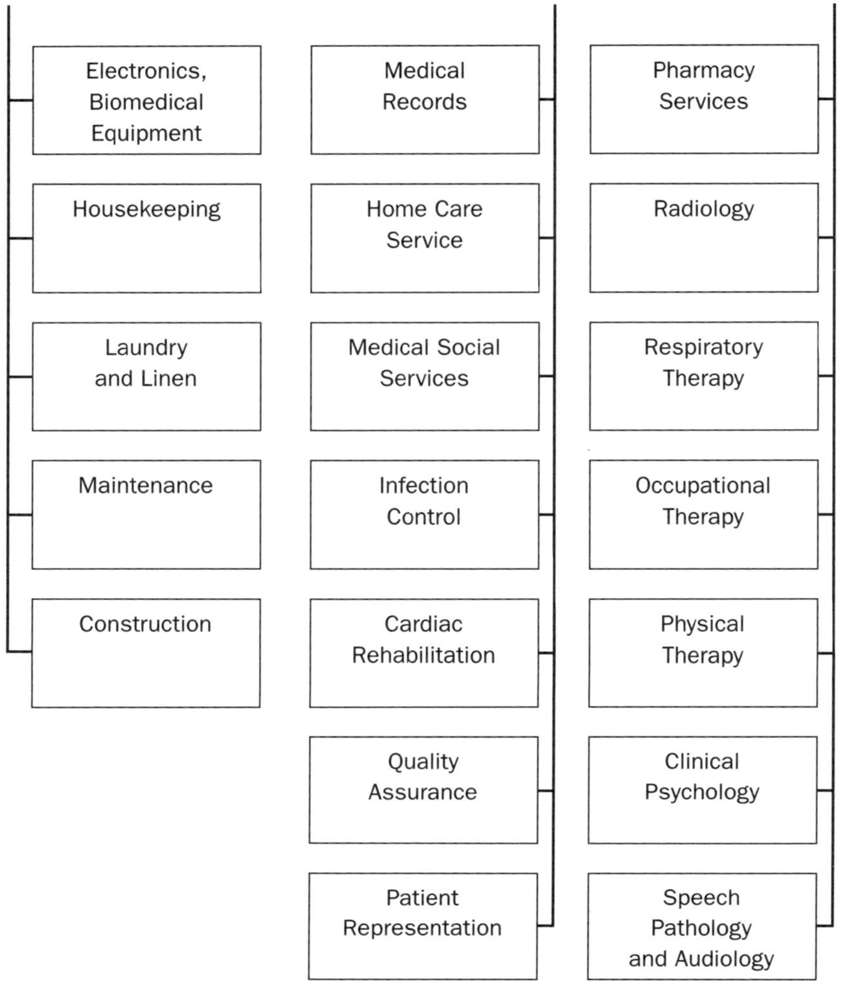

Figure 1.1. Example of an Organizational Structure for a Health Care Facility.

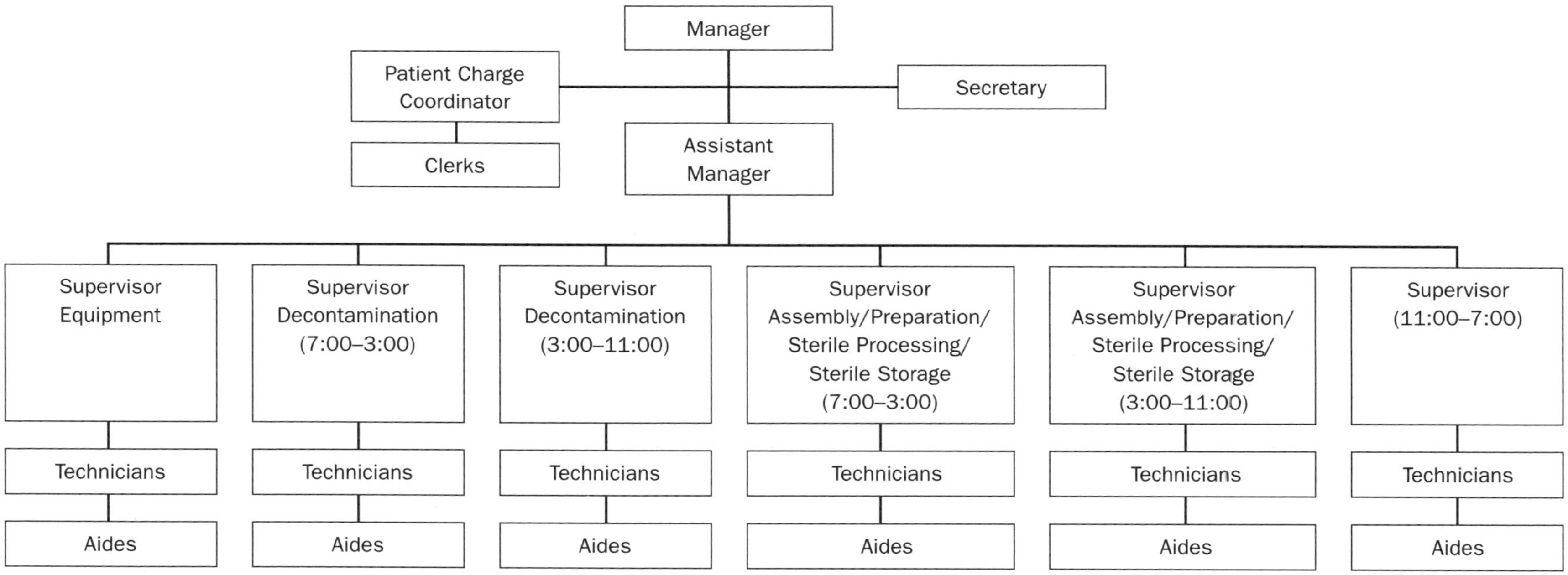

Figure 1.2. Example of an Organizational Structure for a Large CSD.

The sterilizer area of the CSD is where packaged items are subjected to a process that destroys all microorganisms. This can be accomplished through a number of different methods, but most commonly through steam, ethylene oxide (EtO), gas plasma (Sterrad), or peracetic acid (Steris) sterilization. Other means of sterilization include dry heat and liquid chemicals (e.g., 2 percent glutaraldehyde).

Sterile storage is the area of the CSD where items are stored until distributed for use. There may be a separate area for the storage of clean, nonsterile items. The entire storage area must be subject to the principles of sterile storage. These principles include controlled temperature and humidity, limited traffic, ventilation requirements, and mechanisms that ensure that the environment remains as clean and dust-free as possible. Many times sterile trays are stored in this area until needed for surgery. Sterile storage is detailed in Chapter Eight.

Several major CSD functions are performed in the distribution area, including the preparation and delivery of exchange carts, case carts, orders, patient care equipment, and linens. In addition, CSD technicians are often responsible for replenishing stock (par level) of frequently used supplies on patient care units.

The CSD staff members are responsible for furthering the objectives of the department, while performing functions in a timely and conscientious manner and maintaining high standards of ethics, safety, and cleanliness. They must comply with all departmental rules and regulations.

Ethics

In the normal course of their duties, CSD personnel often have access to patient information and have a responsibility to keep all such information confidential. Only the information necessary to perform CSD functions should be discussed within the health care facility, and patient information should never be communicated outside the institution. Not only do patients have a right to privacy, but also inappropriate discussions concerning patients may be overheard and misinterpreted by visitors, patient relatives, or other staff members.

Information or rumors regarding employees and physicians must also be considered confidential. Employees having tests or procedures have the same right to privacy as other patients. Inappropriate discussions concerning employees and physicians may be overheard and misinterpreted.

Central service department staff members have access to many items useful in the home. Just as shoplifting from department stores ultimately increases prices for all consumers, taking these supplies for personal use drives up costs. This action constitutes theft.

All tasks should be performed according to established procedures. Taking shortcuts or breaking protocol may appear to save time; however, supplies may not be prepared correctly and may not be usable. Not following established procedures may also have serious consequences that jeopardize the safety of both patients and staff. Additional time and money may be needed to correct errors or treat injuries resulting from improper work performance. So please check with a supervisor before attempting to make a change.

Safety

Safety is a major concern of the CSD. The primary areas of safety hazards include environmental, electrical, mechanical, chemical, biological, fire, and physical. The work performed in the CSD is complex and requires attention to detail to avoid injury to both patients and employees. Most workplace injuries and accidents are caused by neglect, carelessness, thoughtlessness, or a lack of understanding of the principles of safety. Safety is every employee's responsibility. An understanding and application of basic safety standards will enable the employee to ensure that injuries, accidents, and damage are kept to a minimum.

Environmental Hazards

Workers may suffer cuts or "sticks" from needles, scalpels, other sharp instruments, and glassware in the decontamination area. At *all* times, be alert for these hazards and never reach into any liquid to retrieve items. Always use a forceps or other grasping tool to retrieve items immersed in liquid. The floor may be wet and slippery and can cause falls. Soiled, reusable medical/surgical items are considered to be contaminated with bacteria and other microorganisms, which can cause illness to the staff. Wearing the proper protective equipment as described in Chapter Four helps to prevent this from happening. In the processing and sterilization areas, personnel can be burned when operating steam sterilizers or heat sealers. Be aware that many areas of a steam sterilizer are hot. Use insulated gloves to move carriages and know where hot areas are located on your sterilizers. Employees can be exposed to high levels of EtO. EtO is a known carcinogen and a possible mutagen, but when used properly prevents employee infection. Receiving staff have to contend with heavy boxes, splinters, and large carts, which require the use of proper body mechanics and ergonomically correct equipment. Distribution technicians work with elevators and lifts, bulky patient care equipment, and traction apparatus. All these items pose potential safety problems and require careful, precise use and handling. If workers follow protocols as defined by their department's policies and procedures, these environmental concerns can be minimized. If you have any concerns, be sure to ask your department manager how you can best be protected.

It is important to keep the workplace clean and free of clutter. Work surfaces and equipment must be cleaned and disinfected routinely to retard the growth of microorganisms. Clutter provides fuel for fires and a breeding ground for insects, vermin, and the microorganisms they carry. Passageways must be kept free of boxes and carts, both to prevent injuries and to keep escape routes open in the event of fire or other emergencies. In a health care facility, escape routes must not only accommodate people, but also large transport vehicles such as stretchers and carts. A separate breakout or decasing area should be maintained to hold deliveries until the exterior shipping cartons can be opened and the contents removed in a safe and controlled manner. Exterior shipping cartons have been exposed to many environments (in warehouses, on docks, in trucks), are usually made of corrugated porous material, and must be considered heavily contaminated and should not be brought into the CSD. These procedures all serve to minimize contamination and prevent accidents.

If workers follow the proper protocol as set up by their department these environmental concerns can be minimized. Be sure to ask your department manager how you are protected if you have any concerns.

Electrical Hazards

All electrical devices should be inspected upon arrival in the health care facility to ensure proper grounding and electrical safety, including electrical devices for personal use such as radios, if permitted in the workplace. Routine preventive maintenance of equipment is essential. The health care facility's biomedical or plant engineering staff usually perform these tasks. All maintenance and repairs of equipment issued by the CSD and used in the CSD should be documented and records maintained.

Electrical cords should be kept behind equipment and away from walkways so that personnel will not trip on them. Extension cords should never be used. All cords should have a grounded, three-prong, hospital-grade plug. If a cord is cracked or cut, it must be replaced. Water should never be allowed to collect near an electrical outlet.

For other electrical safety rules, the facility's safety regulations can be consulted.

Mechanical Hazards

Equipment operational safety is very important in the CSD. Large, automated pieces of equipment are used, including several types of washer/decontaminators, ultrasonic washers, scope washers, and sterilizers. To prevent injury (and to avoid damaging expensive equipment), CSD staff must understand and practice the proper operating procedure for each piece of equipment. The equipment manufacturers' written operation and maintenance procedures must be reviewed and followed. As with all in-service education conducted in the department, training on equipment operation should be documented and maintained in each employee's file in the CSD.

Chemical Hazards

A number of hazardous chemicals are used in the decontamination area of the CSD, including detergents, disinfectants, drying agents, and sterilants. During all preparation of cleaning solution, cleaning, and processing procedures, employees must wear gloves to protect their skin. Eye protection should be worn whenever there is potential for splashing and when specified in departmental procedures. Prior to working with or being around these chemicals, each employee must have training on the use and hazards of each chemical. This training is for the employees' safety.

A material safety data sheet (MSDS) for each chemical used must be readily available in the work area. Manufacturers are required to supply users with MSDSs. It is the responsibility of the manager to make sure that employees have access to the MSDS information. The MSDS contains information including hazards, exposure limits, recommended personal protective equipment (PPE), first-aid measures, disposal, and directions for leak or spill situations. Hazards of the chemicals used in the department and use of MSDSs must be a part of the training process, and documentation of this process must be placed into each employee's file.

Biological Hazards

Supplies and equipment arriving in the decontamination area must *all* be considered contaminated with microorganisms that may be pathogenic (disease-producing). Adherence to the department's policy on PPE and correct handling of these items prevents the spread of infection from one person to another. Central service department technicians can also protect themselves from infection by proper attention to their own general health, including proper nutrition and adequate rest. Proper handwashing is one of the keys to preventing infections in the hospital, and is described in detail in Chapter Three.

Fire Hazards

Every employee must comply with the fire safety rules of the CSD and the health care facility. Employees should participate in scheduled safety programs and fire drills and know the proper procedures to follow in the event of a fire. Important considerations include how to respond to a fire you discover, the locations and use of fire alarms and extinguishers, whom to call, and escape routes and exits.

A CSD technician who discovers a fire should get people out of immediate danger, activate the fire alarm, and contact the proper authorities. If feasible, and if staff are trained in fire-fighting procedures, measures may be taken to fight the fire; otherwise, everyone should be evacuated from the immediate area and the doors closed to contain the fire. Most health care facilities have fire doors that close automatically when any type of fire or smoke detection alarm is activated. The doors close to contain the smoke or fire. CSD technicians should know what procedures should be followed if closed fire doors are encountered while supplies are being distributed. Nothing should be stored by the fire doors that would prevent the doors from closing properly. Hallways should always remain clear so that staff can exit without tripping or falling over items in the event of a fire.

Physical Hazards

All CSD technicians should learn and use good body mechanics, including the correct techniques and postures for lifting, pushing, pulling, and reaching. This is especially necessary when moving heavy, bulky, or difficult-to-handle objects such as large carts, heavy trays, or equipment.

CSD technicians should be alert to, and try to correct, any conditions in the work environment that could contribute to injuries. Safe conditions include carts and lifts available to move heavy supplies, work materials within easy access, adjustable chairs, padding for sharp edges and hard surfaces, and tables or desks set at the correct height for easy access to work. Tasks or job assignments should be alternated to avoid repetitive motions and repeated forceful exertions, which can contribute to work-related injuries.

Proper attire can also prevent physical injury. Closed-toe shoes help prevent needle sticks and smashed toes. Open-heel shoes, such as clogs, can be hazardous, especially on wet floors. Loose-fitting clothing and jewelry can get caught in moving equipment and thus should not be worn.

Incident Reports

All accidents and injuries should be reported to a supervisor immediately. At most health care facilities, it is the policy to require an incident report detailing how the accident happened, where and when it occurred, any witnesses to the accident, what medical treatment was necessary, and whether there was any work time lost due to the accident. A description of corrective actions taken to prevent a recurrence of the accident is also required, either in the incident report or in separate documentation.

The incident report is needed for insurance and worker's compensation purposes. This report and ensuing investigation can lead to increased workplace safety by improving procedures, changing environmental design, or correcting identified problems. For example, incidents of skin irritation may indicate that cleaning materials have not been mixed, diluted, or used correctly. Shocks or burns can result from faulty electrical equipment, mishandling of devices, or improper operation of sterilization units. Employees can suffer bruises and strains as a result of using incorrect body mechanics for moving objects or heavy lifting. Falls can result from wet, slippery, or cluttered floors. The investigation of the incident may reveal work practices that need improvement.

Disaster Plans

All health care facilities have internal and external disaster plans. Every employee must understand his or her role in each type of disaster and be able to recognize the various codes that are used to designate the kind of emergency (such as fire, EtO spill, telephone system failure, bomb threat, flood, tornado, earthquake, chemical warfare, biological warfare, or power outage). When the emergency involves substantial numbers of incoming patients (external disaster), the CSD staff are often called on to deliver large amounts of supplies to the triage area. Instead of the word *disaster,* some facilities are using the words *potential injury-creating event* (PICE).

Personal Cleanliness

Personal cleanliness is essential in order to reduce transmission of microorganisms to supplies, patients, and other persons. Personal hygiene, good handwashing technique, and cleanliness of hair and clothing all can help to reduce the spread of infection-causing microorganisms. **Handwashing, in particular, is the single most important method of preventing cross-contamination.**

Proper attire in the CSD also reduces the transfer of microorganisms into or out of the department. Every health care facility has its own policy on attire. In general, CSD personnel are required to wear scrub suits or uniforms, which are provided, laundered, and issued by the health care facility. Laundering by the institution reduces the risk of personnel carrying microorganisms from the home to the workplace and vice versa. Employees generally wear hair coverings, and, in some institutions, shoe covers are worn as well. When working in some of the areas, it is also common practice to prohibit jewelry, except for simple rings (i.e., wedding bands), and nail polish. Rings can harbor microorganisms. Jewelry can get caught in equipment and be a safety hazard, as well as breaking and getting into trays or sets. Nail polish can chip off and get into items being processed. Artificial nails should be prohibited because fungus can grow under the nails or the nails may come off and get into the trays. Nails should be trimmed short to prevent debris from collecting underneath them, which could cause an increase in bioburden and patient infection.

Continuous Quality Improvement

Continuous quality improvement (CQI) is a process designed to improve the quality of products and services provided. The process is continuous because the department should always be striving for the highest level of product and service quality and customer satisfaction. Customers can include patients, physicians, nurses, staff in other departments, visitors, administration, and staff within the CSD. Over time, customer expectations, technology, standards, and costs change. These factors make it necessary to reevaluate the way things are done and determine what changes need to be made to improve the process by which products and services are produced.

Quality means producing a product or service that consistently meets or exceeds customer expectations and standards of practice. The CQI process requires the CSD to achieve standards of practice that meet the expectations of their customers. In other words, the quality of products and services is assessed by the customer.

CQI is a search for the way to *do right things right.* That is, do the *right things* to meet customer expectations and do them in the *right way* to meet the standards of practice and ensure the safety of employees and patients, while maintaining the cost needs of the institution. It also means *not* doing things that are no longer needed, even though they may always have been done, and done well.

It is important that central service professionals be involved in developing a CQI process for the department so the department can provide the best quality of products and services for its customers.

Rules and Regulations

The activities and responsibilities of the CSD are governed by many rules and regulations. Some are established by federal, state, or local government agencies and accrediting bodies, some by the hospital administration, and some by the CSD management. All CSD employees must know the rules and regulations that affect them. Written rules, regulations, policies, and procedures should be available for reference.

Governing Bodies

All health care facilities must meet the standards of federal, state, and local authorities from which flow many of the rules and regulations applicable to the CSD.

The standards of the Joint Commission on Accreditation of Healthcare Organizations (JCAHO) affect most areas of the health care facility. The JCAHO is a voluntary organization, not a government agency, but its standards must be met if the facility is to retain its accreditation and qualify for financial reimbursement by insurers, in particular Medicare and Medicaid. Among the JCAHO standards that specifically affect central service are those for infection control, continuous quality improvement, safety management, sterilization practices, personnel training, leadership, and information management. Policies and procedures in CSD should include these standards.

Several agencies of the federal government regulate hospitals. The regulations of the Occupational Safety and Health Administration (OSHA), the Environmental

Protection Agency (EPA), and the Food and Drug Administration (FDA) are especially relevant to CSD functions. The regulations of OSHA help keep the workplace safe by, for example, establishing and enforcing standards limiting occupational exposure to EtO and other toxic chemicals. The EPA regulates EtO manufacture, labeling, and emissions. The regulations of the FDA are also important to CSD functions. FDA regulations govern the manufacturing and classification of commercially prepared medical devices and provide for a network for tracking purposes and for reporting defective products and user errors (Safe Medical Device Act).

All state governments have one or more departments with jurisdiction over public health, occupational safety, and environmental pollutants. Health care facilities must comply with state regulations as well as with local fire, electrical, and plumbing codes.

Local authorities may regulate waste disposal, including recycling programs, decontamination of contaminated waste, and chemical disposal into sewer systems. The CSD must know what these regulations are and comply with them (e.g., contaminated waste must be kept separate so it can be incinerated or microwaved before being put into a landfill, and chemicals such as glutaraldehyde must be neutralized before going into the sewer system to avoid disturbing the bacterial process used in sewer systems).

Reprocessing Single-Use Medical Devices

In the past many of the medical devices used in health care facilities were manufactured to be used as reusable devices. In the 1960s, manufacturers were using more plastics, technology became more complicated, demand for products increased, and health care facilities encouraged the use of disposable products to meet hospital demand but not increase staffing levels. Manufacturers responded to the demand by making products that were validated for one time use and not tested for multiple uses.

In the 1990s, health care facilities became concerned about the cost of disposable medical devices and their impact on the environment. Using low-temperature sterilization (EtO), health care facilities began to reprocess (collect, clean, inspect, package, sterilize, and distribute) a number of medical devices labeled as single use. Some health care facilities began using third-party reprocessors instead of doing the reprocessing in-house.

The FDA became concerned with the practice of reprocessing used single-use medical devices (SUDs). In August of 2000, the FDA released a document called Enforcement Priorities for Single-Use Devices Reprocessed by Third Parties and Hospitals, which is meant to ensure that reprocessing programs are safe and scientifically based.

According to this document, third-party and hospital reprocessors of single-use devices must adhere to all the same requirements that original equipment manufacturers must follow. In effect, the hospital or third-party reprocessor becomes a manufacturer if they reprocess SUDs. As manufacturers, they are required to

- Register their facility with the FDA and provide a list of all SUDs reprocessed
- Adhere to manufacturer adverse-event reporting requirements as well as user facility reporting requirements already in place
- Establish a tracking system for certain devices specified by the FDA that will enable the facility to quickly locate these devices should they need corrective actions
- Maintain records on and submit a written report to the FDA on device corrections and removals
- Follow good manufacturing practices, including design controls, process validation, controls for manufacture of packaging, proper labeling, storage, and installation, and servicing of devices
- Adhere to labeling requirements, which include name and place of manufacturer and adequate directions for use
- Adhere to premarket submissions and approvals

Most hospitals will find the FDA requirements very costly, time-consuming, and difficult to manage consistently. Therefore, hospitals will be compelled to either identify and stop reprocessing SUDs, adhere to all the FDA requirements if they continue to reprocess SUDs, or use a qualified third-party processor. SUDs chosen to be reprocessed must be identified by a multidisciplinary group that is able to assess the risk, infection-control, ethical, and cost-analysis factors. A third-party reprocessor must be chosen carefully: a site visit is recommended.

CSD and all the other health care areas and facilities must keep up with FDA requirements, changes to those requirements, and changes to the designation of facilities required to abide by them. Belonging to professional organizations, reading magazines and journals, and visiting the FDA Web site are effective ways of keeping current.

General Hospital Policies

The administration of every health care facility establishes policies on general dress code, safety procedures, disaster plans, personnel wages and benefits, budgeting, job classifications, materials purchasing, and many other matters affecting all personnel employed by that institution.

Departmental Rules and Regulations

Some rules and regulations relate specifically to the unique functions of the CSD, especially regarding work flow, air flow, and "people flow."

Work flow refers to the order in which medical or surgical items are received in the CSD, processed, and dispensed for patient use. The department layout and location relative to customer areas varies from facility to facility, as do specific work-flow policies and procedures. Certain general principles of work flow apply to any CSD. The objective is to prevent cross-contamination.

Contaminated reusable items should be transported to the decontamination area in such a manner as to protect people and the environment from contamination. Items should be transported in closed case carts or containers to reduce risk of cross-contamination. After cleaning and decontamination, the items should be taken to the assembly and sterile processing area, where they are inspected, assembled, packaged, and, if necessary, sterilized. They are then transferred to the sterile storage area and maintained until issued. Disposable items should enter the facility through the receiving area. They should be removed from their exterior shipping cartons before they are placed in the sterile storage area. Exterior shipping cartons are porous and a good place for microorganisms to accumulate, especially the fungus organisms. From the storage area, items are dispensed to customers. In summary, work should always flow from "dirty" to clean areas, never the reverse. Deviating from these practices can result in contamination of clean or sterile items and, consequently, may harm patients.

The ventilation system of the CSD must be designed so that the air flow is away from clean areas into "dirty" areas. To accomplish this, the air in the assembly and sterile processing, sterile storage, and distribution areas is maintained under positive pressure, and the air in the decontamination area is maintained under negative pressure. This means that the ventilation system "pushes" air out of clean areas and draws air into "dirty" areas.

People flow refers to the movement of personnel from one area of the CSD to another. Traffic must be controlled so that staff never go from "dirty" to clean areas without putting on a clean uniform. This prevents contamination of clean or sterile items. The correct people-flow pattern is from clean to "dirty" areas, including tours, inspections, and housekeeping tasks.

Policy and Procedure Manuals

Central service department technicians need to be fully aware of all departmental policies and procedures. Policies are general guidelines for action, whereas procedures are the specific steps for performing a task. These manuals are used as constant reference tools and should be kept in a convenient place. Employees should consult these manuals whenever assembling instrument sets or when questions arise, and should help contribute to keeping them current. Policy and procedure manuals are essential tools when assisting in the training of new staff. Computers are beginning to be used for this purpose.

Equipment Manuals

Equipment used for cleaning, sterilization, and other functions in the CSD is quite complex. For each piece of equipment, the manufacturer supplies an information manual that provides instructions for preventive maintenance, troubleshooting, routine care and cleaning, and operation. Such manuals are also supplied for patient care equipment. It is important that the manufacturer's instructions be followed to prolong the useful life of the equipment and ensure that it is maintained in good working condition. Proper care of equipment reduces the operating costs of the CSD and contributes to employee and patient safety.

Communication

Effective communication promotes efficiency, safety, cooperation, and a positive image. Central service technicians interact and communicate not only with each other and with their supervisors, but also with personnel from all other departments, especially those directly involved in patient care. Effective communication requires a conscientious effort to improve and practice.

Four Types of Communication

There are four types of communication: spoken, nonverbal, written, and listening.

People speak in different ways to different people at different times. Social conversation is a way of sounding people out. It is used to get acquainted with people. Avoid emotional interchanges and personal confidences that may interfere with the job. By listening sympathetically to a person's fears, basic feelings, and beliefs you can gain his or her trust. Intellectual conversation deals with facts and ideas, which flow two ways. Talk *to* each other, not *at* each other. Avoid monopolizing the conversation and interrupting the sentences of others. Get feedback and give feedback to make sure the message is understood.

Communication by telephone must be handled with courtesy and efficiency. You have the first three seconds to make a good impression. Important first words when answering the telephone should be a greeting, what department you are with, and your full name. Speak clearly without rushing. People are responsive to the tone of your voice. Convey a feeling of intelligence and helpfulness. Repeat the caller's message to make sure you understand what the caller is trying to communicate. Give complete attention to the caller and avoid conversing with others.

Facial expressions, body language, and voice tone are important parts of nonverbal communication. They can be positive or negative signals. Positive signals, including keeping your eyes on the speaker and standing or sitting erectly, send a message of interest; nodding your head may show active, enthusiastic participation; smiling shows agreement with something and encouragement; and leaning toward the speaker shows approval or a special interest in some point. Crossing arms or legs may signal disinterest or disagreement with the speaker. Restless movements may signal boredom.

Written communication should be specific, accurate, and brief. Gather and analyze facts, then put important pieces together to form a complete picture.

Actively listen. Avoid daydreaming, doodling, or looking out the window. Sift and sort the ideas being presented and ask questions to clarify.

Medical Terminology

All CSD technicians should be able to demonstrate appropriately the use of basic medical terminology in both written and oral communication. Being familiar with terms for medical/surgical items will enable the technician to better understand what is needed when a customer requests supplies. The environment CSD technicians work in requires accurate exchange of information and often quick understanding and reaction to requests. Confusion, errors, and safety hazards can be avoided by the use of correct terminology.

Medical terminology can be simplified by being aware of the meaning of the prefixes, roots, and suffixes used, and building on those parts of words.

All words have a root, which is the main body of the word and gives the primary meaning. Some words can have more than one root, such as hysterosalpingo-oophorectomy (hyster = uterus, salping = tube, oophor = ovary, ectomy = excision), which means the surgical removal of the uterus, fallopian tubes, and ovaries.

A prefix precedes the root and modifies or alters the root's meaning. The word elements in bradycardia are a prefix (brady = slow) and root (cardi = heart); therefore, the meaning would be a slow heartbeat. Another word used often in CSD is *disassemble,* in which the prefix (dis = apart) and root (assemble = put together) would give the meaning to take apart. Not all words have a prefix.

A suffix follows the root and modifies or alters the root's meaning. The word elements in gastrectomy are a root (gastr = stomach) and suffix (ectomy = excision); therefore, the meaning would be the surgical removal of part or all of the stomach. Suffixes such as *ous, eal, ic, ary, al,* and *ac* mean *pertaining to.* Not all words have a suffix.

The letters in word elements (prefix, root, suffix) have to be looked at closely. One letter change or omission can totally change the meaning. Examples include the following:

Prefixes: ante = before
anti = against

Roots: cysto = bladder
cyto = cell
ileo = part of small bowel
ilio = part of hip bone

Suffixes: ostomy = creating a new opening
otomy = incision into

Review the materials in Appendix B carefully before going on to the next chapters in the manual. The study of human anatomy and physiology in Chapter Two will give another opportunity to identify meanings of medical word elements as they relate to body systems.

Summary

Chapter One has introduced the work of the central service technician. The general organizational structure of a health care facility and CSD functions within that facility were discussed. Also addressed were the major physical areas of the CSD and the variety of activities performed in each area.

The importance of ethical behavior and good communication was stressed, along with the many safety precautions necessary in accomplishing daily work. The operation of an efficient support service also depends on personal cleanliness, standards of quality, and other rules and regulations. The medical language used every day in hospitals was also introduced.

Chapter Two will discuss the human body and its functions. By better understanding body structure and how the body works, central service technicians can better appreciate the importance of central service and the responsibilities they have for complete and accurate work.

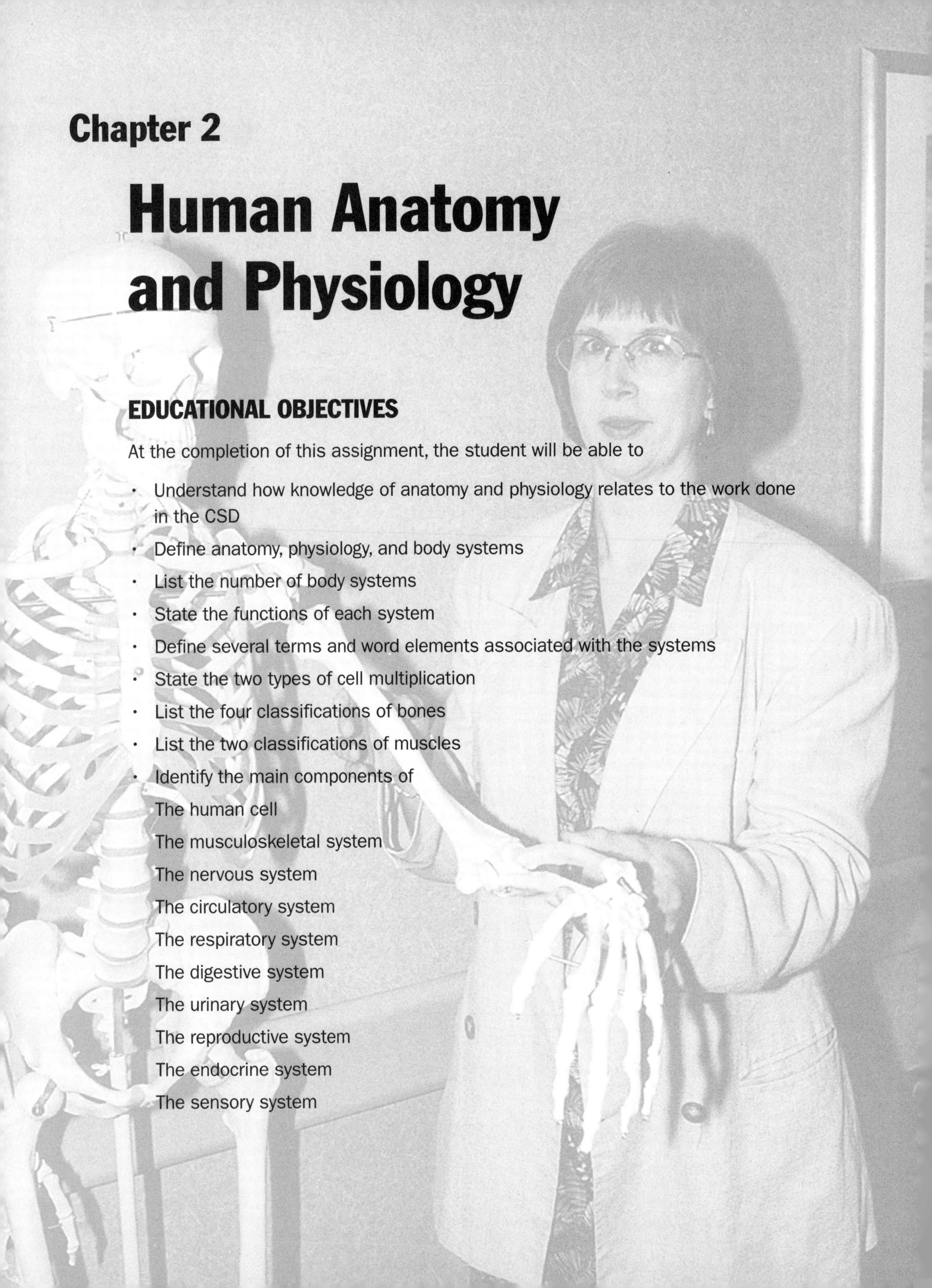

Chapter 2

Human Anatomy and Physiology

EDUCATIONAL OBJECTIVES

At the completion of this assignment, the student will be able to

- Understand how knowledge of anatomy and physiology relates to the work done in the CSD
- Define anatomy, physiology, and body systems
- List the number of body systems
- State the functions of each system
- Define several terms and word elements associated with the systems
- State the two types of cell multiplication
- List the four classifications of bones
- List the two classifications of muscles
- Identify the main components of

The human cell
The musculoskeletal system
The nervous system
The circulatory system
The respiratory system
The digestive system
The urinary system
The reproductive system
The endocrine system
The sensory system

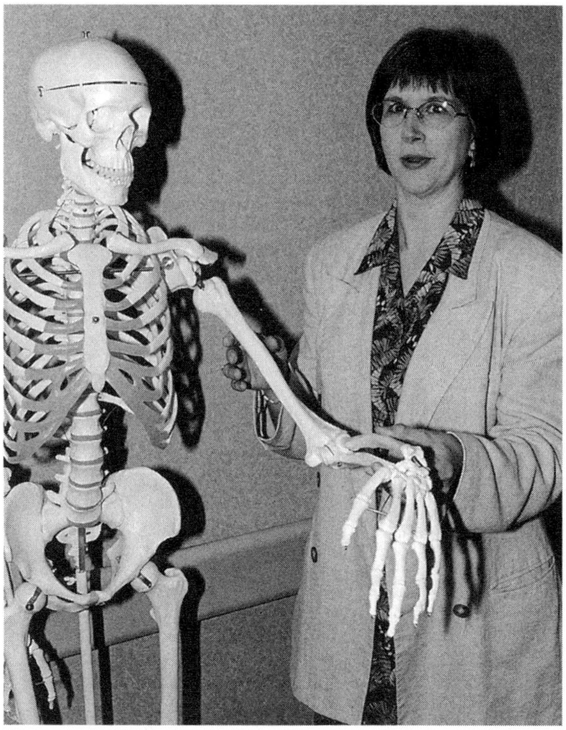

THE CSD TECHNICIAN routinely processes and distributes supplies and equipment used in the treatment and care of patients. A basic knowledge of human anatomy, physiology, and cell biology is important. It enables technicians to better understand the reasons for policies and procedures they are required to follow and provides a framework in which to carry out their duties more efficiently, competently, and safely.

Anatomy is the study of the structure of the human body, and physiology is the study of its functions. The body comprises ten organ systems, each of which consists of a group of structures that work together to perform a specific physiological function. This chapter will review these ten systems: the skeletal, muscular, nervous, circulatory, respiratory, digestive, urinary, reproductive, endocrine, and sensory systems. Examples of related word elements and medical devices will be included. The structure and function of the basic building block of these systems, the cell, will also be reviewed.

Cell Biology

Cells are the building blocks of the body. There are many types of cells, each specializing in a particular function. While each type of cell has unique characteristics related to its specific function, all cells have in common certain structural components and multiply by the same basic process. Together, the cells make up the human body.

Morphology (Cell Structure)

Each cell consists of several parts with specific functions (see Figure 2.1). The nucleus contains the genetic material called deoxyribonucleic acid (DNA), which is organized into chromosomes during cell multiplication. A molecule of DNA consists of two helical or spiral chains connected by bridges of simple amino acids (building blocks). These bridges are arranged in various sequences. All of a person's traits are determined by the pattern of chromosomal arrangements.

The fluid space outside the nuclear membrane (around the nucleus) is called the cytoplasm. It is an incredibly complex maze of membranes and structures where energy is produced for cell functions such as the manufacture of protein.

Metabolism refers to the cellular functions of growth, maintenance, and repair. Surrounding the cytoplasm is the cell membrane.

Multiplication

Early in life, the rapid growth of the body requires multiplication of the cells. Later in life, when body growth stops, cells must still multiply to replace those that die. The entire skeleton changes cells every seven years. Within thirty hours, all of the taste buds are replaced. Red blood cells are constantly being manufactured in the bone marrow. However, some types of cells, such as nerve and muscle cells, are not replaced when they die.

The multiplication process is basic to all normal cells. First, the chromosomes contract and thicken. The 46 chromosomes form 23 pairs and begin to duplicate exact copies of themselves (a process called replication). Then, they line up across the center of the cell and the duplicate pairs go to opposite poles of the cell. A new cell membrane forms across the middle. The chromosomes lengthen as before and two cells are made from one. This multiplication process is called mitosis and re-

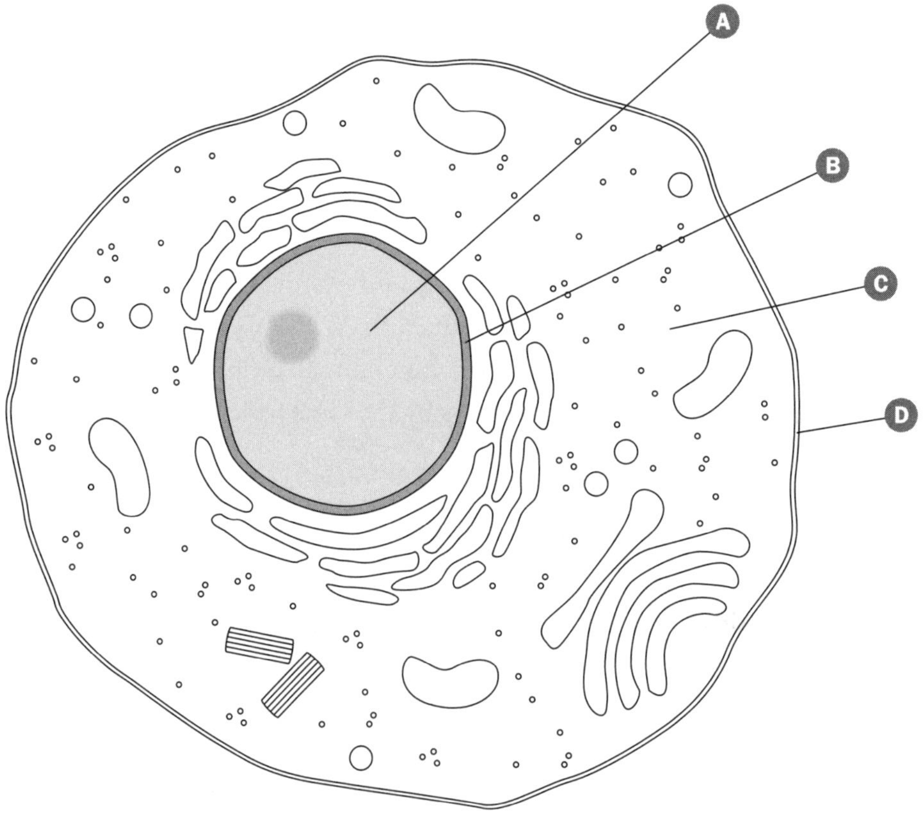

Figure 2.1. Basic Structure of the Human Cell.

Note: a = nucleus; b = nuclear membrane; c = cytoplasm; d = cell membrane.

sults in two identical cells. There is a second type of cell division process, called meiosis. This process is the same as mitosis, except that the pairs of chromosomes do not replicate; so when the chromosomes go to the poles of the cell, only half are in each new cell. These two new cells are not identical and do not have the genetic material necessary to function as normal cells. Instead, these cells are reproductive cells (sperm and eggs), which are produced to unite during reproduction to form a new cell with a full set of chromosomes. This new cell (a fertilized egg) then develops into a human being with unique characteristics.

The Skeletal System

The skeletal system forms the framework for all of the body systems. It has three main functions: to give form and support to various parts of the body, to protect delicate organs such as the brain and spinal cord, and to serve as levers to which muscles are attached, making motion and movement possible.

There are more than 200 bones in the skeleton. They are classified by their shape: long, short, flat, and irregular. The bones of the legs and arms are long. Fingers and toes have short bones. Ribs are flat bones. Some irregular bones are the skull plates and pelvis. Figure 2.2 illustrates the human skeletal system and muscular system (discussed in the next section), and identifies bones and muscles by their medical names.

Bones consist mainly of calcium and phosphorus, which form a very hard and dense material. The long bones and other large bones have a spongy, porous material in the center called marrow. The marrow is where blood cells are formed.

Bones are connected at joints and are cushioned at the ends with cartilage. Some joints are immobile, such as those in the skull. Others, like the knee and elbow, are movable. Ligaments are tough fiber bundles that tie joints together. Joints are covered by a membrane and lubricated by fluid.

Some of the word elements used to describe parts of the skeletal system are as follows:

arthr(o)-	joint
cephal(o)-	head
chondr(o)-	cartilage
crani(o)-	skull
fibr(o)-	fiber, connective tissue
ili(o)-	hip bone
myel(o)-	bone marrow

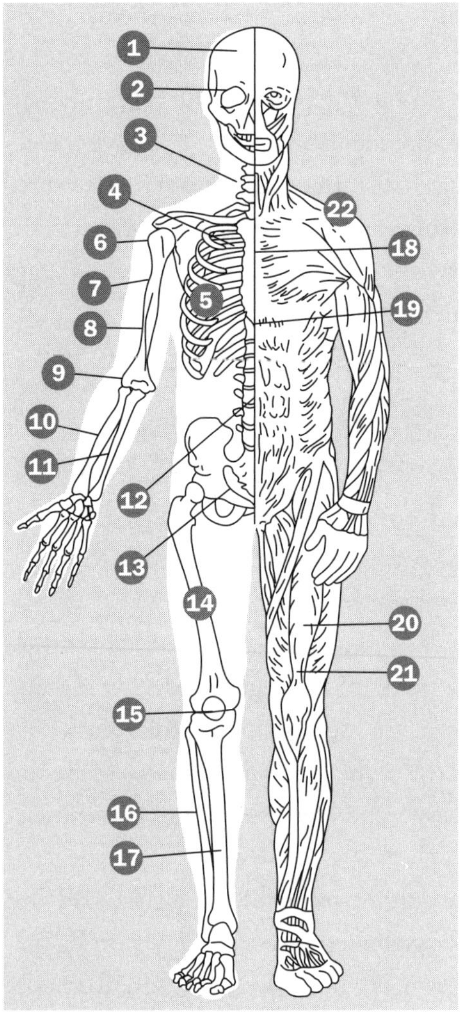

Musculoskeletal System (Anterior View)

Body shape and support, protection of internal organs, and locomotion are but three of the functions of the musculoskeletal system.

1. Cranium
2. Bony orbit
3. Cervical vertebrae
4. Costal cartilage
5. Ribs
6. Humeral epiphysis
7. Humerus
8. Humeral diaphysis
9. Humeral metaphysis
10. Radius
11. Ulna
12. Lumbar vertebrae
13. Pelvis
14. Femur
15. Patella
16. Fibula
17. Tibia
18. Sternum
19. Xiphoid cartilage
20. Rectus femoris muscle
21. Patellar tendon
22. Deltoid muscle

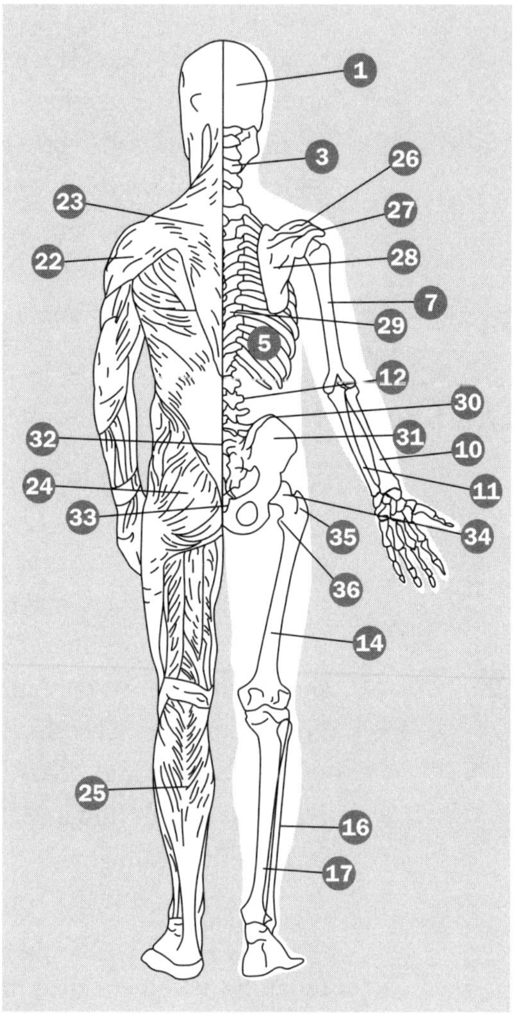

Human Skeleton (Posterior View)

1. Cranium
3. Cervical vertebrae
5. Ribs
7. Humerus
10. Radius
11. Ulna
12. Lumbar vertebrae
14. Femur
16. Fibula
17. Tibia
22. Deltoid muscle
23. Trapezius muscle
24. Gluteus maximus muscle
25. Gastrocnemius muscle
26. Clavicle
27. Acromion
28. Scapula
29. Thoracic vertebrae
30. Iliac crest
31. Ilium
32. Sacrum
33. Coccyx
34. Head of femur
35. Greater trochanter
36. Lesser trochanter

Figure 2.2. The Muscular and Skeletal Systems of the Human Body.

oste(o)-	bone
sacr(o)-	tailbone
synovi(o)-	joint fluid
thorac(o)-	chest

For example, *arthritis* is an inflammation of the joints. A *cranio*tome is an instrument used to cut through the skull. Other terms related to the skeletal system are defined in Appendix B.

A number of types of medical equipment and supplies are used in the treatment of injuries or diseases of the skeletal system. These include arthroscopes, osteotomes, chisels, gouges, mallets, crutches, splints, casts, and various forms of traction. Most often medical problems involving the skeletal system include broken or misaligned bones.

The Muscular System

The muscular system functions to provide motion and movement, maintain posture, produce body heat, and operate involuntary body systems. The muscular system is made up of more than 600 muscles, which are classified as either voluntary or involuntary.

Voluntary (or skeletal) muscles are attached to bones and are under conscious control. Because of its striped appearance when observed under the microscope, voluntary muscle is also called striated muscle. Voluntary muscles consist of bundles of tissue fibers held securely together, something like a bundle of rubber bands. They are attached to bones by tendons, which are cords of firm, white, inelastic tissue. Voluntary muscles are organized into opposing sets, with one set contracting while the other extends, or extending while the other contracts, to allow opposite movements. They contract and extend relatively quickly (compared with involuntary muscles) and are easily fatigued. Figure 2.2 shows some of the voluntary muscles of the human body.

Involuntary (or visceral) muscles operate the automatic functions of the body, such as digestion and blood circulation. They are controlled by the autonomic nervous system and are not under conscious control. Involuntary muscles are found in the walls of the blood vessels and the intestinal tract, the uterine wall, and in the glands. The fibers that make up involuntary muscle are smaller than those that make up voluntary muscle. Because of the way the fibers are connected together, they do not appear striated under the microscope, so involuntary muscle is sometimes called smooth muscle.

Cardiac (heart) muscle is a special type of involuntary muscle. Its structure is different from that of any other muscle. The muscle fibers and cells interlace with one another with very little connective tissue in-between. Cardiac and other types of involuntary muscle alternately contract and relax in a slow, rhythmical fashion when they are functioning normally.

Two of the word elements used to describe the muscular system are *myo-*, muscle, and *teno-*, tendon. A tenomyotomy, for example, is the removal of a portion of a tendon and muscle. A myotome is an instrument used to cut muscle. See Appendix B for other terms related to the muscular system.

Most disease affecting muscles results from damage to nerves that control the muscles. However, sometimes muscle can be damaged by physical activity or can become infected and inflamed due to microorganisms. A variety of medical devices are used in the treatment and diagnosis of muscle diseases and injuries.

The Nervous System

The nervous system is a communication network similar to a telephone system that carries messages between all parts of the body. This system is divided into two anatomical parts: the central nervous system, which consists of the brain and the spinal cord, and the peripheral nervous system, which is made up of nerves and ganglia (groups of nerve cells next to the spinal cord). (See Figure 2.3.) Functionally, the nervous system is made up of two divisions: the voluntary, which is controlled by conscious thought, and the involuntary (or autonomic), which is unconsciously controlled.

Nerves are bundles of nerve cells covered by a sheath. Each nerve cell has several short extensions called dendrites, which act to receive messages from other cells, and a long extension called an axon, which transmits messages some distance to the next nerve cell. Some nerves carry only sensory information, such as pain. Others are motor nerves, transmitting to muscles the instructions to contract or relax. Still others carry both sensory and motor information.

The brain is the control center of the central nervous system. It is organized into three parts, each of which has specific functions. The medulla oblongata is located at the base of the brain. This is where heartbeat, respiration, and body temperature are controlled. The cerebellum controls muscular coordination, body balance, and equilibrium. The cerebrum, the largest part, is involved in memory, thought, voluntary decisions and movements, and interpretation of nervous impulses received from the sense organs.

The spinal cord is a large bundle of nerve cells connecting the brain to all parts of the body. The spinal column of the skeleton protects this very important nerve

Central Nervous System

Messages to and from the brain travel along the spinal cord and nerves seen branching off the cord.

1. Cerebrum
2. Cerebellum
3. Spinal cord
4. Brachial plexus
5. Sacral plexus
6. Peripheral nerve

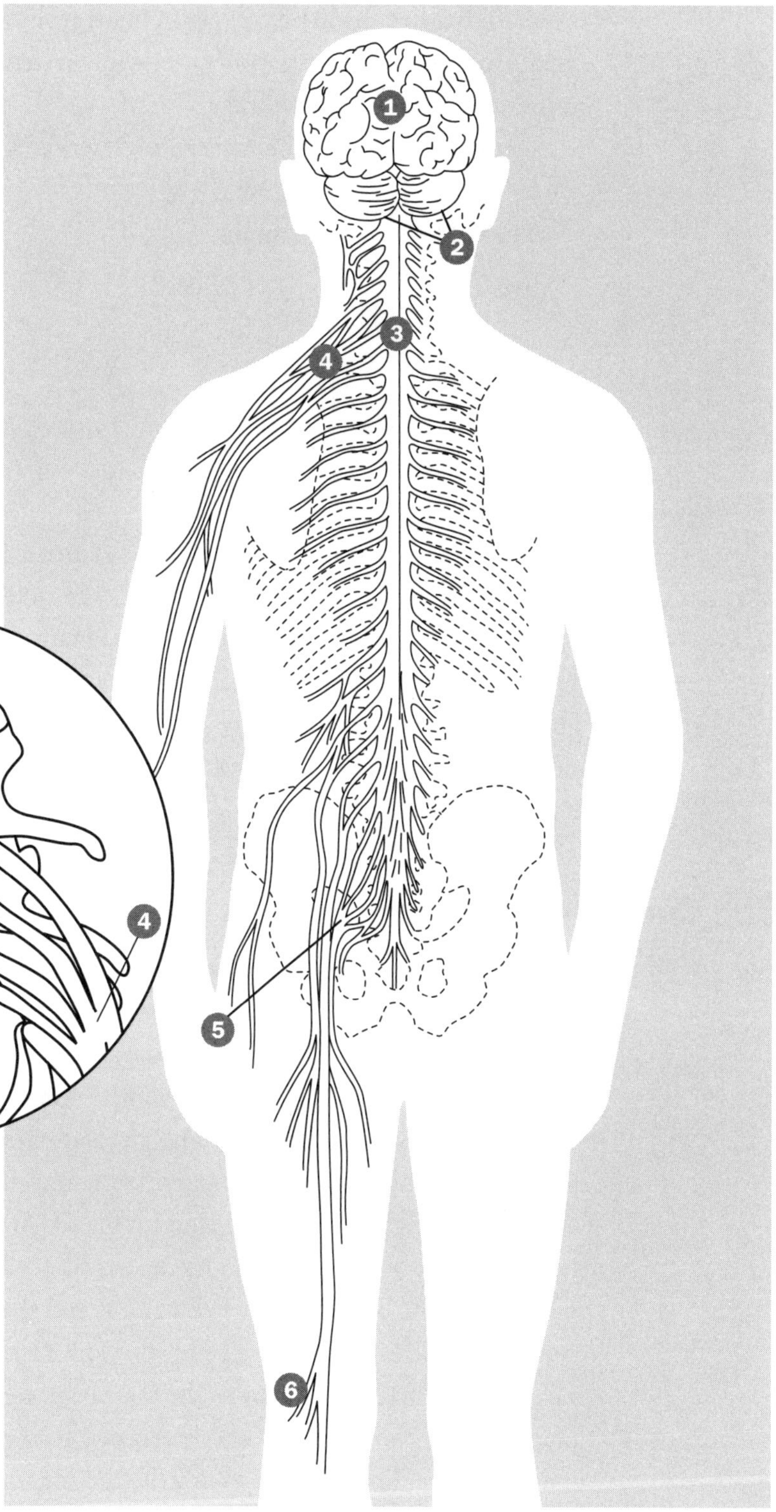

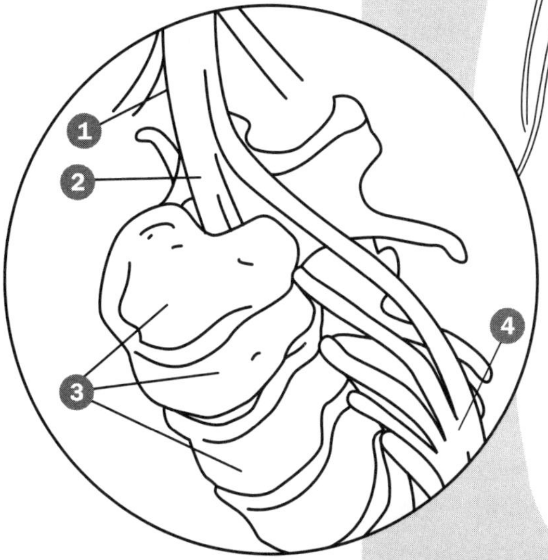

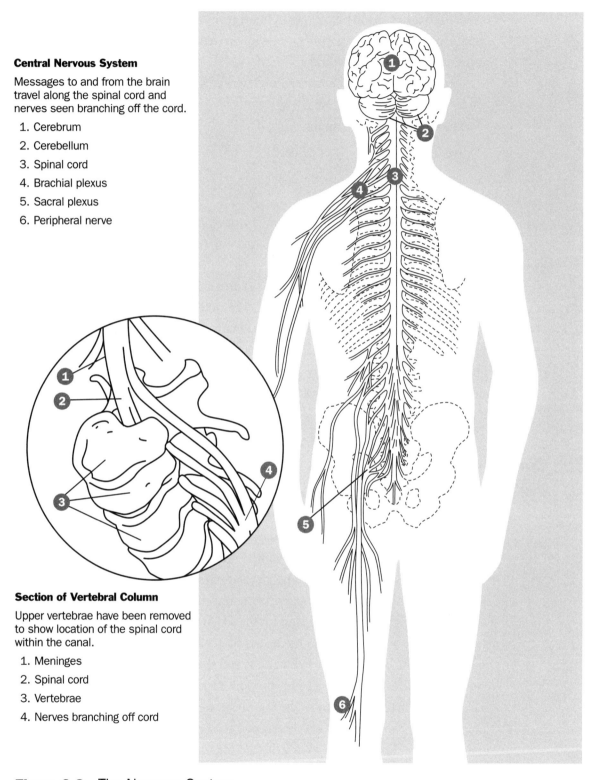

Section of Vertebral Column

Upper vertebrae have been removed to show location of the spinal cord within the canal.

1. Meninges
2. Spinal cord
3. Vertebrae
4. Nerves branching off cord

Figure 2.3. The Nervous System.

center. Individual nerve bundles branch off from the spinal cord at ganglia, which are the beginning of the peripheral nervous system. These peripheral nerves reach to the farthest parts of the body.

Some of the word elements used to describe the nervous system are as follows:

encephal(o)-	brain
myel(o)-	spinal cord
neur(o)-	nerve

For example, an electro*encephalo*graph is a device used to record the electrical activity of the brain. *Neur*itis is inflammation of a nerve. Other terms are defined in Appendix B.

In some diseases or injuries to nerves, regeneration of the nerve cells may take place depending on how severe the disease or injury is. However, brain and spinal cord cells that have separated do not regenerate themselves. A number of medical devices are used to treat and diagnose diseases and injuries to the nervous system. These include electroencephalograms, intracranial pressure monitors, pneumoencephalograms, neurosurgical sponges or patties, hemostatic scalp clips (such as Raney, Adson, and Ligaclip), and spinal needles.

The Circulatory System

The circulatory system transports the oxygen, nutritive substances, immune substances, hormones, and chemicals needed by the organs and tissues of the body. It also carries away waste products and carbon dioxide, equalizes body temperature, and maintains normal electrolyte balance. These functions are accomplished by the blood and lymph networks. The circulatory system consists of the heart and blood vessels, the lymph nodes and vessels, and the blood and lymphatic fluid.

The heart is the pumping station for blood. Arteries carry blood away from the heart; veins carry blood back to the heart. The heart has four chambers: the right atrium, the right ventricle, the left atrium, and the left ventricle. The right atrium collects blood from the largest vein, the vena cava, and pumps it to the right ventricle. The right ventricle pumps the blood through the pulmonary arteries to the lungs, where it is oxygenated and returned to the heart's left atrium via the pulmonary veins. (The pulmonary arteries are the only arteries that carry blood that is not oxygenated; the pulmonary veins are the only veins that carry oxygenated blood.) The blood is then pumped to the left ventricle, the heart's strongest chamber. The left ventricle pumps the blood out through the aorta, the largest artery, to all parts of the body. The heart's chambers contract in pairs, first the atria and then the ventricles. This produces the familiar heartbeat sound of "lub, dub." Figure 2.4 illustrates the structure of the heart and the vessels that enter and leave it. Figure 2.5 shows the arterial and venous systems.

Blood is a fluid containing several vital components:

- Plasma—The liquid part of the blood
- Red blood cells (erythrocytes)—Small, disk-shaped cells rich in hemoglobin
- White blood cells (leukocytes)—Cells of varying sizes and shapes, much less numerous than red cells
- Platelets (thrombocytes)—Irregularly shaped disks that aid in the clotting of blood

The hemoglobin in red blood cells unites with oxygen and carries it to the body's cells. White blood cells mainly destroy disease-producing organisms. Blood carries oxygen, nutrients, and other substances to cells all over the body and picks up the cells' waste products for removal. The exchange of oxygen and nutrients with waste products takes place in extremely small blood vessels called capillaries, which connect arteries and veins.

Adults have approximately 5 quarts of blood in their bodies. The blood makes one complete circuit through the body every minute. In 24 hours, 7200 quarts of blood pass through the heart. The organs and systems of the body vary greatly in the quantity of blood they require at different times. For example, the needs of the brain are constant, but the demands of the muscles are more varied. Heavy physical exertion may increase the rate of blood flow to the muscles to eight times greater than the normal resting rate. In hot weather, a larger percentage of blood flows through the skin to cool the body. After every meal, an extra supply of blood is required by the stomach to help digest and absorb the meal.

Lymph vessels, or lymphatics, constitute another tubal network for body fluids. These vessels carry lymph, a colorless, watery fluid containing cells called lymphocytes. Lymph nodes are filter devices located along the lymph vessels. Together, lymph vessels and lymph nodes make up the lymphatic system. This system drains excess fluid away from the spaces between body cells, transports dead blood cells and some waste products, and serves as another defense system against disease. Lymphatic fluid is drained back toward the heart and collected in the thoracic duct, which empties into the vena cava. Thus, body fluids are kept circulating throughout the circulatory system.

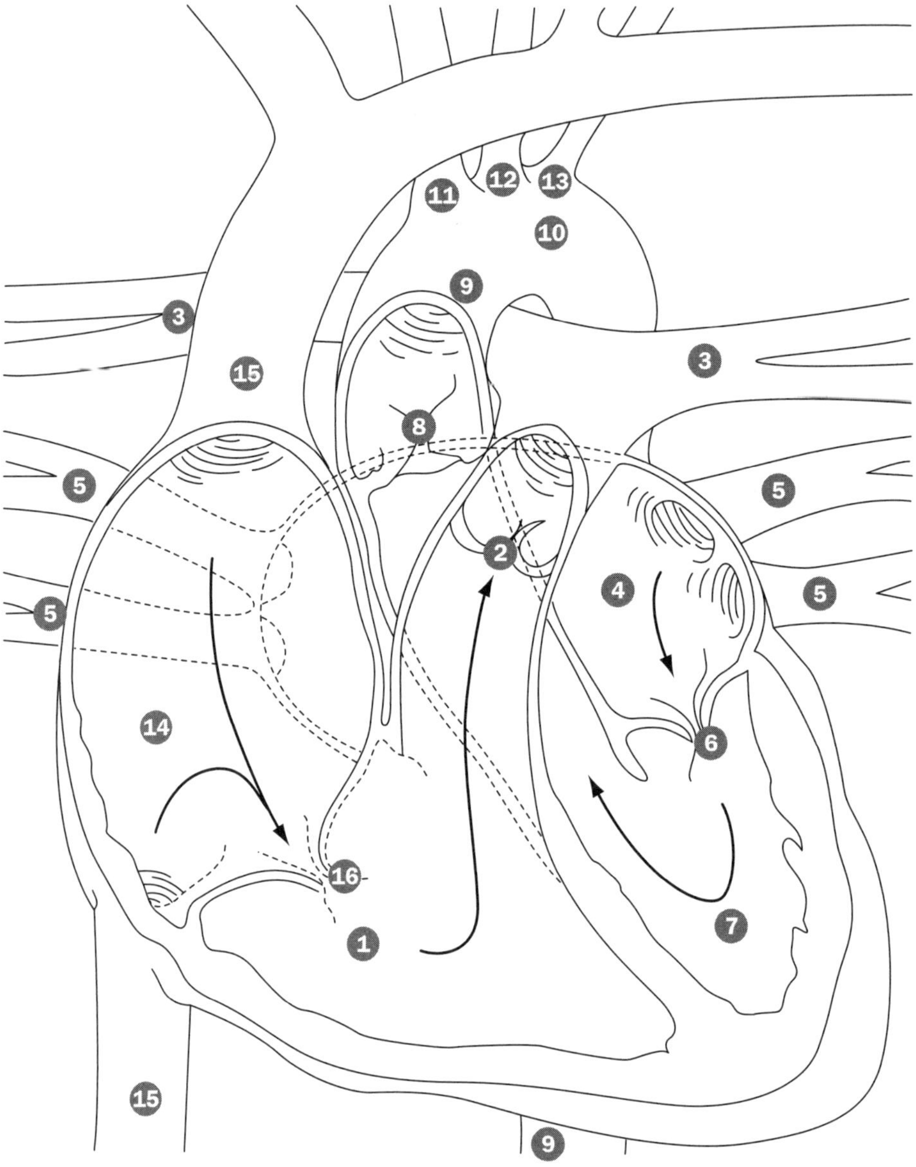

Route of Blood Flow Through the Heart

1. Right ventricle
2. Pulmonary valve
3. Pulmonary artery, right and left
4. Left atrium
5. Pulmonary veins, right and left
6. Mitral (bicuspid) valve
7. Left ventricle
8. Aortic valve
9. Aorta
10. Aortic arch
11. Innominate artery
12. Common carotid artery
13. Subclavian artery
14. Right atrium
15. Venae cavae, inferior and superior
16. Tricuspid valve

Figure 2.4. Blood Flow Through the Heart.

Blood Vascular System

The venous system is illustrated by dark vessels and the arterial system is shown as white vessels. However, both arteries and veins are present all over the body to assure uninterrupted delivery of oxygenated blood and nutrients to cells and their exchange for wastes.

1. Heart
2. Aortic arch
3. Innominate artery
4. Common carotid artery
5. Right subclavian artery
6. Axillary artery
7. Brachial artery
8. Radial artery
9. Ulnar artery
10. Thoracic aorta
11. Abdominal aorta
12. Bifurcation of aorta
13. Common iliac artery
14. Femoral artery
15. Profundus femoris
16. Popliteal artery
17. Anterior and posterior tibial arteries
18. Superior vena cava
19. Internal jugular vein
20. External jugular vein
21. Brachial vein
22. Basilic vein
23. Cephalic vein
24. Median cubital vein
25. Inferior vena cava
26. Common iliac vein
27. External iliac vein
28. Femoral vein
29. Saphenous vein
30. Popliteal vein
31. Tibial vein

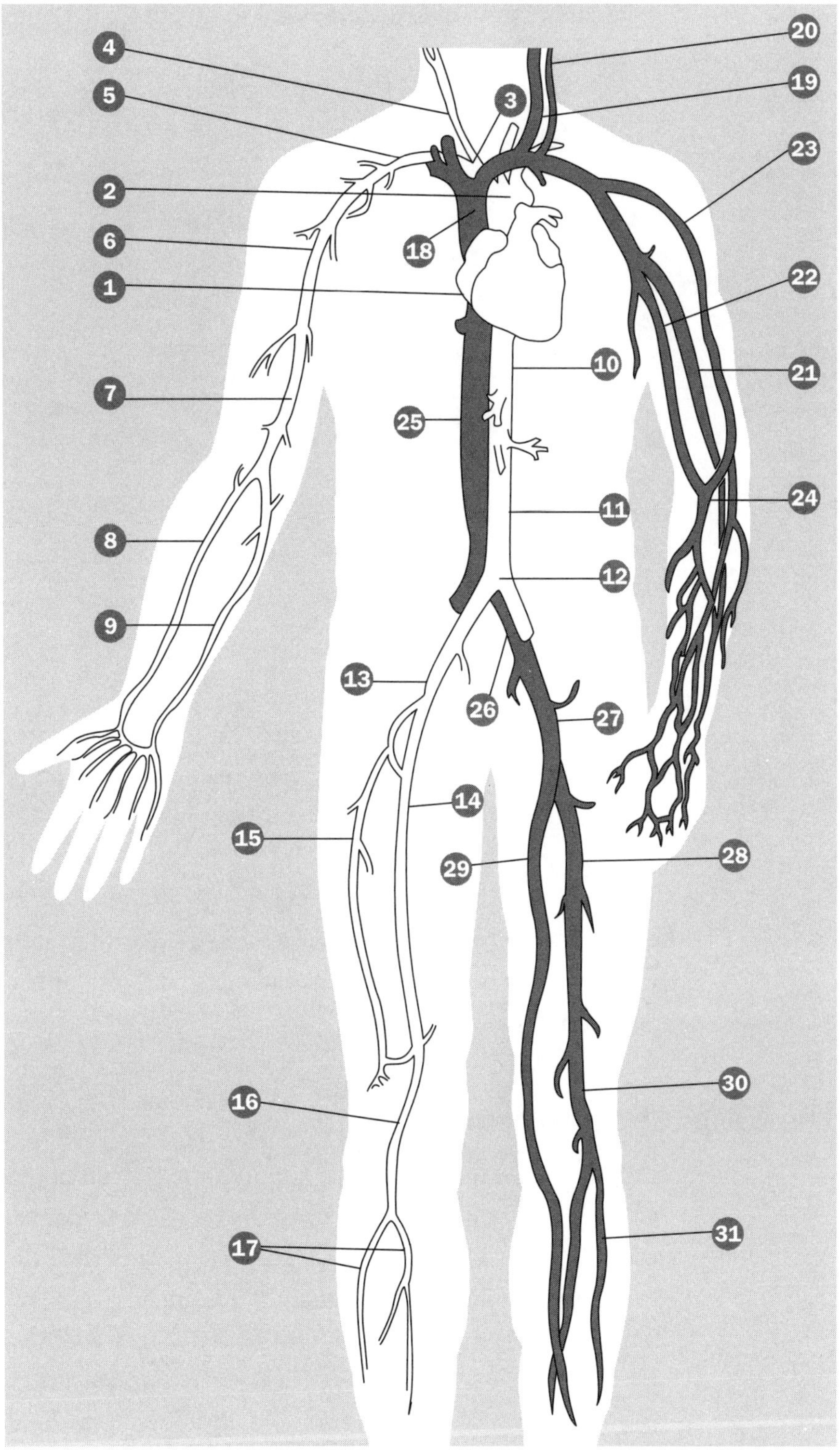

Figure 2.5. The Circulatory System.

Some of the word elements used to describe parts of the circulatory system are as follows:

angi(o)-	vessel, channel
arterio-	artery
cardi(o)-	heart
cyan(o)-	blue
-cyte-	cell
erythr(o)-	red
hemat(o), hemo-	blood
leuk(o)-	white
lymph(o)-	lymphatic
phleb(o)-	vein
vas(o)-	vessel, duct

For example, a *hemo*stat is a surgical clamp used for constricting blood vessels to prevent bleeding during surgery. An electro*cardio*graph is a device used to record the electrical activity of the heart. Other medical terms related to the circulatory system are defined in Appendix B.

A number of medical devices are used in the treatment and diagnosis of diseases of the circulatory system. These include cardiac monitors, pacemakers, various intravenous and central line catheters, infusion pumps, and patient-controlled analgesia devices.

The Respiratory System

Respiration is the process that supplies the oxygen necessary for the production of energy in the body and removes the carbon dioxide that results from the body's use of oxygen. This exchange of gases is accomplished through the two phases of breathing: inspiration and expiration. During inspiration (inhalation), air is drawn into the lungs; during expiration (exhalation), it is pushed out of the lungs.

The main organs of the respiratory system are the nostrils (nose), pharynx, larynx, trachea (windpipe), bronchi, and lungs (see Figure 2.6). During the inspiration phase of breathing, air enters the body through the nostrils, where it is filtered, moistened, and warmed. It then passes through the pharynx and the larynx and enters the trachea, or windpipe, which divides into the right and left bronchi. Each bronchus divides many times, like the limbs of a tree, to form smaller tubes called bronchioles. Each bronchiole ends in a cluster of tiny air sacs called alveoli. The walls of the alveoli are very thin and are surrounded by capillaries. This is where the transfer of oxygen into the blood and of carbon dioxide out of the blood takes place. The carbon dioxide is then exhaled back out of the body through the same network of tubes, and the oxygenated blood is circulated throughout the body via the heart.

Some of the word elements that refer to the respiratory system are as follows:

aer(o)-	air, gas
naso-, rhin(o)-	nose
pharyng(o)-	pharynx
pneum(o)-	air, gas, lung
spir(o)-	breath, breathing
thorac(o)-	chest
tracheo-	trachea

For example, a tracheotomy is the creation of an opening into the trachea through the neck, usually for the purpose of removing an airway obstruction or of inserting a tracheotomy tube to facilitate breathing. In a thoracostomy, an incision is made in the chest and a chest tube is inserted for the purpose of draining fluid. A spirometer is an instrument used to measure the efficiency of breathing. Other terms related to the respiratory system are defined in Appendix B.

Most diseases of the respiratory system involve the lungs and their ability to inhale and exhale properly. These diseases include pneumonia, tuberculosis, emphysema, and cancer of the lung. A number of medical devices are used in the treatment and diagnosis of diseases of the respiratory system. These include chest x-rays, various masks and cannulas, tracheotomy tubes, airways, bronchoscopes, and suction catheters.

The Digestive System

The digestive system breaks down food from large, complex elements into simple ones that can be absorbed into the bloodstream and carried to the body's cells. This system consists of the alimentary canal and accessory glands and organs (see Figure 2.7).

The alimentary canal of an adult is about 30 feet long. Its components are the mouth, esophagus, stomach, small intestine, large intestine, rectum, and anus. The accessory glands produce digestive fluids containing enzymes that are the primary means by which food is broken down into components that can be absorbed into the blood stream. Some secretions of the accessory glands act mainly on specific

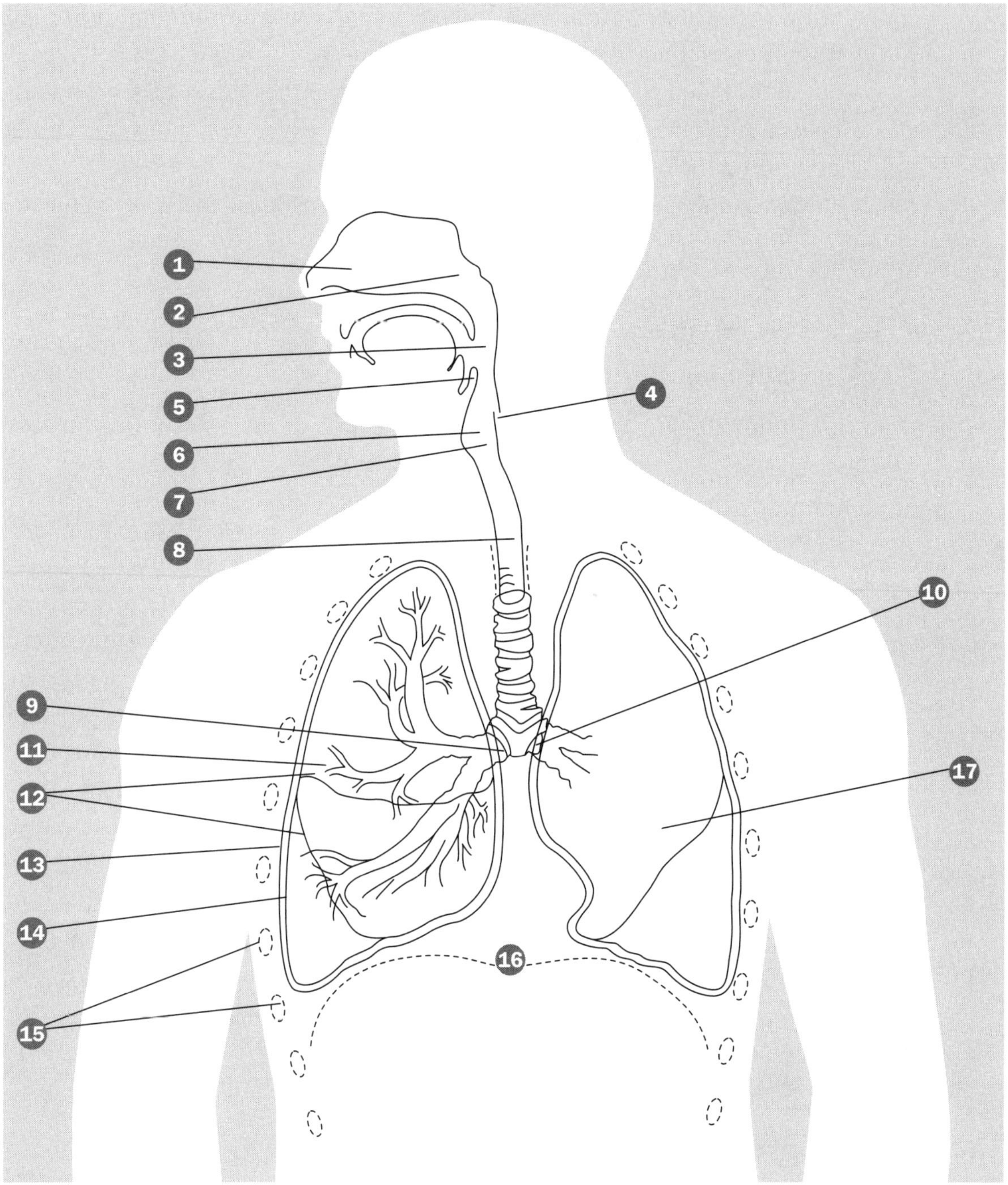

Respiratory System

Supplying oxygen, which is vital to tissue cells, and eliminating carbon dioxide wastes from the cells are the major tasks of this body system.

1. Nasal cavity
2. Nasopharynx
3. Pharynx
4. Esophagus
5. Epiglottis
6. Vocal cords
7. Larynx
8. Trachea
9. Right main stem bronchus
10. Left main stem bronchus
11. Right lung (Lobar and segmental bronchi exposed)
12. Lobe divisions
13. Parietal pleura
14. Visceral pleura
15. Ribs
16. Diaphragm
17. Left lung

Figure 2.6. The Respiratory System.

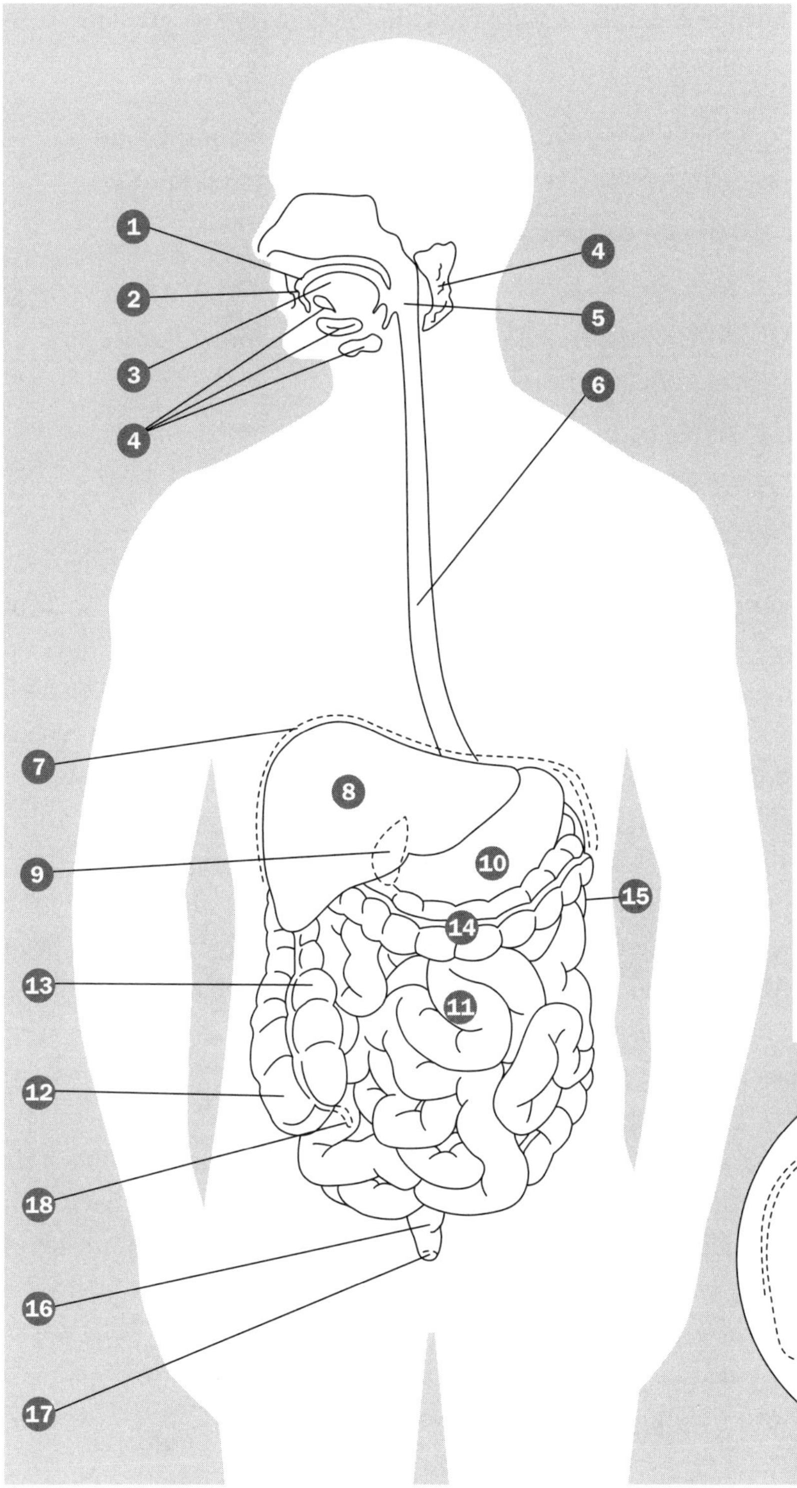

Digestive System

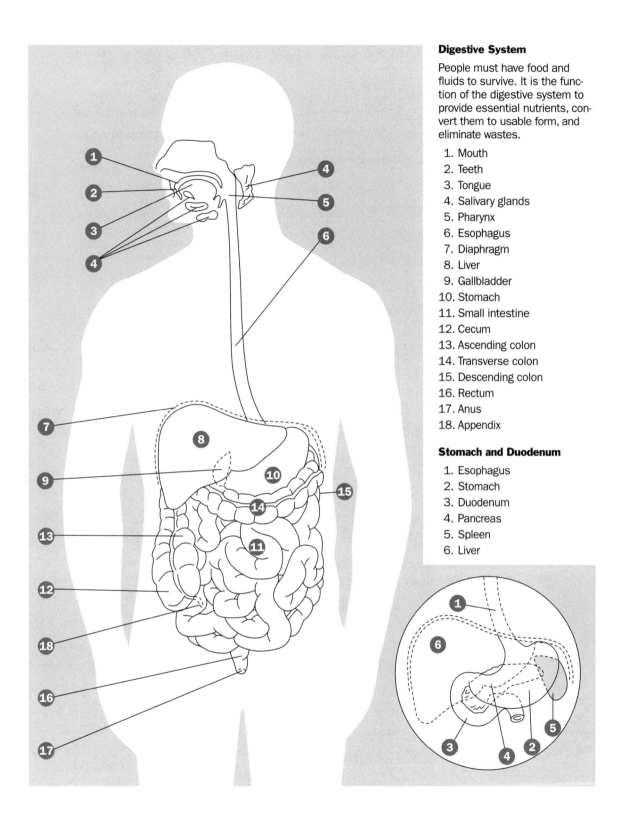

People must have food and fluids to survive. It is the function of the digestive system to provide essential nutrients, convert them to usable form, and eliminate wastes.

1. Mouth
2. Teeth
3. Tongue
4. Salivary glands
5. Pharynx
6. Esophagus
7. Diaphragm
8. Liver
9. Gallbladder
10. Stomach
11. Small intestine
12. Cecum
13. Ascending colon
14. Transverse colon
15. Descending colon
16. Rectum
17. Anus
18. Appendix

Stomach and Duodenum

1. Esophagus
2. Stomach
3. Duodenum
4. Pancreas
5. Spleen
6. Liver

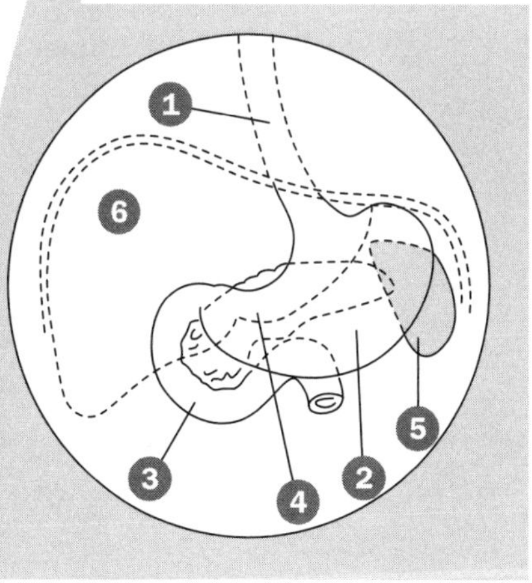

Figure 2.7. The Digestive System

types of food; bile, for example, aids primarily in the digestion of fats. The accessory glands are as follows:

- The salivary glands of the mouth, whose secretions moisten the food, making it easier to chew and swallow and begin the digestion process
- The gastric glands of the stomach
- The intestinal glands of the small intestine
- The liver (which secretes bile and performs a variety of other metabolic functions, such as the detoxification of blood)
- The gall bladder (which stores bile)
- The pancreas

Food moves through the alimentary canal by means of *peristalsis,* the slow, synchronized contraction of the involuntary muscles that make up the walls of the canal. Valves in the canal prevent food from moving "backwards."

Food is taken in through the mouth, chewed into smaller pieces, mixed with saliva (from the salivary glands), and swallowed. It then passes through the esophagus into the stomach, a muscular reservoir where the food is acted upon by the gastric juices (from the gastric glands) and converted into a semiliquid called chyme. From the stomach, the chyme enters the small intestine, which is functionally divided into three sections: the duodenum, jejunum, and ileum. In the duodenum, the food is mixed with bile from the liver and digestive fluids from the pancreas. Also, the duodenum contributes other digestive fluids. The small intestine is the principal center for absorption and is by far the longest segment of the alimentary canal (about 23 feet long in adults). Most of the nutrients and water needed by the body are absorbed there.

The remaining material moves on to the large intestine, which consists of six portions: the ascending colon, transverse colon, descending colon, sigmoid colon, rectum, and anus. The appendix is an unused pouch located near the junction of the small and large intestines and is sometimes the site of infection. More water is removed from the material as it travels through the colon, leaving fecal waste. This waste is collected in the rectum and eliminated through the anus.

Word elements used to describe the digestive system include the following:

chole-	bile
colo-	large intestine
dent(o)-	tooth
enter(o)-	small intestine

gastr(o)-	stomach
hepato-	liver
proct(o)-	rectum
stomat(o)-	mouth

For example, *procto*scopes and *gastro*scopes are instruments used to view the inside of the rectum and the stomach, respectively. *Hepat*itis is an inflammation of the liver. Other medical terms related to the digestive system are defined in Appendix B.

Numerous disorders and diseases can affect the digestive system. These may include colitis, ulcers, gastritis, and gastroenteritis. Various medical devices are used to treat and diagnose problems in the digestive system. These devices include nasogastric tubes, proctoscopes, sigmoidoscopes, gastroscopes, colonoscopes, gastrostomy tubes, feeding tubes, and colostomy supplies.

The Urinary System

The urinary system filters waste products (primarily those produced by the breakdown of protein) out of the blood and eliminates them from the body. It is often referred to as the genitourinary system or urogenital system because of its close relationship with the reproductive organs. It also sometimes called the renal system (*renal* means "pertaining to the kidneys"). The urinary system consists of four parts: the kidneys, ureters, bladder, and urethra (see Figure 2.8).

The kidneys are two bean-shaped organs located in the back upper portion of the abdominal cavity, one on each side of the spine. Each kidney contains a vast network of tiny filtering units called nephrons, which filter liquid wastes and other substances from the blood circulating through them. These substances make up the fluid called urine. As urine is formed, it leaves the kidneys and drains out through tubes called ureters, which are connected to the bladder. The bladder is a hollow, muscular bag that stores the urine until it is eliminated through the urethra (a tube connecting the bladder with the outside of the body).

Besides filtration of wastes, another important function of the kidneys is the reabsorption of water, salts, sugar, and protein from the blood. This selective absorption regulates the acid-base balance of the blood and helps maintain a relatively constant concentration of water, salts, proteins, and electrolytes (such as potassium). This delicate balance is essential for proper body function.

About 1.5 quarts of urine are excreted daily by the average adult. The efficiency of the kidney is one of the most remarkable aspects of the body. The normal kidney has a filtering capacity of a quart of blood a minute, 15 gallons an hour, or 360 gallons a day.

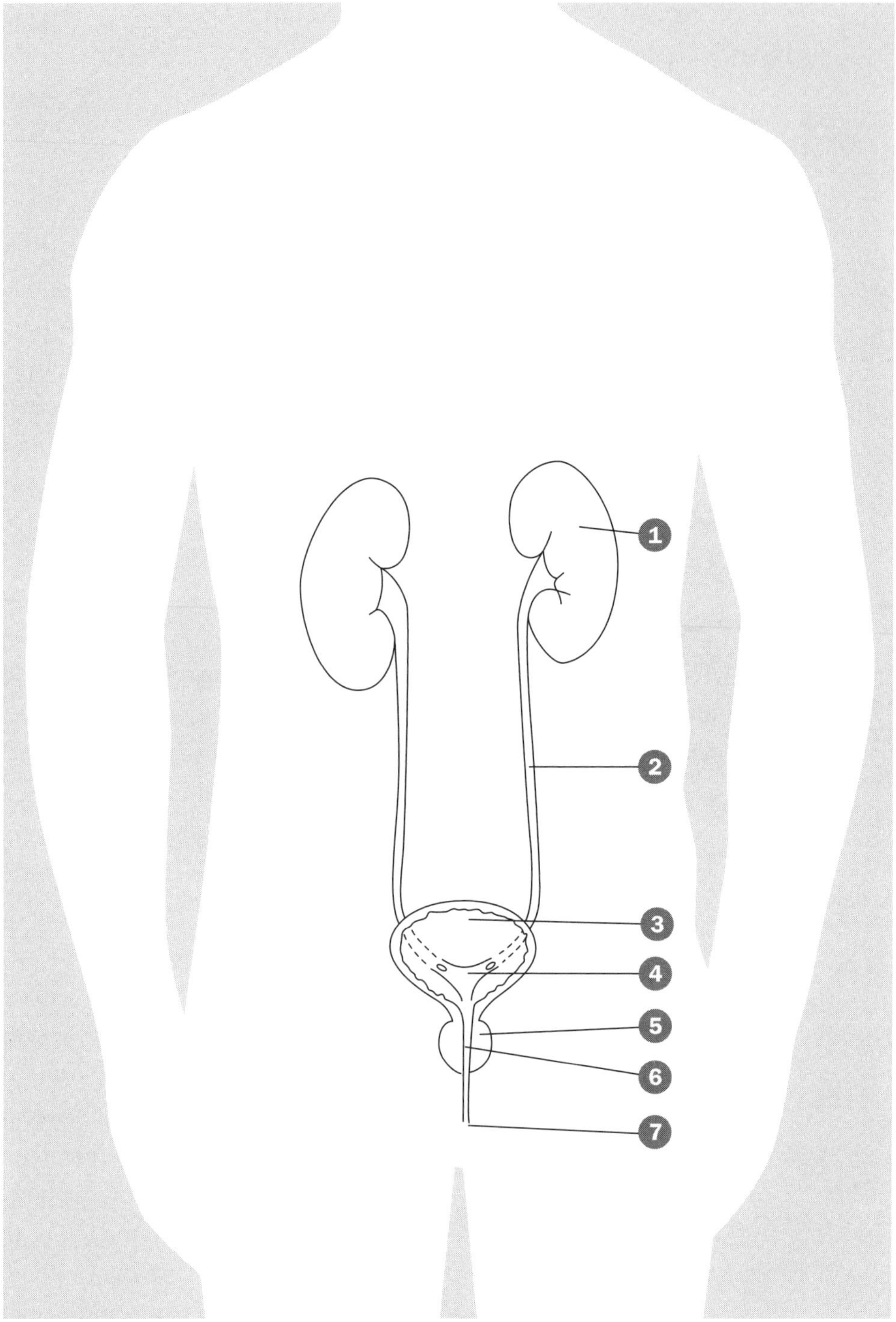

Urinary System

Organs of the urinary system extract certain wastes from the bloodstream, convert them to urine, transport the urine to the bladder reservoir, and eliminate it at appropriate intervals.

1. Left kidney
2. Left ureter
3. Bladder
4. Trigone of the bladder
5. Prostate (male)
6. Urethra
7. Meatus of urethra

Figure 2.8. The Urinary System.

Some of the word elements used to describe parts of the urinary system are as follows:

cyst(o)-	bladder
nephr(o)-	kidney
pyel(o)-	pelvis of the kidney
ureter(o)-	ureter
uro-	urine

For example, a *cysto*scope is an instrument used to view the inside of the bladder. *Nephr*itis is an inflammation of the kidney. A *uro*pathy is any disease of the urinary tract. Other terms related to the urinary system are defined in Appendix B.

Various medical devices are used in the treatment and diagnosis of problems that affect the urinary system. These include Foley retention catheter, ureteral catheters, Pezzer or mushroom catheter, Phillips filiforms and followers, cystoscopes, and resectoscopes.

The Reproductive System

The reproductive system has two main functions in both sexes: to produce the hormones that influence the development of masculine or feminine characteristics and to reproduce human life.

The principal male organs that perform these functions are the testes (testicles), the penis, and the prostate gland. The testes produce spermatozoa, the sex cells carrying male genes. They also produce the hormone testosterone, which is responsible for male secondary sex characteristics (such as facial hair). The penis is the external male organ of urination and coitus. The prostate gland secretes a watery alkaline fluid that carries the sperm and protects them from the acid secretion of the female vagina.

The principal female organs of reproduction are the ovaries, the fallopian tubes, the uterus, the vagina (birth canal), and the mammary glands. The ovaries produce ova (eggs), which carry the female genes. They also produce hormones, chiefly estrogen and progesterone, which cause the development of feminine characteristics and regulate the menstrual cycle. The fallopian tubes connect the ovaries with the uterus, a large muscular organ that holds and nourishes the growing fetus during pregnancy. The vagina is a canal extending from the lower portion of the uterus (the cervix) to the exterior of the body.

Reproduction is the process of fertilization, pregnancy, and birth. The male sperm and female egg unite in one of the fallopian tubes. The fertilized egg travels to the uterus and attaches to the uterine wall. The uterus protects the developing fetus. The ovaries produce special hormones that control the body changes during pregnancy. Labor begins the birth process. The cervix and the birth canal open to allow passage of the baby from the uterus. The baby can be nourished from the mother's breasts, which, under the control of special hormones, have filled with milk.

Among the word elements used to describe the reproductive system are:

andr(o)-	male, masculine
colp(o)-	vagina
gyne-, gyno-	female, feminine
hyster(o)-	uterus
masto-	breast
oophor(o)-	ovary
orchi(o)-	testis
salping(o)-	oviduct, fallopian tube

For example, a *hyster*ectomy is the removal of the uterus. An *orchi*ectomy is the removal of a testicle. A *gyne*cologist is a physician who studies the diseases of women. Other terms related to the reproductive system are defined in Appendix B.

A number of medical devices are used to treat and diagnose problems with the reproductive system or to aid in the birth process. Some of these are vaginal speculums, uterine dilators, uterine curettes, and penile implants.

The Endocrine System

The endocrine system is made up of glands that produce chemical substances called hormones. The endocrine glands are sometimes called ductless glands because they release their hormones directly into the bloodstream, which carries them throughout the body.

Some endocrine glands secrete more than one hormone, but each hormone only affects specific cell types located some distance from the gland. Hormones have a considerable influence on growth, body functions, and even personality. The most important endocrine glands are the pituitary, the thyroid, the four parathyroids, the two adrenals, the numerous pancreatic islets, the two ovaries, and the two testes (see Figure 2.9).

The pituitary gland coordinates the activities of all the other endocrine glands and is therefore called the "master gland." Its secretions also regulate skeletal growth as well as some muscle, blood, and reproductive functions.

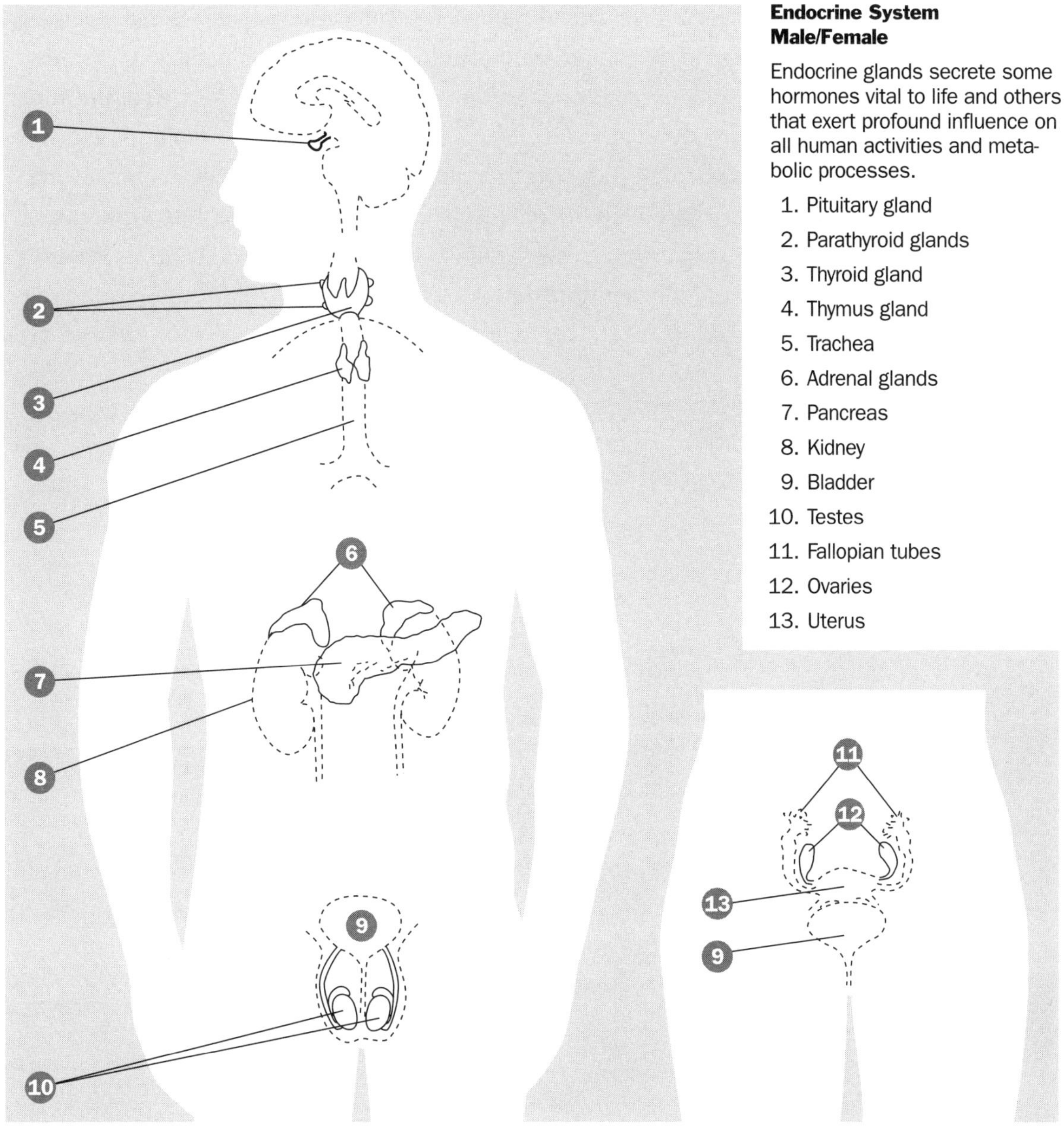

Endocrine System Male/Female

Endocrine glands secrete some hormones vital to life and others that exert profound influence on all human activities and metabolic processes.

1. Pituitary gland
2. Parathyroid glands
3. Thyroid gland
4. Thymus gland
5. Trachea
6. Adrenal glands
7. Pancreas
8. Kidney
9. Bladder
10. Testes
11. Fallopian tubes
12. Ovaries
13. Uterus

Figure 2.9. The Endocrine System.

The thyroid gland regulates the body's general metabolism and growth. The hormones produced by the parathyroid glands regulate the metabolism of calcium in the body. The adrenal glands respond to emotional excitement by secreting adrenaline. Adrenaline stimulates muscles for action in emergency situations, which explains why the adrenal glands have been nicknamed the "glands of combat or stress."

The pancreas has many small clusters of endocrine tissue, known as the islet of Langerhans or pancreatic islets, that secrete insulin, which controls the use of sugar in the body. As mentioned previously, the ovaries and testes produce eggs and sperm and secrete hormones that control the development of female and male sex characteristics.

Some of the word elements used to describe aspects of the endocrine system are as follows:

adren(o)-	adrenal gland
endo-	within
thyro-	thyroid

For example, *endo*crine means to secrete internally. A *hyro*parathyroidectomy is the removal of the thyroid and parathyroid glands. Other terms related to the endocrine system are defined in Appendix B.

Injury and disease can cause a variety of problems to occur in the endocrine system. Most of these problems are treated with medication or surgery. No common medical devices are solely associated with the treatment and diagnosis of problems related to the endocrine system.

The Sensory System

The sensory system consists of the organs governing the five senses of sight, sound, smell, taste, and touch. Modern scientists also consider the sensations of pressure, heat, cold, and pain to be distinct elements of the sensory system.

The eye is the organ of vision. It is shaped like a globe or ball and has three layers, called the sclera, choroid, and retina (see Figure 2.10). The sclera is the white, outer coat that protects the eye. The choroid is the middle layer. Light enters the eye through the pupil, which is surrounded by a colored ring called the iris, and opens and closes to control the amount of light entering. The lens focuses the light onto the retina. The rods and cones receive the light impressions and transmit them to the brain via the optic nerves. Here the images are put together and interpreted.

The ear is the organ of hearing (see Figure 2.11). Sound waves enter the outer ear, which directs them through the auditory canal and against the eardrum. The eardrum conducts the waves into the middle ear, where three small, connected bones (the hammer, the anvil, and the stirrup) transmit them into the inner ear. The eustachian tube is connected to the middle ear and the pharynx, thereby equalizing the pressure on both sides of the eardrum. In the inner ear, sound waves are converted into nerve impulses, which are carried to the brain via the auditory nerve.

The nose contains numerous sensory cells, which are located in the mucous membrane that lines the upper part of the nasal cavity. As air passes through the nose, smells and odors stimulate these cells. The sensory cells are connected to the olfactory nerve, which goes to the brain.

The tongue is the organ of taste. Its surface is covered with tiny buds (receptors) that are capable of distinguishing four kinds of taste: sweet, sour, bitter, and salt.

The major function of the skin is to protect the body against infection, injury, and loss of fluids. In addition, it plays a vital role in maintaining normal body temperature and eliminating waste materials. Because the skin contains many special nerve endings, it also acts as a sensory organ for pain, touch, heat, cold, and pressure.

There are also sensors in other organs of the body, such as the stomach, for sensations of stretch or pressure. These sensations are translated as pain.

The following word elements describe parts of the sensory system:

dermat(o)-	skin
gloss(o)-	tongue
naso-, rhin(o)-	nose

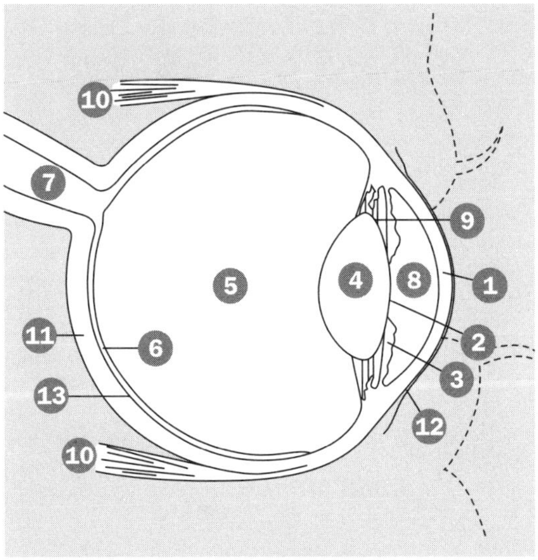

The Eye

Eyes convert light rays into nerve impulses, enabling people to see.

1. Cornea
2. Pupil
3. Iris
4. Crystalline lens
5. Vitreous body
6. Retina
7. Optic nerve
8. Anterior chamber
9. Posterior chamber
10. Muscle
11. Sclera
12. Conjunctiva
13. Choroid

Figure 2.10. The Structure of the Eye.

ocul(o)-, ophthalm(o)-	eye
ot(o)-	ear

For example, *ophthalmo*scopes and *oto*scopes are instruments used to view the eye and ear, respectively. Other terms related to the sensory system are defined in Appendix B.

A number of medical devices are used in the treatment and diagnosis of injuries to or diseases of the sensory system. These include otoscopes, ophthalmoscopes, eye glasses, eye dressings, eye shields, and hearing aids.

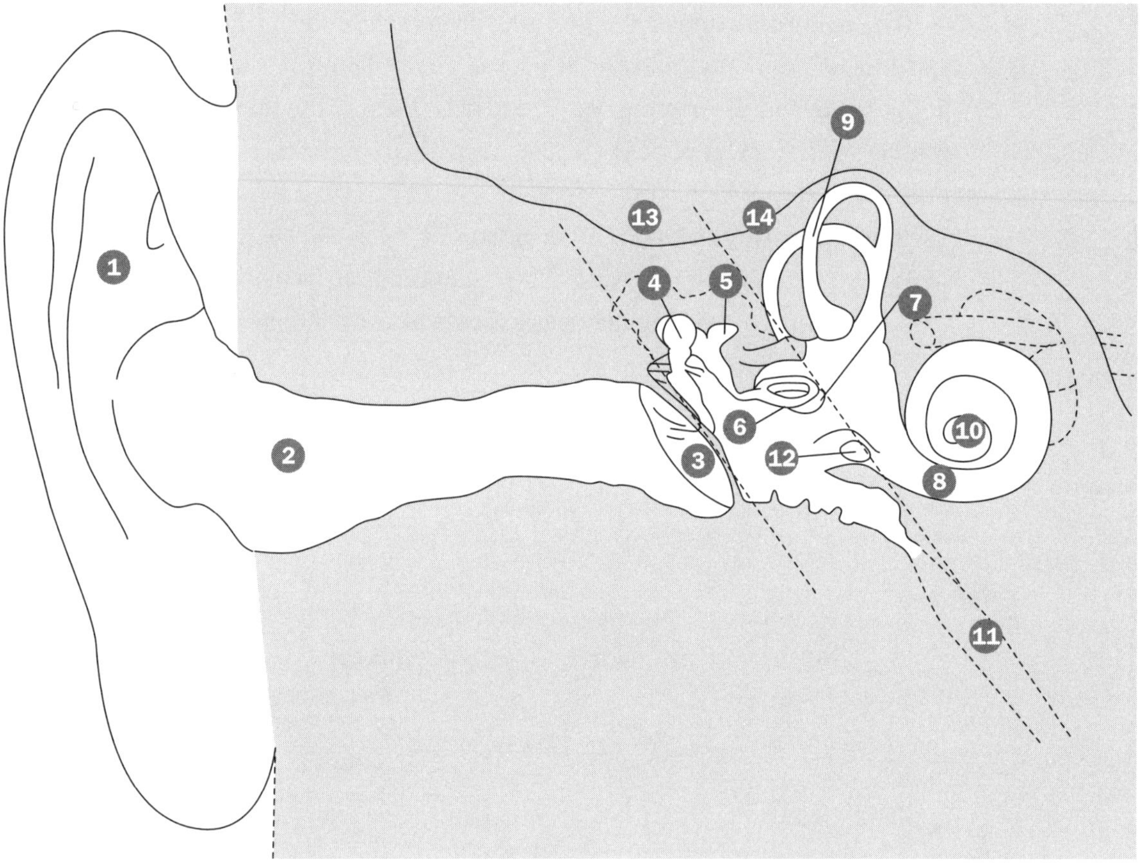

The Ear

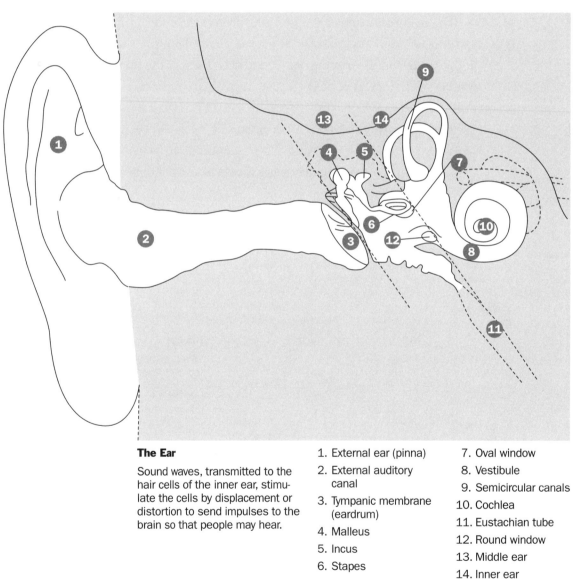

Sound waves, transmitted to the hair cells of the inner ear, stimulate the cells by displacement or distortion to send impulses to the brain so that people may hear.

1. External ear (pinna)
2. External auditory canal
3. Tympanic membrane (eardrum)
4. Malleus
5. Incus
6. Stapes
7. Oval window
8. Vestibule
9. Semicircular canals
10. Cochlea
11. Eustachian tube
12. Round window
13. Middle ear
14. Inner ear

Figure 2.11. The Structure of the Ear.

Summary

This introduction to the structure and function of the cells and organs that make up the body provides background necessary to understanding the mechanisms of disease transmission and the challenges of infection control.

Chapter Three will discuss how diseases are transmitted and the challenges in controlling the spread of infection. It will also clarify the importance of handling instruments and equipment properly based on where they are being used in or on the body.

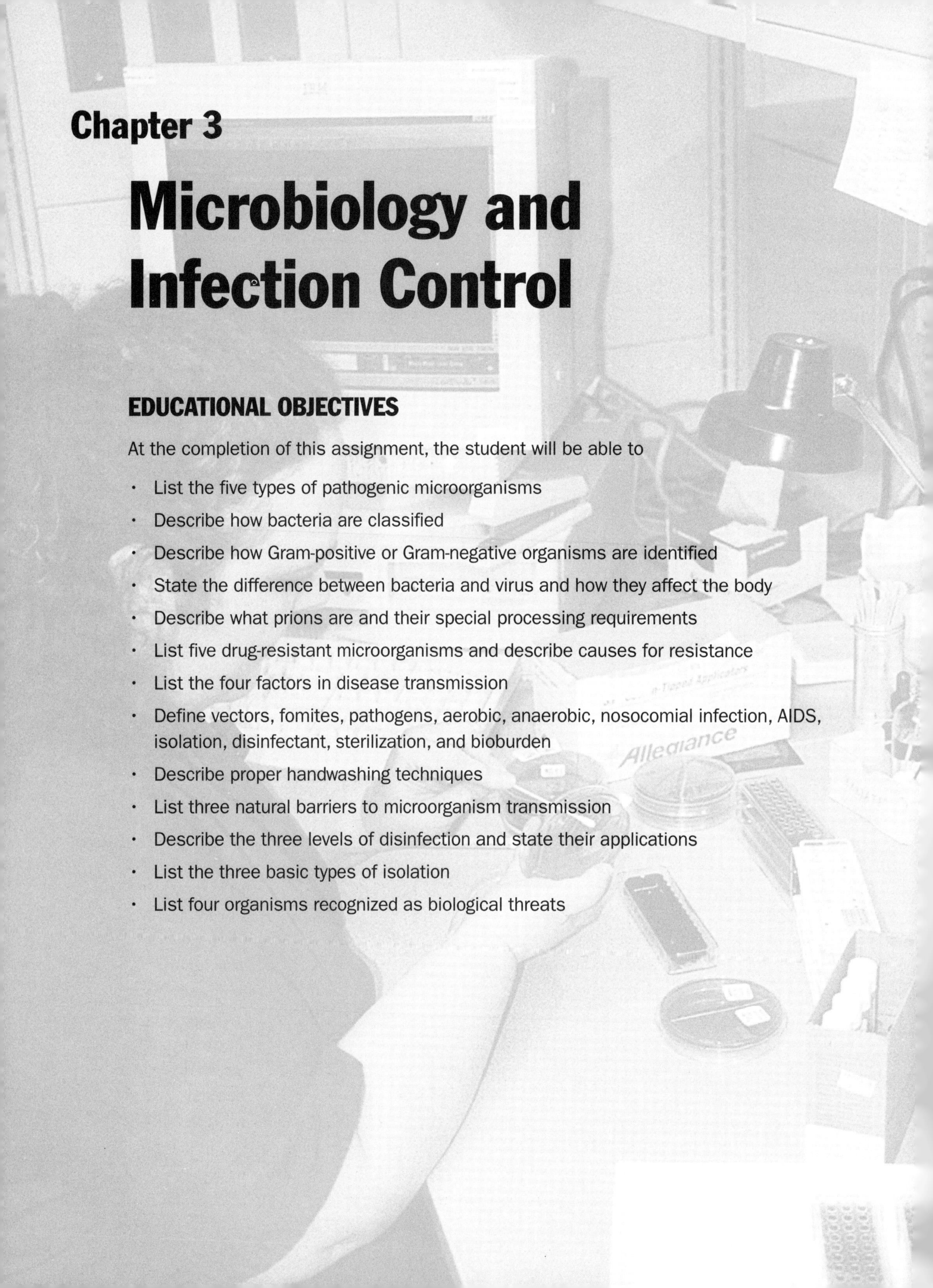

Chapter 3

Microbiology and Infection Control

EDUCATIONAL OBJECTIVES

At the completion of this assignment, the student will be able to

- List the five types of pathogenic microorganisms
- Describe how bacteria are classified
- Describe how Gram-positive or Gram-negative organisms are identified
- State the difference between bacteria and virus and how they affect the body
- Describe what prions are and their special processing requirements
- List five drug-resistant microorganisms and describe causes for resistance
- List the four factors in disease transmission
- Define vectors, fomites, pathogens, aerobic, anaerobic, nosocomial infection, AIDS, isolation, disinfectant, sterilization, and bioburden
- Describe proper handwashing techniques
- List three natural barriers to microorganism transmission
- Describe the three levels of disinfection and state their applications
- List the three basic types of isolation
- List four organisms recognized as biological threats

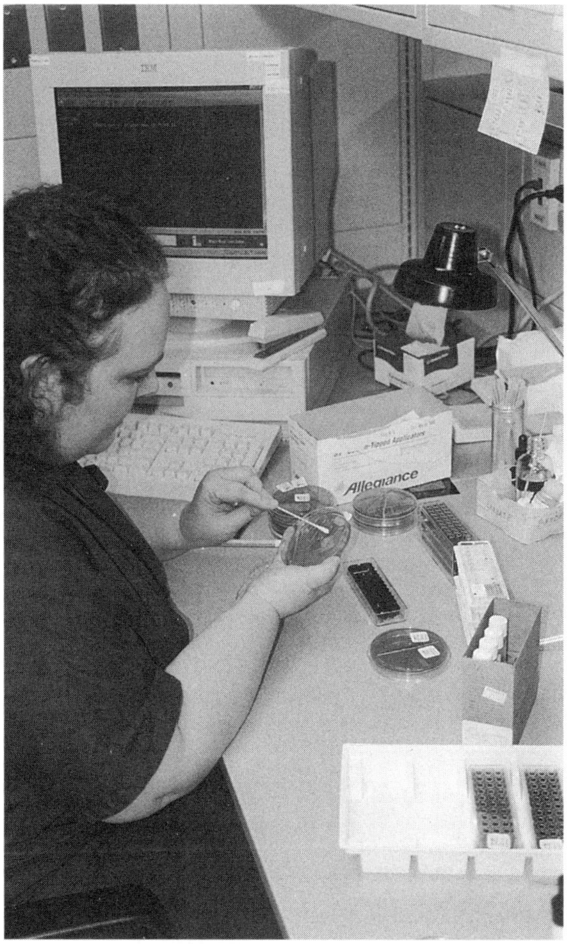

Basic Microbiology

Microorganisms (microscopic organisms) are everywhere in our world. Most are helpful, but some are potentially pathogenic (disease-producing). Hospital personnel must be aware that pathogenic microorganisms are prevalent in health care facilities due to the large number of patients with transmittable diseases. Understanding the microscopic world and the mechanisms of disease transmission is essential for central service technicians, for their own safety and for that of patients. The CSD technician must assume responsibility for following standards, policies, and procedures for decontamination, sterilization, storage, and handling, which will be explained in later chapters of this manual.

This chapter reviews the basic types of microorganisms and how they cause disease. It also discusses important concepts of infection control and introduces the principles of disinfection and sterilization.

The types of microorganisms of most concern in medicine are bacteria, viruses, rickettsiae, fungi, and protozoa. Another type of microorganism that is not common but can cause serious diseases in humans is prions.

Bacteria

Bacteria are single-celled organisms ranging from 1 to 10 microns in length and from 0.2 to 1 micron in width (a micron is a millionth of a meter or 1/25,000 of an inch). Like animal cells, bacteria have a cell membrane surrounding cytoplasm. Rather than a defined nucleus, however, bacteria have a diffuse nuclear region and, in addition to the cell membrane, a cell wall. Because of this latter characteristic, bacteria are classified as part of the plant kingdom. Like all living things, the genetic material of bacteria consists of chromosomes made up of DNA molecules.

Bacteria are classified by shape, by their spore-forming capabilities, by their biochemical and physiological characteristics, by their staining properties, and by their pathogenicity (tendency to cause disease). Classified by shape, there are three basic types of bacteria: the rod-like bacilli, the spherical or ovoid cocci, and the spiral corkscrew (spirochete). Some bacteria have whip-like cellular outgrowths which can help the bacterial cell travel distances quickly in a suitable liquid environment.

If the projections are few and are long in relation to the size of the cell, they are called flagella; if the projections are numerous and short, they are called cilia.

Most bacteria need the following environmental conditions for growth:

- Moisture—acting as a vehicle to transport food into, and wastes out of, the cell
- Food
- Warmth—preferably 98.6°F
- Slightly alkaline environment—7.1 to 7.4
- Free oxygen—aerobes (Some bacteria are anaerobes, which do not need free oxygen.)
- Indirect light
- No accumulation of wastes

Certain gram-positive bacteria, such as *clostridium* and *bacillus,* have the ability to become dormant when their environment becomes unfavorable (for example, very dry or lacking in nutrients). The cell loses water and shrinks. It remains this way until moisture is again available. Other species form spores to survive in extremely hot, dry, or cold environments. The cell shrinks and forms a new, thicker wall inside the old one.

This form of the cell (the spore) can withstand a harsh environment (extreme heat, lack of water, exposure to many toxic chemicals and radiation). When conditions are more favorable, the spore can absorb moisture, break out of its inner shell, and become a typical bacteria cell (vegetative stage). Some spores have been shown to survive for thousands of years in their dormant state. Spores discovered in the tombs of Egyptian pharaohs are still capable of becoming active bacteria. As another protective technique, a few types of bacteria, such as the bacterium that causes tuberculosis, have the ability to produce a waxy protein layer, called a capsule, on the outside of the cell wall. This outer layer protects them from unfavorable environments. Even without the thickened wall or capsule some cells can mend themselves, unless exposed to an adequate destructive process.

Most bacteria require free oxygen to function. These are called aerobic. Those that do not require free oxygen are anaerobic. (In fact, oxygen inhibits the growth of anaerobes.) The bacterium that causes tetanus (lockjaw), for example, is anaerobic. In a deep cut or puncture wound (as might be caused by a needle stick), where there is no air, it will find favorable conditions for growth and can cause illness. Examples of aerobic bacteria are *Staphylococci* and *Streptococci,* which will multiply in air if suitable nutrients (such as blood or pus) are available.

Bacteria can often be identified by their shape, colony structure, and color when stained with the method devised by the Danish physician Christian Gram. Gram staining is useful because it divides bacteria into two large groups, gram-positive and gram-negative. Gram-positive bacteria such as *Staphylococcus* and *Streptococcus* have cell walls that take on a characteristic color (purple-blue) from the Gram stain. Gram-negative bacteria such as *Pseudomonas* and *Klebsiella* resist the Gram stain, but can be colored by other dyes (pink-red).

Bacteria reproduce asexually. Each cell divides individually by a process called binary fission, which is similar to the mitotic process of higher organisms. Bacteria can multiply at remarkable speed. Reproduction becomes self-limited through depletion of needed nutrients; therefore it is important for the CSD technician to use thorough cleaning processes to maintain an environment in which it is difficult for microorganisms to survive. Some species grown in laboratory conditions can divide every 20 minutes. Without interference, a small number can grow to 250,000 bacteria within 6 hours. This explains why the entrance of only a few pathogenic bacteria into a human being can result so quickly in the symptoms of disease. Especially important is that the same bacteria may be nonpathogenic to some people, but extremely pathogenic to others.

Any type of bacteria that destroys tissue or produces toxins is pathogenic. Pathogenic bacteria cause diseases, such as staphylococcal infections (food poisoning, carbuncles), streptococcal infections ("strep throat"), tuberculosis, typhoid fever, tetanus (lockjaw), syphilis, and many others.

Bacteria can be useful as well as harmful. Some produce chemicals such as ethanol, acetic acid, butanol, and acetone. Others are used in the synthesis of drugs. Bacterial action is used in the curing of tobacco and in preparing animal hides for tanning. Bacteria also play a role in the production of cheese, sauerkraut, and other foods. In addition, they are used to break down raw sewage in sewage treatment plants.

Several types of bacteria are essential to normal body functions and, if confined to the appropriate area, do not produce disease. *Escherichia coli* (*E. coli*), for example, is found in the intestinal tract, where it helps in the formation of substances needed for proper intestinal function. If *E. coli* invades a wound or incision, however, it can become a pathogen and cause a severe infection. *E. coli* is also a common cause of urinary tract infections. *Clostridium perfringens,* when outside the intestine, causes gas gangrene. Tetanus is caused by *Clostridium tetani.*

Rickettsiae

At one time rickettsiae were classified as a separate type of microbial life, intermediate between bacteria and viruses because of features they share with both. However, they are now recognized as Gram-negative bacteria. Some are spherical and others are rod-shaped. Like viruses, they are intracellular parasites; that is, they can only multiply when they are inside living cells. As many as 50 different kinds of rickettsiae are harmless parasites in the intestinal tracts and salivary glands of insects such as lice, bedbugs, and ticks. A few of these rickettsiae, when transmitted to humans by insect bites, will multiply within human cells and produce the symptoms of disease. Only six kinds of rickettsiae are known to produce human disease. Examples of the diseases caused by rickettsiae are typhus fever, Rocky Mountain spotted fever, and Lyme disease.

Viruses

Viruses are much smaller than bacteria. Indeed, they are scarcely larger than some single molecules of protein. In one sense, viruses are not living organisms but large nucleoprotein particles, which enter specific kinds of animal or plant cells and multiply to form new virus particles. Viruses outside the host cell are inactive, since they rely on the metabolism of living cells to multiply. Each virus particle is a bit of genetic material enclosed within a protective coat of protein that permits it to pass from one cell to the next.

Viruses are the infective agent in many human diseases, including human immunodeficiency virus (HIV), smallpox, rabies, poliomyelitis, measles, warts, fever blisters, herpes, influenza, hepatitis, and the common cold. Also, research suggests that some forms of cancer may be caused or transmitted by viruses.

Each kind of virus usually attacks some specific part of the host's body. Apparently, the virus particles can reproduce only in certain cells and not in all cells of the body. The viruses of smallpox, measles, and warts attack the skin. Those of polio and rabies attack the brain and spinal cord, and those of yellow fever attack the liver. It is fortunate that many of the infections caused by viruses create a lasting immunity against reinfection (by triggering the body to produce antibodies, which kill virus particles before they multiply). Inoculating people with antibodies, or with mild forms of viruses that cause the production of antibodies, has been highly successful in preventing smallpox, measles, rabies, and yellow fever. Smallpox has been, for the most part, eliminated through immunization.

Fungi

Fungi are larger than bacteria and are more complex in structure and higher in evolutionary development; they are similar to simple plants. The most common types of fungi are yeasts and molds. Fungi may have one or many cells. Fungal cells have rigid outer walls and many have tubular, branching filaments called hyphae. The presence of fungi is often visible as an amorphous mass of fibers, as in the case of bread mold.

Fungi grow best in a dark, moist environment and have a strong resistance to environmental changes. They can either grow on their own or as parasites. The spores of aquatic fungi typically move about by means of flagellae. On land, fungal spores are dispersed by the wind or by animals. Before any health care facility undertakes renovations or repairs that would involve breaking into walls or ceilings, the area must be sealed off to avoid the spread of fungus (e.g., *Aspergillus*).

After remodeling or repairs are completed the area should be thoroughly cleaned before removing the barriers.

Fungi cause a variety of diseases in humans, domestic animals, and crop plants. These include poisoning (by certain mushrooms), ringworm, and athlete's foot in humans, and Dutch elm disease, brown rot, and timber rot in plants. Fungi are also a source of lysergic acid, or LSD, a hallucinogenic drug. In addition, fungi can cause the deterioration of wood, leather, cloth, and similar materials. However, some fungi are beneficial. There are edible mushrooms, penicillin is derived from fungi, and fungi are used in the production of some cheese, beers, wine, bread, and litmus.

Diseases caused by fungi are of great concern because there are limited antibiotics available for treatment and those that are available are highly toxic.

Protozoa

Protozoa are single-celled animals with no cell wall or with one composed of chitin (a carbohydrate material that also makes up the outer coat of insects). Some protozoa live as parasites in the blood or tissue fluids of humans and animals. Most live in fresh or salt water. Several diseases are caused by protozoa, including African sleeping sickness, amoebic dysentery, and malaria.

Prions

Prions are virus-like agents that can cause serious disease in humans and animals, and that cause chronic, fatal diseases of the central nervous system. Little is known about prions, but they are thought to differ from viruses in that they contain only protein (no DNA or RNA). They are not common, but they may become a problem in the future as more becomes known about current or orphan (rare) diseases. Prions are extremely resistant to destruction by methods that destroy other microorganisms.

Three diseases caused by prions are known in humans; an example is Creutzfeldt-Jakob disease (CJD). Extreme care must be taken to avoid contact with tissues of the brain, cornea, and spinal cord. At this time, it is recommended that instruments exposed to prions be wiped off at the site of use and steam sterilized in a prevacuum steam cycle at 270°F for 18 minutes exposure. They then should be put through the regular decontamination and disinfection process before terminal sterilization. Low-temperature sterilization methods, such as ethylene oxide and gas plasma, are ineffective in killing prions. Prions can remain in contaminated meat even after thorough cooking, can survive high temperatures, and can cling to surgical instruments even after they have been sterilized. Instruments have been known to transmit prions from one patient to another. The Centers for Disease Control (CDC) are developing guidelines for processing devices exposed to prions. CSD technicians must become familiar with their facility's policy on processing devices exposed to prions.

Antiobiotic-Resistant Microorganisms

Over the years there have been antibiotics developed that were able to fight off the infections caused by certain microorganisms. However, in the past few years some microorganisms have developed resistance to being killed by antibiotics. Some of these are methicillin-resistant *Staphylococcus aureus* (MRSA), drug-resistant tuberculosis (TB), drug-resistant *Streptococcus pneumonia,* Beta-lactam-resistant *Klebsiella pneumonia,* and Vancomycin-resistant Enterococcus (VRE). Some causes for resistance may be the misuse and indiscriminate use of antibiotics, and the mutation of microorganisms to create different enzymes or to change their cell wall structure. It becomes increasingly important for the CSD technician to understand how microbes are transmitted, to follow proper handwashing techniques, to understand the concept of microbial disinfection, and to adhere to all other infection control procedures.

Bioterrorism

Use of chemical and biological agents has become the weapon of choice for those that would like to destroy life. Health care facilities should have a readiness plan of response to bioterrorism events. CSDs should have a plan that partners with the housewide plan and includes such things as a disaster call list, means of acquiring additional supplies, ways of getting supplies in and out of the facility, a reserve supply of caregiver personal protective equipment, and cooperation with area health care facilities.

Four diseases with recognized bioterrorism potential are anthrax, botulism, plague, and smallpox.

Anthrax is an acute infectious disease caused by *Bacillus anthracis,* a spore-forming, gram-positive bacillus. Humans can become infected through skin contact, ingestion, or inhalation of the spores from infected animals or animal products. Person-to-person transmission of inhalation disease does not occur. Direct exposure to secretions of anthrax lesions may result in cutaneous infection. Pulmonary anthrax is associated with bioterrorism exposure to aerosolized spores.

Botulism is caused by *clostridium botuinum,* which is an anerobic gram-positive bacillus that produces a potent neurotoxin. Foodborne botulism is the most common form of disease in adults. An inhalational form of botulism is also possible. Botulinum toxin exposure may occur in both forms as agents of bioterrorism.

Plague is an acute bactierial disease caused by the gram-negative *bacillus Yersinia pestis.* It is usually transmitted by infected fleas, resulting in lymphatic and blood infections. A bioterrorism-related outbreak may be expected to be airborne, causing pneumonic plague.

Smallpox is an acute viral illness caused by the *variola* virus. Smallpox is a bioterrorism threat due to its potential to spread rapidly in a nonimmune population and because it can be transmitted via the airborne route. Smallpox is transmitted via large and small respiratory droplets and by contact with skin lesions or secretions.

All patients in health care facilities should be managed using standard precautions. Standard precautions are designed to reduce transmission from both recognized and unrecognized sources of infection in health care facilities, regardless of their diagnosis or presumed infection status. Principles of standard precautions should be applied for the management of all used patient-care equipment. CSD should be prepared for extra personal protective equipment usage, especially when smallpox or plague is the bioterrorism agent used.

Disease Transmission

To produce symptoms of a disease, microorganisms must have a fertile host. The term *cross-infection* indicates that they move from one host to another.

The following four basic factors are involved in disease transmission:

- There must be a portal of exit for microorganisms and a means by which they can travel to the next host.
- The host (potential recipient of an infection) must be susceptible.
- There must be a portal of entry for microorganisms into the new host.
- There must be a sufficient number of pathogenic microorganisms to cause an infection.

All these factors must be present for an infection to be acquired and to spread. With the knowledge of how microorganisms are transmitted, how they leave the body, and how they enter the body to cause an infection, CSD technicians can better protect patients and themselves.

Portals of Exit and Pathways of Transmission

The portals of exit are the means by which organisms leave one host and travel to the next host or patient. The portal of exit is not necessarily the same as the portal of entry. The hepatitis virus, for example, leaves the body by means of the intestinal tract (in the feces), urinary tract (in the urine), or blood (via a needle). To cause hepatitis in a technician or in another patient, the virus has to enter the body via either the mouth or the bloodstream (for example, a technician is pricked by a needle used on a hepatitis patient).

The transmission of pathogenic microorganisms from one human host to another occurs through four main pathways: direct contact, airborne particles or droplets, vectors, and fomites. Most pathogens cannot survive for very long outside their hosts. Thus, breaking the transmission cycle will destroy the microorganism and stop the spread of the disease.

Direct contact between humans transmits many diseases. Often, microorganisms travel across mucous membranes in the mouth from kissing or via the genitals (reproductive organs) from sexual contact. Sometimes transmission can occur on the skin due to hand contact or other skin-to-skin contact.

Airborne transmission occurs when a pathogen such as a spore is carried in the wind, on air currents, or on a dust particle from one host to a new host. The pathogen then enters the body through the respiratory tract or through a mucous membrane, such as the eye. Water droplets also carry microorganisms between people. This occurs through sneezing, through splashing of fluids, or through body secretions.

Many of the most difficult-to-control diseases are spread through vectors and fomites. Vectors are necessary to carry pathogens from the blood of one person to another. Living vectors are animals, usually ticks, fleas, and lice (also known as arthropods). Other arthropod vectors are insects such as mosquitoes and flies. Insects and animals are vectors when they host human pathogens and then infect humans through bites. Mosquitoes and rats, for example, are vectors for several diseases. In general, vectors are not harmed by the pathogens they carry.

Fomites are inanimate objects or materials on which disease-producing agents may be conveyed. Examples of fomites in the hospital environment are bedding, bandages, dressings, surgical instruments, patient care equipment, and eating utensils. Vectors and fomites are difficult to control, because the organisms they carry are spread rapidly. CSD technicians play an important role in the prevention of transmission of microorganisms by thoroughly cleaning patient care equipment, decontaminating surgical instruments, and keeping all work areas clean and dry at all times.

Susceptibility of the Host

A person's general health will affect his or her vulnerability to infection. Adequate nutrition, in particular, is essential in maintaining the body's natural defense mechanisms. The body's ability to recognize and combat foreign substances (by means of the antibodies of the immune system) and the numbers and capabilities of the white blood cells are two key factors in preventing disease. Maintaining their own general health is the single most important way that central service technicians can defend themselves against the microorganisms they will confront every day.

The patients who are most susceptible to infection include the elderly, the very young, and those whose general condition is compromised from a long-term illness or malnutrition. Sometimes a patient's defense mechanisms are impaired as a result of receiving chemotherapy for cancer or medication given to prevent rejection of a transplanted organ.

Certain types of cancer directly affect the immune system, making the patient highly vulnerable to infection. In fact, patients with lymphoma (cancer of the lymphatic system) may die not of the cancer itself but of a minor infection that ordinarily would not be life-threatening. The same is true of patients with leukemia, cancer of the bone marrow, which interferes with the production of healthy white blood cells.

One of the most devastating diseases of the immune system is acquired immunodeficiency syndrome (AIDS), a disease caused by a virus in which the body's defense mechanisms completely collapse, leaving it unable to fight infection at the cellular level. Similar in its catastrophic consequences is severe combined immunodeficiency syndrome (SCIDS), a congenital disease in which babies are born with almost totally nonfunctional immune systems. A famous SCIDS patient was "the boy in the bubble," a child who was kept in a sterile environment for more than 12 years in the hope that his immune system would eventually mature and he would be able to resist infection. However, soon after he left his "bubble," he died of a minor infection.

Portals of Entry

There are certain routes by which microorganisms normally enter the body and cause infections. The most common portals of entry are the respiratory tract, the eyes, the mouth and gastrointestinal tract, the genitourinary tract, and cuts or abrasions of the skin. Many disease organisms can cause an infection only if they enter through a specific portal. The bacterium that causes dysentery, for example, would probably not cause a problem if rubbed into a wound in the skin. If the same organism is swallowed, however, fatal dysentery may be the result. Some organisms can enter through almost any portal and cause a disease. From various portals of entry, organisms may pass into the circulating bloodstream and cause a secondary infection. A *Streptococcus* infection of the tonsil, for example, may secondarily cause endocarditis, an inflammation of the lining of the heart.

Microbial Population and Probability of Infection

Even if there is a portal of exit and means of transmission, a susceptible host, and a portal of entry, the symptoms of an infection will not develop until the microorganism is present in sufficient numbers. The number of microorganisms required to cause illness varies greatly. For example, one tubercle bacillus in the lung of a susceptible host can cause tuberculosis. On the other hand, hundreds of staphylococcal bacteria in a wound may not cause a problem. However, if the number of staphylococcal bacteria increases to thousands or hundreds of thousands, the body's defenses may be overwhelmed. The relationship between the number of microorganisms and the probability of infection is one reason why there is so much emphasis on cleanliness in the CSD.

$$\text{Infection} = \frac{\text{\# of microbes} \times \text{virulence}}{\text{host resistance}}$$

Disease Prevention

In order to prevent a disease from occurring, at least one of the factors involved in disease transmission must be eliminated. All infection control policies in the health care facility are aimed at eliminating these factors.

The rule to follow in eliminating the portal of exit involves blocking the exit. This requires such basic actions as covering the mouth when coughing or sneezing. Employees working in sterile areas of the CSD should be required to wear masks when they have a cold. This will reduce the possibility that any pathogens will be deposited on or in supplies that are being prepared for sterilization or that have already been sterilized.

Environmental cleaning of the health care facility is extremely important in preventing the spread of infection. Limiting the amount of dust and lint in the environment inhibits the movement of microorganisms.

Eliminating the portal of entry involves blocking these portals and preventing infective agents from coming into contact with them. This is the premise upon which standard precautions, OSHA's Bloodborne Pathogen Standard, and OSHA's Respiratory Exposure Control Plan are based. Employees are required to wear personal protective equipment that will protect them from exposures.

One of the areas with the highest probability of exposure to body fluids is the decontamination area of the CSD. In this area the following personal protective equipment is required to be worn: hair covers, eye protection or a face shield, masks that cover the mouth and nose, gowns or other attire (bunny suits) that are impervious, gloves, and shoe covers.

There are many ways in which people can protect themselves from becoming susceptible hosts. One of the primary ways involves maintaining general health. Adequate nutrition, sufficient rest, and good personal hygiene are essential to maintaining the body's natural defense mechanisms. The body's ability to recognize and combat foreign substances (by means of the antibodies in the immune system) and the number and capability of the white blood cells are two key factors in preventing disease.

Vaccination against disease is another method by which people can protect themselves from becoming susceptible hosts. Vaccines stimulate the formation of antibodies upon introduction into the body. These antibodies will fight the disease and the person will not become ill. Vaccines are disease-specific; that is, they will provide immunity only to a particular disease and not to general types of diseases. Many vaccines provide a permanent immunity. Other vaccines have to be repeated at intervals to remain effective. Diseases for which vaccines are available include polio (all three forms), typhoid fever, rabies, measles, mumps, rubella, pertussis, tetanus, and hepatitis B.

Reducing the bioburden (the number of microorganisms on an item) is one of the major ways in which the CSD assists in the health care facility's infection control program. This process begins when the item is picked up in the nursing area and is transported to the decontamination area, where medical devices are cleaned and disinfected. If necessary, the cleaned and disinfected items are then prepared for sterilization. Proper handling, storage, and distribution of these items can prevent bioburden buildup. Some of the ways CSD technicians avoid adding bioburden to clean and sterile supplies are proper handwashing prior to handling items, keeping storage areas clean and dry, and handling items as little as possible.

Nosocomial Infections and Cross-Contamination

Nosocomial infections are health care–acquired or health care–associated infections; that is, an infection that the patient did not have before entering the hospital but does have before leaving or shortly after discharge.

Nosocomial infections are a great expense and a source of suffering for patients. A longer hospital stay may be required to adequately treat the patient's infections, which means the patient spends more time away from family, work, and other obligations. Costly pharmaceuticals and additional supplies may be needed, thus increasing expense to the patient or the health care facility. There are an estimated 2 million nosocomial infections per year in the United States. Extra medical expenses due to nosocomial infections are estimated to cost as much as $5 billion per year.

Cross-contamination, the transmission of infection-causing microorganisms, is a major cause of nosocomial infections. Infection can be carried from person to person, or from one person to an object to another person. It is the responsibility of CSD staff to reduce cross-contamination (and thus help minimize the nosocomial infection rate) by doing the following:

- Using proper handwashing techniques
- Maintaining good hygiene
- Following good housekeeping practices
- Adhering to required work-flow patterns
- Maintaining barriers to contamination
- Following standard precautions
- Cleaning and decontaminating items properly

- Ensuring the sterility of processed items
- Correctly handling, storing, and transporting clean and sterile items

Three of these points warrant special emphasis: handwashing, barriers to contamination, and standard precautions.

Handwashing

Frequent and thorough washing of the hands by hospital personnel is the single best way to prevent nosocomial infections (Figure 3.1). Employees should wash their hands before going on duty, before and after meals, after using the bathroom, after handling soiled items, before entering clean areas or handling clean items, after blowing nose or sneezing into hand, after touching face, after removing protective gloves, and before going off duty. Good handwashing technique is as follows:

1. Remove rings.
2. Expose the forearms.
3. Turn on faucet and secure a steady stream of warm water.
4. Lather hands thoroughly to the wrist with a CSD-approved handwashing agent. Soap helps suspend the soil.
5. Vigorously rub all surfaces of hands for at least 10 seconds. Friction helps loosen the soil. Don't forget to clean areas around nails, between fingers, and back of hands.
6. Thoroughly rinse the hands under a stream of running water.
7. Dry hands thoroughly with a paper towel, taking care not to scrape the skin surface and cause irritation.
8. Discard the paper towel in a designated container.
9. Turn off the faucet with a clean, dry paper towel.
10. Discard the paper towel in a designated container.

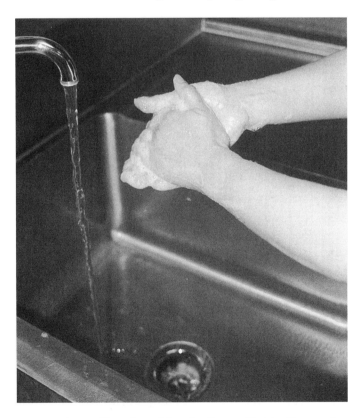

Figure 3.1. Handwashing Is Essential in Preventing Cross-Contamination.

11. Use hand lotion to soften the skin and discourage the shedding of skin flakes harboring microorganisms. Hand lotion should not be used when handling sterile supplies or surgical instruments. Lotion can keep hands moist, get on packaging, and cause contamination of the package. Lotion that gets on cleaned surgical instruments can harbor microorganisms and increase the bioburden. It could also be considered a foreign material inside a patient's body.

Alcohol-based, waterless hand hygiene agents may be used to clean hands, but only when they are not visibly soiled, such as after blowing a nose or sneezing. Apply to the palm of the hand, cover all areas of hands with the gel, rub lightly until dry, and do not rinse hands. Oil-based lotions should be avoided when wearing latex gloves; oil breaks down the gloves' protection.

Barriers to Contamination

Throughout the hospital, potentially contaminated areas are usually separated from clean areas by barriers. In most CSDs, there are physical barriers between the decontamination area and the rest of the department. The best barriers between such areas are solid walls. Anything less may allow airborne pathogens or droplets carrying pathogens to gain access to clean areas.

Air flow must be controlled to minimize the travel of microorganisms from "dirty" areas to clean areas. This is accomplished by designing the ventilation system so that air is drawn into some areas and drawn out of others. In the CSD, air is drawn from clean areas (positive air pressure) into the decontamination area (negative air pressure), thereby helping to confine microorganisms in the latter area.

Fans should not be allowed in CSD. They create turbulent air flow, changing the downward air flow of the ventilation system. Air flow created by fans can recirculate dust and microorganisms from work surfaces and the floor.

Another important barrier to contamination is traffic control. People carry microorganisms on their bodies and clothing. Therefore, to minimize contamination, only authorized, properly attired personnel are allowed into the CSD. Also, the traffic patterns within the CSD should be designed so that the "people flow" is always from clean to "dirty areas."

Standard Precautions

Standard precautions are an approach to infection control required by OSHA's Bloodborne Pathogen Standard. Standard precautions synthesize the major features of universal precautions (blood and body fluid precautions) and body substance isolation (designed to reduce the risk of transmission of pathogens from moist body substances) and apply them to all patients receiving care in the health care facility, regardless of their diagnosis or presumed infection status. Standard precautions apply to blood, all body fluids and secretions and excretions except sweat (regardless of whether or not they contain visible blood), nonintact skin, and mucous membranes. Standard precautions are designed to reduce the risk of transmission of microorganisms from both recognized and unrecognized sources of infection. Articles contaminated with blood or body fluids must be discarded, bagged as infectious in a red bag, or placed in an impervious container and labeled with a biohazard logo before being sent to the CSD. All sharps should be handled with care. Disposable sharps should be discarded at point of use in leakproof, puncture-resistant containers. Reusable sharps should be separated from other instruments and contained for transport in an impervious container.

Employees are to wear personal protective equipment (PPE) whenever performing procedures that put them at risk of exposure. Personal protective equipment includes gloves, masks, eye protection, hair covering, shoe covers, and a barrier such as impervious gowns and aprons. More details on standard precautions and PPE are presented in Chapter Four.

Disinfection Principles

Disinfection is the process of killing most pathogenic microorganisms, but not necessarily spores, on an item or surface. Disinfection is usually accomplished with chemicals, although physical agents, such as hot water, may also be used. The chemicals used to disinfect hard surfaces or inanimate objects are called disinfectants. Those used on body surfaces are referred to as antiseptics. Items must be thoroughly cleaned before the disinfection process. Some soils can decrease the effectiveness of disinfectants.

Microorganisms can be grouped according to their resistance to physical or chemical germicidal agents. The descending order of microorganism resistance to germicidal chemicals is bacterial spores, mycobacteria (TB), nonlipid or small viruses, fungi, vegetative bacteria, and lipid or medium-sized viruses. Prions are not listed here because they cannot be destroyed by any chemicals. It is important for the CSD technician to know what microorganisms are currently a problem in health care facilities so that they can evaluate which disinfectants should be used. As was explained earlier, the list of microorganisms of concern can change from year to year.

The process of disinfection can be thought of as having three levels of effectiveness: low, medium, and high. The nature and amount of contamination and the intended use of an item determine which level is appropriate. The chemicals used for disinfection vary in their level of effectiveness, depending on their properties and on the concentration and manner in which they are used. The major classes of disinfectants are described in Chapter Four.

Low-level disinfection removes or kills some types of vegetative bacteria and some fungi and lipid viruses. It is ineffective against TB, spores, and nonlipid viruses. This level is usually appropriate for general cleaning of environmental surfaces in noncritical areas, such as floors and work counters.

Medium or intermediate-level disinfection kills most pathogenic microorganisms, but may not remove some viruses and does not kill bacterial spores. This level is usually appropriate for general patient care equipment, such as stethoscopes and blood pressure cuffs, and for hospital laundry.

High-level disinfection kills all microorganisms except a large number of spores. This level of disinfection is appropriate for items that have been in contact with infectious tissue or body fluids. It is also used for medical devices that will come in contact with a patient's mucous membranes when in use (such as a gastroscope passed through the mouth and esophagus to allow examination of the inside of the stomach).

For items that will penetrate skin or mucous membranes, or that will be in contact with the vascular system of a patient, it is necessary to go even further in eliminating microorganisms. These items must be sterile, that is, free of all microbial life. Examples of items that must be sterilized before use are surgical instruments and cardiac catheters. The principles of sterilization are discussed in the next section of this chapter. The various sterilization techniques used in hospitals are described in Chapter Seven.

As noted earlier, physical agents can also be used for the disinfection of surfaces. Pasteurization is usually thought of as the process that makes milk safe to drink, but it is also used in some hospitals to disinfect respiratory therapy and anesthesia equipment. The process involves immersing cleaned items in water heated to 160–180°F for at least 30 minutes. Pasteurization produces high-level disinfection, which kills most bacteria, viruses, and fungi, but does not eliminate all spores.

Sterilization Principles

Sterilization is the process of killing all forms of microbial life. In health care facilities, this is accomplished by subjecting items to a sterilizing agent under prescribed conditions for a specified time.

Proving that a particular item is sterile is difficult. Even if an item is immersed in culture media and incubated for days, and then shows no evidence of microbial growth, it is still possible that some microorganisms have survived. The surviving microorganisms might have required different conditions for growth than those established in the culture test (for example, a higher incubation temperature or different nutrients). Surviving bacteria may have required anaerobic conditions, and viruses require living cells of another organism in order to reproduce. Some proof of the probability of sterility can be gained by testing a few items from a sterilized group, but there still might be surviving microorganisms on untested items.

Microorganisms differ in their resistance to being killed under adverse conditions. Some types can resist high temperatures. Some are relatively resistant to poisonous chemicals. Even within the same species or type of microorganism, some individuals are "hardier" than others and take longer to die.

Because of these complexities, sterilization processes are designed to provide a very high probability or assurance that no microorganisms will survive on any item in the load. This probability is usually accepted to be about a one-in-a-million chance that any microorganisms will survive after the sterilization process. To achieve this level of sterility assurance, the sterilization process must create conditions that will kill even the most highly resistant microorganisms (bacterial spores) and must maintain these conditions until all areas of the load are penetrated and all microorganisms destroyed. Reusable items exposed to prions require extremely extended sterilization time (270°F for 18 minutes' exposure in a prevacuum steam sterilizer).

The fewer the number of microorganisms on an item (the lower the bioburden), the better the assurance that the item can be sterilized. Therefore, items should be cleaned thoroughly before being sterilized. Longer sterilization processing time is also required for items with complex structures that slow down the penetration of the sterilizing agent (for example, air-powered surgical instrumentation).

Pyrogens (fever-inducing substances) are another reason it is important to reduce the bioburden on an item to be sterilized. When bacteria and other microorganisms die, their cell walls may rupture. The cellular material released may be highly toxic to patients if it comes into contact with the bloodstream, even though the bacteria themselves are dead. The cellular debris left behind after sterilization can cause illness that is usually manifested by fever. Reducing the bioburden before sterilization reduces the amount of cellular debris left after processing and thus reduces the risk of introducing pyrogens into patients.

Five basic sterilization techniques are used in health care facilities: steam sterilization, EtO gas sterilization, dry-heat sterilization, gas plasma, and chemical immersion. These basic techniques are discussed in detail in Chapter Seven. Other low-temperature sterilization technologies are being developed. The CSD technician should keep up on what technologies have been cleared for use.

Radiation sterilization is used extensively in industry for those items that can withstand this process. Only large quantities of items are sterilized in this manner because of the high cost of a radiation sterilization facility. Because of the size of the loads, however, the cost per item is quite economical, which explains the use of radiation sterilization by manufacturers of sterile hospital supplies.

Making the choice to sterilize or disinfect patient care instruments and devices and deciding which level of disinfectant should be used are made easier by categorizing the items. CDC guidelines classify patient care items, by risk of infection associated with use of the item, as critical, semicritical, and noncritical.

Critical items are those instruments or objects that are introduced into the body, either into normally sterile areas or the bloodstream. They pose a high risk of infection if contaminated; therefore the use of sterile items is required. Examples of critical items are surgical instruments, implants, intravenous (IV) infusion items, and catheters.

Semicritical items are those that come in contact with intact mucous membranes. Use of sterile items is desirable; however, high-level disinfection of these items is acceptable. Examples of semicritical items are anesthesia and respiratory therapy equipment, endotracheal tubes, and flexible endoscopes.

Noncritical items are those that come in contact with intact skin. Intermediate to low-level disinfection can be used. Examples of noncritical items are blood pressure cuffs, bedpans, IV pumps and poles, and linens.

Isolation

Central service department technicians may have to supply various areas in the health care facility with isolation precaution items, such as respirators, masks, gloves, and gowns. Direct patient care givers use isolation precautions as a type of barrier to contamination aimed at reducing the opportunity for transmission of certain pathogens. The types of precautions for which PPE is used by care givers are airborne, contact, and droplet. Since CSD technicians must consider all used items as having harmful microorganisms, no special handling or cleaning techniques are used for items having been used on patients in isolation. Standard precautions (explained earlier and in Chapter Four) must be practiced for all used reusable items that have been exposed to the patient and then are returned to the CSD department.

Summary

Chapter Three has reviewed the structure, types, and mode of action of microorganisms that cause disease and the means by which disease can be transmitted from one person to another. Ways in which infections are acquired in hospitals have been discussed, along with some of the basic techniques for preventing cross-contamination. The principles of disinfection and sterilization were presented.

The following chapters present in greater depth the role of the CSD in infection control and its major processing and distribution functions.

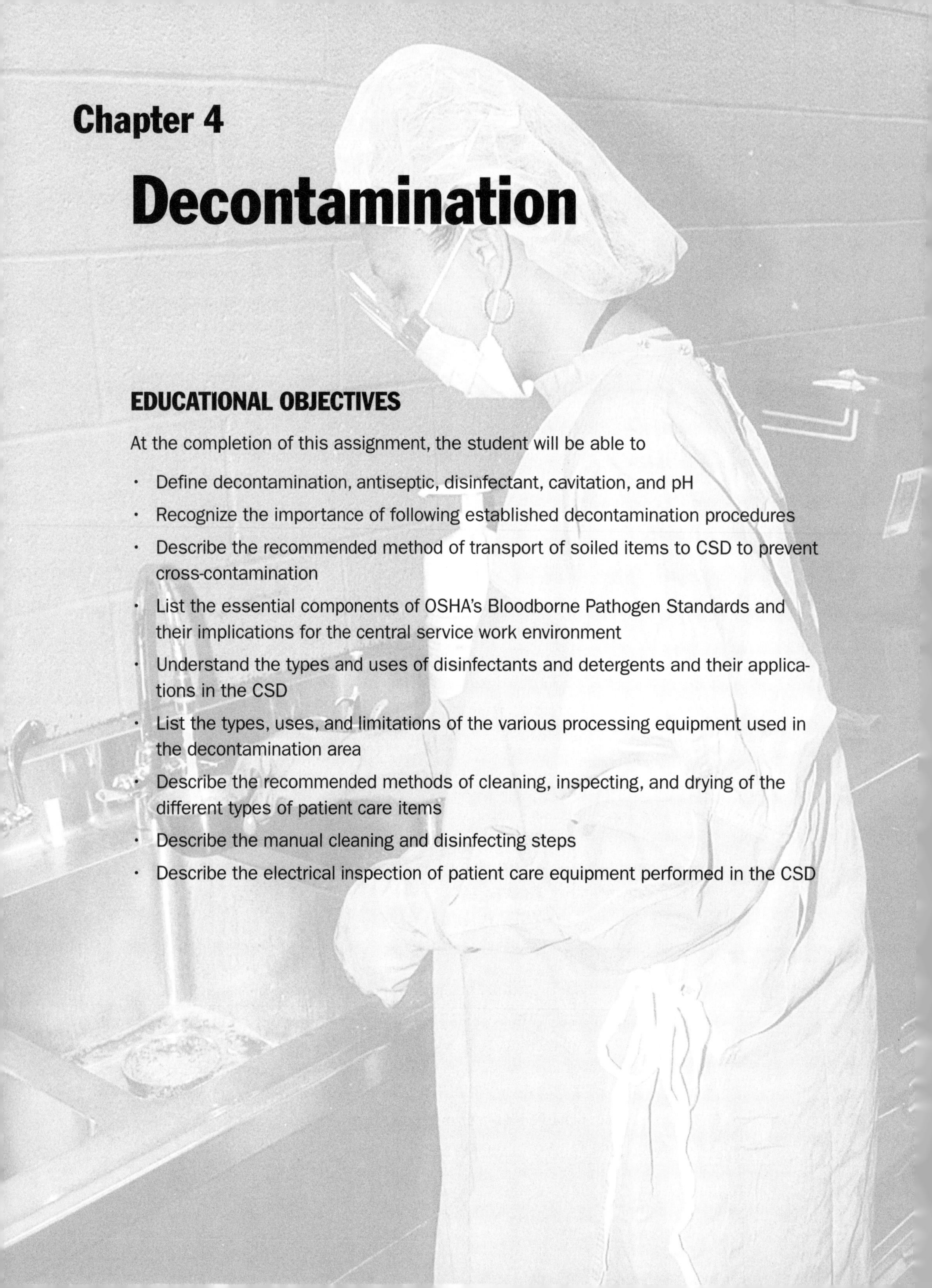

Chapter 4

Decontamination

EDUCATIONAL OBJECTIVES

At the completion of this assignment, the student will be able to

- Define decontamination, antiseptic, disinfectant, cavitation, and pH
- Recognize the importance of following established decontamination procedures
- Describe the recommended method of transport of soiled items to CSD to prevent cross-contamination
- List the essential components of OSHA's Bloodborne Pathogen Standards and their implications for the central service work environment
- Understand the types and uses of disinfectants and detergents and their applications in the CSD
- List the types, uses, and limitations of the various processing equipment used in the decontamination area
- Describe the recommended methods of cleaning, inspecting, and drying of the different types of patient care items
- Describe the manual cleaning and disinfecting steps
- Describe the electrical inspection of patient care equipment performed in the CSD

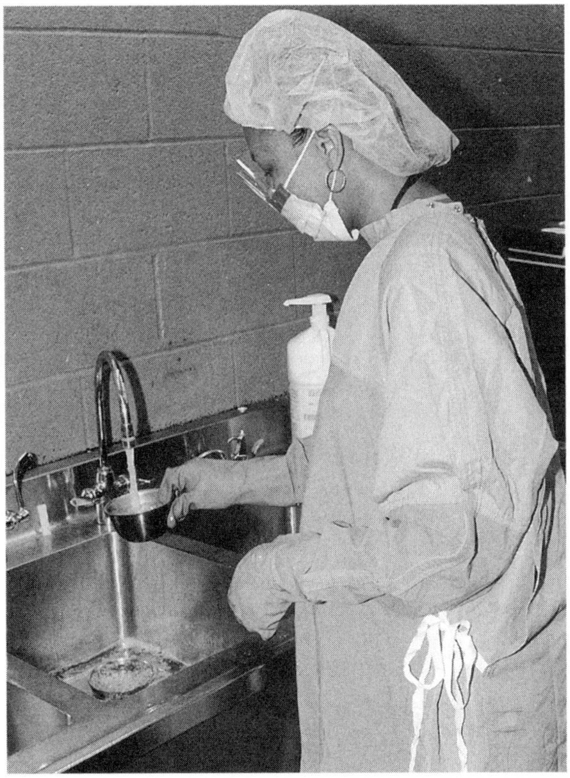

DECONTAMINATION IS THE PROCESS by which contaminated items are rendered safe for handling by personnel who are not wearing protective attire. It is the first and most critical step in breaking the chain of disease transmission. The decontamination process can range from manual cleaning and disinfection to cleaning equipment and supplies. This process does not necessarily mean items such as medical instruments or devices are ready for patient use. It is essential that central service technicians understand and comply with the policies and procedures that have been established for the protection of patients and themselves, because the decontamination process also presents the greatest biological hazard to personnel.

This chapter addresses decontamination area design, personal protective equipment (PPE), and recommended materials-handling techniques. The major types of cleaning and processing equipment, detergents, and disinfectants will be discussed, as well as general guidelines for their consistent use.

Collection and Transport of Used Supplies and Equipment

All used supplies and equipment are considered contaminated and should be collected and transported to the decontamination area in a manner that minimizes the potential of contamination of staff, patients, or the environment. Equipment should be covered. Supplies should be contained. Covered carts, closed totes, containers with covers, or closed plastic bags may be used to contain contaminated supplies during transport (Figure 4.1).

Some instrument sets are not owned by the facility. They are brought to the facility by instrument manufacturers as needed. These are called loaner instruments. Loaner instruments should always be opened and decontaminated even if they are brought into the facility wrapped. How the instruments were previously cleaned and sterilized is unknown; therefore loaner instruments should be processed according to the facility's policies and procedures for all instruments. A system must be established for verifying loaner instruments coming into and leaving the facility. As discussed in the preceding chapter, diseases such as CJD that contain prions have special instrument-processing requirements to destroy the prions. For this reason, the facility should have specific policies and procedures in place that address how loaner neurosurgical and ophthalmic instruments will be processed when they are brought into the facility. Some facilities may require long-exposure-time sterilization of these types of instruments before regular processing steps.

Whenever possible, equipment and carts should be taken to the decontamination area in designated elevators, cart lifts, or dumbwaiters, so that contact with patients, staff, or visitors can be avoided. Liquids should be disposed of at the point of use in the nearest designated sanitary sewer or septic system. If liquids cannot be disposed of at the point of use they must be contained and secured for transport to prevent spilling or splashing. Personal protective equipment must be worn when disposing of liquid waste. Pour liquids gently to minimize splashing. Some hospitals do have equipment that can be hooked to suction containers to empty them and lower potential for employee contact with blood or other infectious materials. The hazardous waste policy at each hospital may vary and should be reviewed (during initial orientation and then yearly) and followed.

The decontamination area should be directly accessible from outside the CSD through either corridor doorways or dedicated automatic lifts, cart lifts, or dumbwaiters, and it should be physically separated from all other hospital and CSD areas. Air in the decontamination area must not be allowed to flow into clean areas of the CSD. This is accomplished by keeping doors closed and by exhausting more air from the area than is supplied by the air ducts, which results in negative air pressure. These design and ventilation arrangements help ensure that contaminants will not be spread to other areas of the department, which must remain clean. Testing of this air-handling system should be done annually for the protection and safety of the workers. There should be at least 10 air exchanges per hour. The temperature should be kept between 60°F and 65°F, and humidity should be kept between 35 percent and 60 percent. These parameters help control the spread and growth of microorganisms and allow some comfort for those wearing protective equipment.

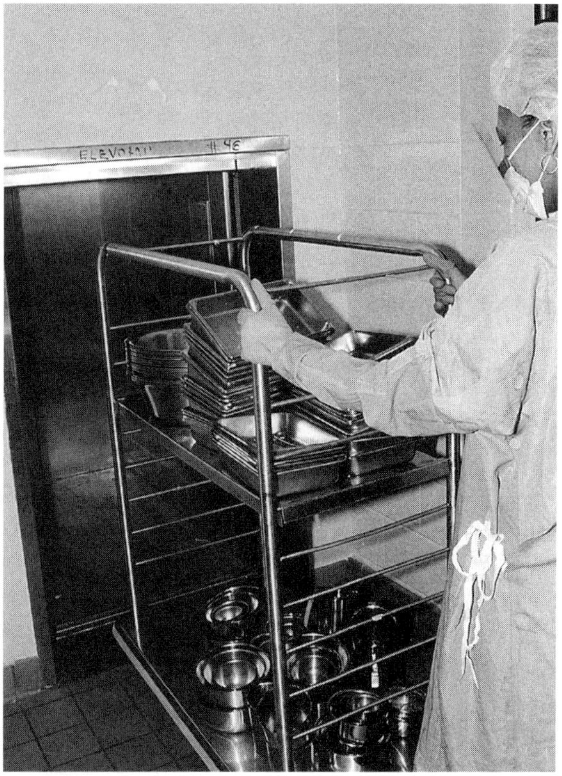

Figure 4.1. A Dedicated Dumbwaiter May Be Used to Transport Supplies from the Operating Room to the Decontamination Area.

Decontamination Area

The decontamination area must be kept clean to reduce the risk of infection to employees and to minimize the bioburden on items as they enter the assembly/ preparation area. All horizontal surfaces (floors, work counters) and sinks should be cleaned and disinfected with an environmental disinfectant at least once a day, preferably every shift, and as necessary due to gross contamination of an area from splashing or a spill. Cleaning the floors and hand sinks is usually the responsibility of environmental services, and CSD staff are responsible for work surfaces and sinks. Only the supplies needed for cleaning and disinfection should be stored in the decontamination area and only in small quantities.

Personnel working in the decontamination area should wear surgical scrubs laundered by the hospital. In addition, employees assigned to decontamination must wear PPE, which includes disposable hair covering, an impervious barrier (a jumpsuit, apron with sleeves, or gown), shoe covers, heavy-duty latex-free or plastic gloves, a face mask, and safety glasses that wrap around the eyes, or a face shield whenever there is potential for splashing, spraying, or aerosolization of blood or other potentially infectious materials (Figure 4.2). When personnel leave the decontamination area, PPE must be removed. If gloves are reusable they must be washed inside and outside and then hung inside-out to dry. Hands must be washed after removing protective attire and gloves. Remember that a warm, moist environment is conducive to microbial growth, and skin is always shedding microorganisms. Any reusable protective equipment, such as a face shield, must be cleaned thoroughly and disinfected. Clean protective attire should be donned upon return to the area. Surgical scrubs must be changed whenever they become wet or contaminated.

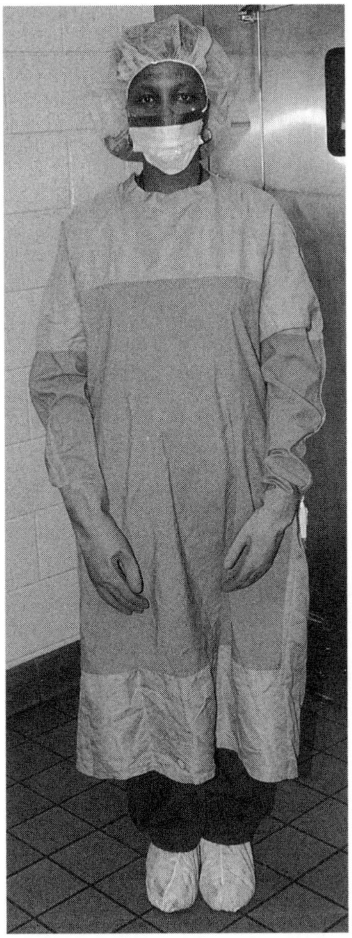

Figure 4.2. An Example of Protective, Impervious Attire.

Requirements for PPE are in place to protect workers and are mandated by the OSHA rule for bloodborne pathogens. This rule also contains information on handling and containment of contaminated items and hazardous waste, safe work practices, environmental controls, response to spills, and training requirements. All CSD technicians must know and follow the parts of the rule that apply to their work areas.

Standard Precautions

On December 6, 1991, the U.S. Occupational Safety and Health Administration (OSHA) published the final federal rule for *bloodborne pathogens.* Bloodborne pathogens are pathogenic microorganisms that are present in human blood and can cause disease and death in humans. These pathogens include, but are not limited to, hepatitis B virus (HBV), hepatitis C virus (HCV), and human immunodeficiency virus (HIV).

This rule is to help protect workers from all occupational exposures to blood or other potentially infectious materials (OPIM). The rule requires the use of an approach to infection control called *standard precautions.* Standard precautions require that all human blood and all body fluids, secretions, and excretions except sweat regardless of whether or not they contain visible blood; all nonintact skin; and all mucous membranes be treated as if they are infectious. This standard requires all workers to follow OSHA guidelines while doing their jobs.

Background

The U.S. Congress was asked by health care worker unions to pass the bloodborne pathogens standard. As the concern over the AIDS epidemic increased, health care workers became more concerned about work-related exposure to bloodborne diseases. Needle-stick and sharps injuries, in particular, have drawn attention because, despite safety guidelines and staff education, the incidence of these injuries still exist. Infection with HIV, which causes AIDS, is unusual but can occur after a needle stick.

Prior to the AIDS epidemic, little attention was focused on the highly contagious hepatitis B virus and other diseases that are spread through the blood. The CDC reports that about 200 to 300 health care workers die each year as a direct or indirect result of work-related injuries when the employee is infected with hepatitis B. As many as 12,000 health care workers per year become infected with the hepatitis B virus. Studies show that at least 20 types of microorganisms that can cause disease are spread by needle-stick injuries.

The OSHA standards on bloodborne diseases were based on guidelines already written by the CDC and the National Committee for Clinical Laboratory Studies. The CDC is not a regulatory agency.

However, the Infection Control Program of the CDC does have a *guideline* containing general considerations for methods and indications for handwashing, disinfecting, and sterilizing of medical instruments and environmental surfaces, and for protection from harmful microorganisms. The CDC does not test, evaluate, or recommend specific products.

Exposure Control Plan

Each health care facility must have an exposure control plan that provides a basic framework for how the facility will follow the bloodborne pathogens rule. Some departments, such as CSD, will have additions to the plan to meet personal protection in the work area. The plan must be accessible to all staff 24 hours each day.

Exposure Determination

Employees who perform jobs in which there is a reasonable likelihood of exposure are covered by the bloodborne standard. An exposure incident may result from contact with human blood or other potentially infectious materials, which include cerebrospinal fluid, synovial (joint) fluid, pleural (lungs) fluid, pericardial (heart) fluid, peritoneal (abdominal) fluid, amniotic (uterine) fluid, saliva in dental procedures, semen, vaginal secretions, any body fluid that is visibly contaminated with blood, and all body fluids in situations where it is difficult or impossible to tell the difference between body fluids.

Exposure of an employee to blood or other potentially infectious materials may occur in the following ways: percutaneous (needle stick or sharp under the skin); exposed skin (dermatitis, cuts, abrasions, hangnails, etc.); broken skin (human bite); eye (splash); or mucous membrane (splash into mouth or eyes).

Examples of CSD tasks that may involve potential exposure to bloodborne pathogens include cleaning medical, surgical, or diagnostic equipment; cleaning up a blood or body fluid spill; or handling contaminated waste or linen. Any person doing these activities is responsible for understanding and abiding by the OSHA Bloodborne Pathogen Standard.

Engineering Controls

Engineering controls will be used when possible to avoid or reduce staff exposure to blood and body pathogens. Examples of engineering controls are sinks for handwashing in an immediate work area, a separate decontamination area with negative air pressure relative to surrounding areas, temperature and humidity controlled to allow workers to wear required protective equipment, surfaces (counters, shelves, tables, floors, walls, ceiling) in the decontamination area made of material that can be cleaned, adequate floor drains, and safety shields that prevent staff from being splashed or splattered.

Safe Work Practices

Safe work practices will be used by CSD technicians to avoid or reduce exposure to blood and body fluid pathogens. These practices can be defined as how work is done and the following of policies, procedures, rules, and regulations. All CSD technicians must be constantly alert to, and must change, practices that may contribute to injury and contamination of self and others. Work practices defined in the OSHA Bloodborne Pathogen Standard that apply to CSD are explained in the following paragraphs.

NEEDLES AND OTHER SHARPS When moving trash or soiled linen, pick up bags from the top (not the bottom) and hold the bags away from the body. Sharps may have inadvertently been put in a bag.

Staff must not place needles and other sharps in their pockets or attempt to catch sharps or glassware that have been dropped.

Recapping of contaminated needles using a two-handed method, removal of contaminated needles from disposable syringes by hand, and bending, shearing, or breaking of contaminated needles are *NOT* allowed.

If recapping must be done, a one-handed scoop technique or a mechanical device must be used.

Contaminated disposable needles and other sharps must be put into facility-designated, disposable, puncture-resistant, leakproof sharps containers right away or as soon as possible after use. Sharps containers are put as close to the area of use as possible and in areas such as central service where contaminated needles and sharps are likely to be found. Sharps containers must be labeled with the biohazard symbol or word (Figure 4.3) and have a lid that can be closed and cannot be reopened. Never reach into or overfill sharps containers.

Contaminated reusable needles and sharps are placed in containers that are puncture-resistant, leakproof, and labeled with the biohazard sign. Reusable sharps must not be stored in a manner that would require staff to reach with hands into the containers where these sharps have been placed.

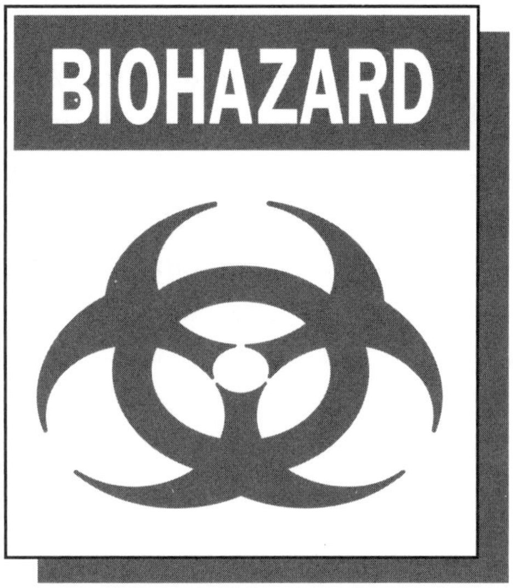

Figure 4.3. Biohazard Symbol.

INSTRUMENTS TRAY Never reach with the hand into reusable surgical or procedure instrument containers. Forceps should be used to retrieve instruments. Approved dirty instrument containers (perforated containers that fit inside solid containers) could be used for instruments that require soaking in a solution. Solutions can be drained so that each instrument can be identified as it is picked up. After use, instruments should be placed back in a tray with hinged instruments open and multipart instruments apart. This minimizes the handling of used items from the point of use to completion of decontamination. The instruments are then ready to be put in the mechanical cleaning equipment without additional handling.

BROKEN GLASSWARE Broken glassware must not be picked up with the hands. Use brushes and dust pans. Broken glassware should be placed in regulated waste containers after being picked up.

EATING AND DRINKING Eating, drinking, putting on make-up or lip balm, and handling contact lenses are not allowed in areas where contact with blood and other potentially infectious materials may occur. Food and drink must not be stored in or on shelves, cabinets, or countertops where blood and other potentially infectious materials may be present.

HANDWASHING Handwashing areas should be available in the work area. An antiseptic hand cleaner that is bactericidal should be available for use in areas where handwashing facilities are not available. Hands must be washed after exposure to any body fluid and right after removing protective gloves.

PREVENTION OF SPLASHING, SPRAYING, AND SPLATTERING Any procedure involving blood, body fluids, or infectious materials—for example, emptying a suction unit, disposing of a solution that instruments have been soaking in, or using a spray or brush—must be performed in a way that greatly lowers the risk of splash, spray, or splatter. Gently pour the solution down the side of the sewer receptacle. When using compressed air to dry lumens, direct spray away from everyone.

CONTAMINATED EQUIPMENT All contaminated equipment and instruments are to be decontaminated prior to being inspected or repaired in the facility or sent to the manufacturer. If the equipment or instrument cannot be fully decontaminated, a biohazard symbol must be placed on the equipment and the portion of the equipment that remains contaminated must be identified. In addition, if a contaminated item is being sent to the manufacturer, a biohazard symbol must be placed on the outside of the shipping package. Each facility should have guidelines on shipping biohazardous materials.

PERSONAL PROTECTIVE EQUIPMENT The health care facility must provide staff, who are at risk for exposure to blood and OPIM, with the right PPE. The equipment must be supplied in the right sizes and without cost to the employees. It must be cleaned, and repaired or replaced by the institution if the equipment is damaged or for some other reason can no longer be used. Staff who are at risk are required to use these barriers, such as gowns, masks, eye protection, and gloves, and to remove them prior to leaving the decontamination work area. If any PPE is penetrated by blood or OPIM, it must be replaced as soon as possible. Gloves that become torn or punctured must be replaced immediately. Disposable gloves should never be decontaminated and reused.

Staff must be trained to use PPE in the correct way and to select barriers appropriate for the task. The PPE for staff working in decontamination is described earlier in this chapter.

HOUSEKEEPING, LAUNDRY, AND REGULATED WASTE A routine schedule for cleaning and decontamination of all equipment, work surfaces, sinks, cupboards, floors, walls, air vents or HVAC vents, and ceilings must be established and maintained. Each health care facility must designate, in its exposure control plan, the staff who are responsible for cleaning specific surfaces and equipment. The CSD-specific plan must contain information on their areas of responsibility.

Reusable linen that has touched moist body substances must be contained in labeled (by word, symbol, or color), leakproof bags. Used linen must not be rinsed or sorted in the area of use. Staff must wear gloves and other protective equipment as needed when collecting or transporting soiled linen.

Regulated waste (contaminated) must be placed in labeled (by word, symbol, or color), leakproof bags or containers. These bags or containers must be accessible to all areas in which staff handle contaminated waste. Only regulated waste should be put in these designated bags or containers because it is disposed of in a more costly manner (e.g., burned or microwaved) than regular trash (e.g., landfill). CSD technicians must follow state and local waste disposal regulations.

RETRIEVING REUSABLES ACCIDENTALLY PUT INTO CONTAMINATED WASTE, LINEN, OR SHARPS BAGS OR CONTAINERS This procedure must be carried out in a "soiled" area (e.g., decontamination, soiled utility room, disposable holding area). Person(s) inspecting waste, linen, or sharps for reusable items must wear PPE. An impervious material can be placed on the floor or work surface and the contents *gently* dumped onto it. *Never* reach into the bag or container. Pickup forceps must be used to retrieve the reusable item and to put the rest of the contents back into a bag or container. Dispose of the impervious material and PPE in an appropriate bag or container.

SPILLS OF BLOOD OR OPIM PPE must be worn. Spills should be contained and gross soil picked up with an absorbent material, such as paper towels. Contaminated absorbent material must be handled like regulated waste. The area is then cleaned with the disinfectant designated in the facility's exposure control plan.

Compliance

CSD technicians must comply with the personal protective measures and safe work practices described. Staff who do not comply must be subject to corrective action. Supervisors are responsible for ensuring compliance of their staff.

Training and Continuing Education Requirements

Supervisors will ensure that all staff with the potential for an occupational exposure attend a training program, which should be given at no cost to the staff during work hours. Introduction to OSHA's Bloodborne Pathogen Standard and the facility's exposure control plan must be given during employee orientation. A CSD-specific plan for PPE and safe work practices should be part of the training at the time tasks are introduced in which exposure to contaminated items may take place.

Documentation of all training must be placed in each employee's file. Training and education records for all employees must be kept for a period of three years. Retraining should occur at least once a year, covering changes in task performance or procedures, or new tasks or procedures that may affect the staff's occupational exposure risks or a review. The training must be documented in the employee's file. Educational materials should be appropriate to the education level, literacy, and language of the staff.

The person leading the training should be knowledgeable about the topic as it relates to the workplace under discussion.

The training program should contain at least the following:

- A copy of the text of OSHA's Bloodborne Pathogen Standard and details about its contents
- Information about the epidemiology and symptoms of bloodborne diseases
- Information about the ways bloodborne pathogens are spread to people
- Information about the exposure control plan and how staff can get a copy of the plan
- Information about safe work practices, engineering controls, and appropriate PPE for different tasks or activities that might involve exposure to blood and potentially infectious materials
- Information about how to pick out PPE and on the types, proper use, location, removal, handling, decontamination, and disposal of protective gear
- Information about hepatitis B vaccine
- Information about the right actions to take and persons to contact after a spill with blood or potentially infectious materials

- Information about the procedure to follow if an exposure incident occurs, including the way to report the incident and the medical follow-up that will happen
- Information about the postexposure evaluation and follow-up that is required after an exposure incident
- Information about the signs, labels, or color coding required and used
- Time for questions and answers with a qualified instructor

Detergents and Cleaning Agents

Cleaning items manually or mechanically is the first step in the decontamination process. Detergent solutions are used for cleaning. Detergents are agents that lower surface tension, break down fat, oil, and grease, break soil into fine particles, and suspend particles during the cleaning process. This aids in the rinsing off of soil. Before using the detergent solution, gross soil should be rinsed off with cool water. Warm or hot water may coagulate the protein in the organic material and make it harder to remove.

Detergents used in the decontamination area are selected for their suitability for the cleaning job to be done. Always follow the manufacturers' instructions for correct dilution, solution temperature, water hardness, and use. A germicide and detergent combination may be used to clean and disinfect equipment. There are specific detergents designed for use in washer/sanitizers, washer/sterilizers, washer/decontaminators, ultrasonic washers, laboratory dishwashers, and cart washers, and for manual cleaning. Some detergents can be used for manual as well as ultrasonic washing of instruments. Proteolytic enzymatic cleaners facilitate the process of removing protein materials (blood and body fluids). Lipolytic enzymatic cleaners facilitate the process of removing fatty materials (bone marrow and adipose tissue). Proteolytic or lipolytic enzymatic cleaners are generally used to soak instruments that have hard-to-remove or dried-on protein or fatty materials on them. It is essential to know the maximum temperature of the water when using enzymatic detergents. Temperatures exceeding 140°F can inactivate the enzyme activity. Always read the manufacturer's written instructions for use. It is best to use a detergent designed specifically for the particular application (e.g., type of soil, type of mechanical equipment, manual cleaning, the material the item is made of, water hardness). A detergent with neutral pH should be used for surgical instruments, because they can be damaged by harsher detergents. Manual cleaning requires a nearly neutral pH (7–8) solution and friction on the item surface to loosen and suspend the soil. A more alkaline detergent is generally used with mechanical equipment to compensate for the lack of friction used with manual cleaning in loosening soil. Low-sudsing detergents must be used in mechanical equipment to avoid damaging the equipment.

The pH is a measure of the acidity or alkalinity of a substance. A pH of 7 is considered neutral. A liquid with a low pH is acidic; a liquid with a high pH is caustic or alkaline (see the display). Examples of acidic substances are blood, vinegar, and lemon juice. Soap is an example of an alkaline substance. Substances that have either a high pH (very alkaline) or low pH (very acidic) can be damaging to tissue, metal, rubber, and plastics.

pH

1	2	3	4	5	6	7	8	9	10	11	12	13	14
acidic						neutral							alkaline

Soap has little value in the CSD for cleaning purposes because it is a strong alkaline material with fatty substances, rinses off poorly, leaves a film that will interfere with germicidal action, and interferes with the action of some disinfectants. Some manufacturers of implantable devices and specialty materials recommend washing in organic soap, not a synthetic detergent because the implant material (e.g., mammary sizers) can absorb the detergent and the patient can have an unpleasant reaction. Therefore, the CSD may need to keep a supply of organic soap (e.g., Ivory flakes) on hand for these specialty items. Items washed with organic soap require thorough rinsing because soaps are more difficult to remove.

Disinfectants

A disinfectant is an agent that destroys vegetative forms of pathogenic microorganisms but not bacterial spores on inanimate objects. Environmental disinfectants are low to medium level and are used to disinfect work surfaces and equipment. High-level disinfection is typically used for medical devices. High-level disinfection is accomplished by immersing the device for a specified period in a chemical agent that has been registered by the FDA as a high-level disinfectant/sterilant.

General Guidelines for Using Disinfectants

Items must be *thoroughly cleaned* before being disinfected because dirt, blood, mucus, and tissue will interfere with the action of the disinfectant. The disinfectant, in sufficient concentration and at the correct temperature, must remain in contact with all surfaces for a specific period to allow penetration of all the microbial cell walls and deactivation. The necessary concentration, temperature, and exposure period are different for each disinfectant, and the manufacturer's directions for use must be followed carefully.

Disinfectants should not be mixed with each other or with detergents, since this may inactivate their disinfecting properties. Disinfectants should be mixed with distilled or deionized water. Tap water contains minerals that may interfere with the action of disinfectants. If air is entrapped under or within an item, the disinfectant cannot completely contact all the surfaces. Items should be dried after cleaning to prevent dilution of the disinfectant. When indicated, it is essential that the disinfectant be thoroughly rinsed from items before the items are used. Follow manufacturers' instructions carefully. When evaluating disinfectants, keep in mind that the necessary concentration, type of water used to make a solution, appropriate temperature, and exposure period differ, so always check the label for specific information for using that product correctly. For example, the microbiocidal activity of the disinfectant will be rendered inactive when used in combination with hard water. The label will specify whether the disinfectant needs to be mixed with distilled or demineralized water.

Several types of disinfectants are commonly used. Only those whose labels indicate approval by the EPA for hospital use (or FDA for high-level disinfectants) are acceptable for CSD applications. The CSD technician must understand the properties and appropriate uses of each type of disinfectant. Some disinfectants are more effective than others against particular pathogens. Some bacteria are harder to kill than others. The tubercle bacillus, for example, which causes tuberculosis, has a waxy coating that protects the cell wall and makes it harder to penetrate. Some disinfectants are harmful to certain materials. The label on the disinfectant container will indicate the type of microorganisms it is effective against (tuberculocidal, virucidal, bactericidal, fungicidal, sporicidal, etc.). Follow the *label* information and directions. Labeling requirements are strict. Other printed materials do not have any restrictions.

Always remember that if disinfectants will kill microorganisms, they can also be harmful to the cells of the human body, so personnel should take precautions to avoid direct contact with these chemicals. These chemicals should always be used in well-ventilated areas. Material safety data sheets (MSDSs) should be readily available for review or reference. OSHA's Hazard Communication Standard requires that workers must be informed of the hazards of the chemicals with which they work. Information must include PPE (gloves, goggles), exposure limit, and review of MSDS for chemicals used in the work area. Review chemical hazards under "Safety" in Chapter One. Documentation of this training must be placed in the employee's file. The label on the disinfectant container also contains information on hazards, PPE, spill and disposal and first-aid steps.

Types of Disinfectants and Antiseptics

Quaternary ammonium compounds (QUATS) are most commonly used as low-level disinfectants for environmental cleaning. They are effective against Gram-positive bacteria, but ineffective against some Gram-negative bacteria, *M. tuberculosis,* lipid viruses, and spores. Some QUATS have additives that make them effective against more types of microorganisms. Check the label on the container carefully. QUATS are relatively nontoxic to humans. Concentrated quaternary ammonium compounds, which must be diluted, should be mixed with distilled water to achieve the proper concentration, because certain minerals commonly found in tap water will interfere with their action. Quaternary ammonium compounds are inactivated by inappropriate dilution and organic matter. QUATS are neutralized or absorbed by gauze, cotton, and wool; therefore, these can decrease the concentration of the solution. It is especially important to remove moisture and gross debris from surfaces to be disinfected to ensure effectiveness. In addition, QUATS are somewhat corrosive to metal, so care must be taken in their use.

Chlorine and iodine belong to the chemical group called halogens and are the active ingredients in several commonly used disinfectant solutions. Because these elements are gaseous at room temperature, they are mixed with other chemicals or compounds to keep them in solution. Sodium hypochlorite (household bleach) is used in the laundry as a low-level to medium-level disinfectant, depending on concentration. It is also used to clean environmental surfaces, especially when they may be contaminated with hepatitis viruses or HIV. Surfaces must be clean and gross soil and contaminants removed so that the active chlorine can contact all surfaces. Hypochlorites are inactivated by organic matter. Chlorine deteriorates with age and corrodes stainless steel. Disinfection level and the type of microorganisms that can be destroyed depend on the concentration of free chlorine (e.g., dilutions of 1:10 to 1:100 chlorine are acceptable for use with blood spills).

Iodine is used primarily as an antiseptic on skin. Tincture of iodine (iodine combined with alcohol) is used on cuts and abrasions. Iodophor compounds also contain iodine and are less harsh to skin than tincture of iodine. They are commonly used as the final preparation of the skin before injections or surgical incisions. Also, when combined with a detergent, iodophors are used as handwashing agents. The concentration of iodine used for these purposes is inadequate for hard-surface disinfection. To produce effective medium-level or high-level disinfection, the concentration of available free iodine must be at least 450 parts per million (ppm) (the concentration will be stated on the product label). The product must be registered with the EPA as a hard-surface disinfectant iodophor at the recommended dilution. Some individuals are allergic to the iodine in iodophors. (An allergy to shellfish may indicate an iodine allergy.) Iodine is corrosive to metal and damages rubber and some plastics.

Phenolic compounds are derived from carbolic acid (phenol) and are more effective disinfectants than the original form. Most phenolics are effective against vegetative bacteria, fungus, and *M. tuberculosis.* They are not effective against bacterial spores and some viruses such as Coxsackie virus and echovirus. Because of their long-lasting action (leaves a residual film), phenolic compounds are good for disinfecting walls, floors, exterior surfaces, and equipment in areas where hepatitis or other viral disease is not a concern. Before phenolic compounds are used, all detergent residuals must be rinsed thoroughly from the items to be disinfected, or else the disinfectant may be totally inactivated. (However, there are commercially prepared mixtures of phenolics and detergents. These mixtures should be used according to the manufacturer's instructions.) Carefully read label directions for preparing the phenolic solutions because small changes in the dilution make a big difference in the disinfecting action. To disinfect there must be wet contact for a specific period. Follow label directions.

Because phenolic compounds are quite toxic, they should not be used in food preparation areas, in the nursery or on nursery equipment, or in the operating room. Nor should they be used on porous materials (such as anesthesia or respiratory therapy tubing), because the phenolic may be absorbed, and rinsing does not remove the chemical. The chemical could cause skin or mucous membrane irritation if the materials come into prolonged direct contact with patients or staff. Prolonged contact may cause irreversible depigmentation of the skin (loss of color), so CSD personnel should wear plastic or latex-free gloves when using phenolic disinfectants. Rubber gloves should not be worn when using phenolics. Infants exposed to phenols may develop hyperbilirubinemia; therefore, phenolics should not be used to clean infant bassinets and incubators.

Hexachlorophene is a phenol-based skin antiseptic used for handwashing. It is effective only against Gram-positive bacteria and is relatively slow-acting compared to other skin antiseptics. Hexachlorophene is absorbed through the skin and can cause damage to the nervous system of infants. Therefore, it should not be used on infants or by pregnant women (because it will cross the placental barrier).

Alcohols are effective antiseptics and sanitizers that will kill a variety of bacteria, viruses, fungi, and *M. tuberculosis,* but not bacterial spores and some hydrophilic viruses. It is not always practical to use alcohols as disinfectants because of the prolonged wet contact time (5 to 10 minutes) needed, and alcohol evaporates rapidly. Isopropyl alcohol is the alcohol most commonly used for antisepsis and sanitizing, and its most effective concentration is 70 percent alcohol to 30 percent water by volume. More frequently, 70 percent isopropyl alcohol is used to dust surfaces because it removes dust and quickly evaporates. Alcohol can damage rubber, plastics, and lensed instruments. It is inactivated in the presence of organic soil.

Glutaraldehyde is an effective high-level disinfectant commonly used for medical devices that can withstand complete immersion in the solution. Because the solution must contact all surfaces, how items are immersed (e.g., air displaced by solution in lumens) is critical. Examples of items that might be disinfected in this way are rigid and flexible endoscopes and some anesthesia and respiratory therapy equipment. Glutaraldehyde is noncorrosive to rubber, plastic, and metal.

Glutaraldehydes have both a shelf life and a use life. The shelf life is a predetermined time that has been established by the manufacturer between activation (i.e., adding an alkaline buffer to the solution) and disposal. This period is usually 14 days for products without surfactants and 28 days for products with surfactants (agents that lower surface tension). Use life is affected by events such as temperature, organic soil, and in-use dilution. The use life cannot exceed the shelf life, but may be less depending on the events. The concentration of glutaraldehyde should be tested frequently during the 14 or 28 day period to determine if there has been in-use dilution to a point where it should no longer be used. There are test strips available to test the concentration, which should remain close to 2 percent (refer to the label for minimum effective concentration). To avoid dilution, dry items before immersing in the glutaraldehyde. In 2 percent concentration, glutaraldehyde is effective against all vegetative bacteria, viruses, *M. tuberculosis,* and fungi when items are immersed for 10 hours. (Chapter Seven describes the use of glutaraldehyde as a sterilant.)

There are conflicting label claims and lack of consistency in the published literature on the time and temperature required for high-level disinfection using glutaraldehyde. Some mycobacterium, including *M. tuberculosis,* requires a longer high-level disinfection exposure time than most organisms. A minimum of 20 minutes at 68°F or 20°C (room temperature) exposure is generally required *when items have been cleaned prior to disinfection.* The Association for Professionals in Infection Control (APIC) endorses this recommendation. The FDA has cleared some aldehyde products requiring an exposure of 45 minutes at 77°F to 25°C (requires heating the solution) and some at 20°C. The manufacturer's instructions on the label regarding shelf life, dilution, immersion time, and temperature should be followed.

Glutaraldehyde can be very toxic. All items disinfected with glutaraldehydes must be rinsed *thoroughly,* preferably with sterile distilled water. Using tap water will add bioburden again. Personnel must take precautions to protect themselves. Goggles or protective glasses and butyl or nitrile rubber gloves should be worn when mixing or using glutaraldehydes. Not all rubber gloves are protective against aldehydes. The vapors can cause severe irritation of the eyes, nasal passages, and upper respiratory tract. Liquid contact with skin and mucous membranes can cause irritation. If liquid contacts skin or eyes, flush with water immediately. In fact, some individuals become allergic to glutaraldehyde and cannot tolerate being in a room where there is even a tiny amount of vapor in the air. Glutaraldehyde must be stored in a covered container and used only in a well-ventilated area, preferably under a self-contained fume hood.

Employee exposure to glutaraldehyde is regulated by federal and state agencies. OSHA has set a ceiling limit of 0.2 ppm as a regulatory requirement for exposure to glutaraldehyde. The American Conference of Governmental and Industrial Hygienists (ACGIH) has made an official recommendation to lower the ceiling limit to 0.05 ppm. A ceiling limit is the maximum air concentration of a substance to which anyone should be exposed, even momentarily. (Do not confuse ceiling limit with time weighted average [TWA], which is the amount of exposure averaged from an eight-hour period.) The ACGIH is not a regulatory agency; however, OSHA often adopts recommendations from ACGIH. CSD technicians must keep up with changing regulations. There are instruments that can measure real-time glutaraldehyde levels in the work environment. As mentioned earlier, some manufacturers require a temperature of 25°C when using their product. This requires heating of the solution, which releases vapors, therefore potentially increasing the level of glutaraldehyde in the work environment.

Ortho-phthaldehyde 0.55 percent is a non–glutaraldehyde-based high-level disinfectant that can be used for medical devices that can withstand complete immersion in the solution. It is compatible with many metals, adhesives, plastics, and elastomers. After a thorough cleaning and drying, the device is immersed in the solution for 12 minutes at room temperature. Thorough rinsing at least three times with fresh water each time is required. The solution has a tendency to stain protein and tissue. An advantage to this is that devices that have not been thoroughly cleaned will be identified by the stain.

The concentration of this liquid chemical disinfectant should be tested daily to determine if there has been in-use dilution to a point where it should no longer be used. The manufacturer of the chemical has test strips available to verify minimum effective concentration. The in-use life of this chemical is 14 days.

Cleaning and Processing Equipment

Many types of mechanical cleaning equipment are available. The CSD technician must be familiar with the specific applications, limitations, and procedures for using each piece of equipment used in their work environment.

General instruments can be processed through mechanical equipment, such as a washer/sterilizer, washer/decontaminator, or ultrasonic washer. It is essential that instruments and other items being processed in a mechanical cleaner be loaded correctly, to ensure that all surfaces get exposed to the detergent and rinse water. Instruments must be placed into perforated or wire-mesh trays, if not already done so by the user. These types of trays are used so that there is no interference with the proper mechanical action of the equipment. The heaviest instruments should be placed on the bottom of the tray to avoid damaging lighter instruments. Hinged instruments must be open and arranged in a manner to allow water, detergent, and steam to contact all surfaces. Instruments consisting of two or more parts should be disassembled unless the instrument manufacturer recommends otherwise. Items with concave surfaces should be placed on their side or upside down to allow adequate cleaning, rinsing, and steam contact. Cups, bowls, etc., should not be placed over instruments. Doing so can prevent the detergent solution from reaching all surfaces of instruments. The trays should not be stacked or overloaded in washers, to ensure that all surfaces are exposed to the detergent and rinse water. Sets should never be stacked in ultrasonic washers, to avoid the action of the cavitation process being blocked. Other types of mechanical equipment are available to clean glassware, carts, utensils, and respiratory therapy items.

Washer/Sterilizers

The washer/sterilizer is used to clean heat-tolerant items. After removal of gross soil, surgical instruments are often processed through a washer/sterilizer. It is very important that washer/sterilizer manufacturers' directions be followed concerning the arrangement of instruments in the trays. If soil is dried on instruments or they are not arranged properly before processing, some soil may remain after the wash phase and be baked on during the sterilization phase, which may damage the metal, require special cleaning processes to remove the dried-on soil, interfere with subsequent sterilization processes, contaminate clean processing areas, or cause a pyrogen or allergic reaction in the next patient. For some washer/sterilizers, detergent must be manually added with each load; others have a system that feeds the detergent automatically when it is needed. The cycle consists of several washes and rinses, followed by a steam sterilization cycle appropriate for the types of items contained in the load (Figure 4.4).

Although subjected to a cycle designed to sterilize clean items, items processed in a washer/sterilizer should not be assumed to be sterile at the end of the process. The reason for this is that items enter the washer/sterilizer with an unknown, but probably very high, level of microbial contamination, which the sterilization cycle may not be able to completely destroy. In addition, items should not be used as sterile, because there may be residual soil, which can cause pyrogenic reactions.

Stainless steel instruments should not be processed close to instruments made of other metals, such as nonanodized aluminum, brass, copper, or chrome plating. It is possible for a reaction known as electrolytic conduction to occur in the wet, hot chamber of the washer/sterilizer; this results in one metal plating onto another. Although this is not a common reaction, the separation of stainless steel instruments from other metals will prevent permanent damage should this reaction occur.

Delicate instruments can be damaged in one type of washer/sterilizer due to the agitation of solution during the wash phase. In this type the chamber fills with solution, steam is injected through the solution, and the turbulent action of the solution loosens the soil. Another type of washer/sterilizer has rotating sprayer arms that spray the detergent solution from several directions during the wash phase.

It is extremely important to use the recommended amount of a low-sudsing, free-rinsing detergent with a pH of between 7 and 10 in these machines. Use of a high-sudsing detergent or too much detergent will result in residue on the instruments. Detergents with a pH below 6 or much above 9 will damage the surface finish of the instruments. Never use abrasive cleaners, as they can also cause damage to instruments.

Biological control testing should be performed on the washer/sterilizer at least once a week, preferably daily, to test its kill power. A glass ampoule biological test is the product of choice for this testing.

Washer/Sanitizers

The washer/sanitizer is similar to a washer/sterilizer, except that after the dirty items have been subjected to several washes and rinses, they are exposed to live steam at at-

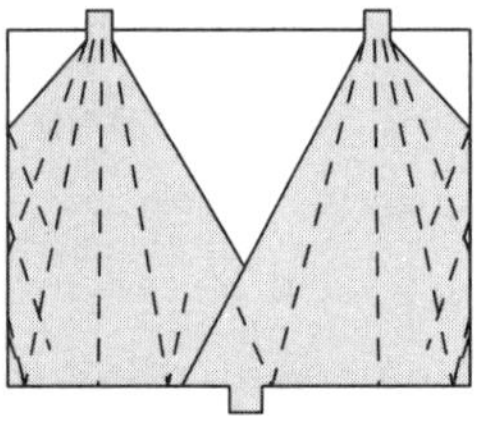

Pre-rinse aids removal of heavy protein soil deposits such as blood and tissue by continuous spray rinse in the chamber.

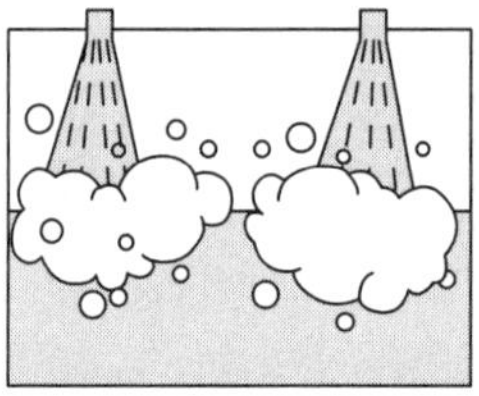

Automatic detergent injection measures the amount of detergent needed and eliminates hand dispensing. This predetermined quantity provides economical detergent use and reduces foaming. Injection is adjustable to meet varying water conditions.

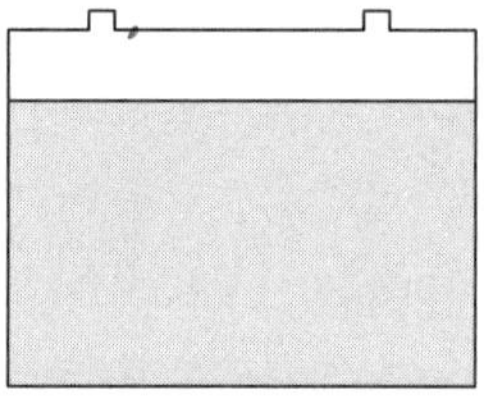

During the fill phase water level control assures instrument immersion for effective cleaning. A computer-controlled timer monitors lapsed fill time and communicates potential low pressure in the water supply, which is important to the cleaning process.

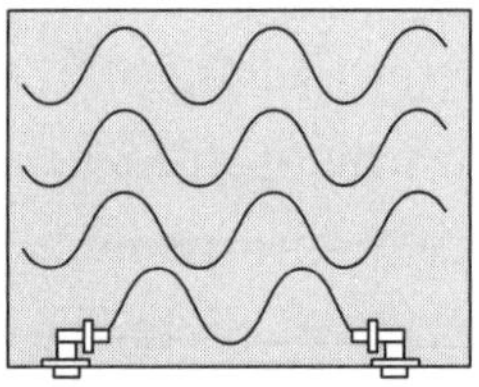

Wash phase is computer designed to maximize agitation for soil removal. Water temperature is carefully controlled, which is also important in the removal of protein soil.

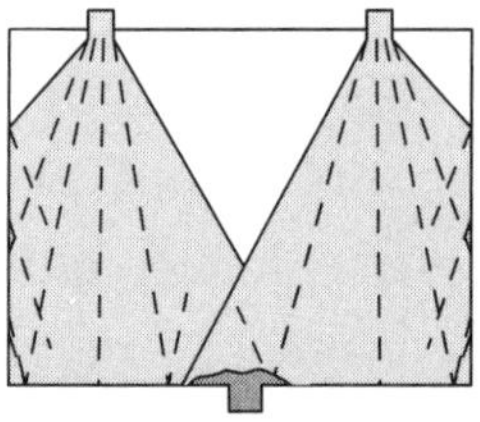

Post-rinsing rids instruments of loose residual soil and detergent film. This final phase of the cleaning process effectively prepares instruments for sterilization.

Figure 4.4. The Wash and Rinse Cycles of One Type of Washer/Sterilizer.

mospheric pressure rather than to a steam sterilization cycle. At atmospheric pressure the steam does not reach the temperature it would in a sterilizer (steam under pressure). Sanitization is a process that reduces the number of microorganisms to safe levels as judged by public health requirements. The process is not designed to kill spores, and it may not destroy highly resistant microorganisms, such as anthrax, bubonic plague, or gas gangrene. The end result is medium-level disinfection only.

Washer/Decontaminators

Washer/decontaminators use a cycle of pre-rinsing (with an enzymatic solution in some models), cleaning with a detergent solution, rinsing with a final rinse using very hot water (180° to 195°F), and drying at a high temperature. Some models have an ultrasonic cleaning phase after a general cleaning phase, some have a chemical disinfectant rinse, and some use a very high-alkaline detergent, which is neutralized after a short time. They can be single-chamber units or multichamber units. Washer/decontaminators use rotating sprayer arms at the top and bottom, and between each layer of instruments (Figure 4.5).

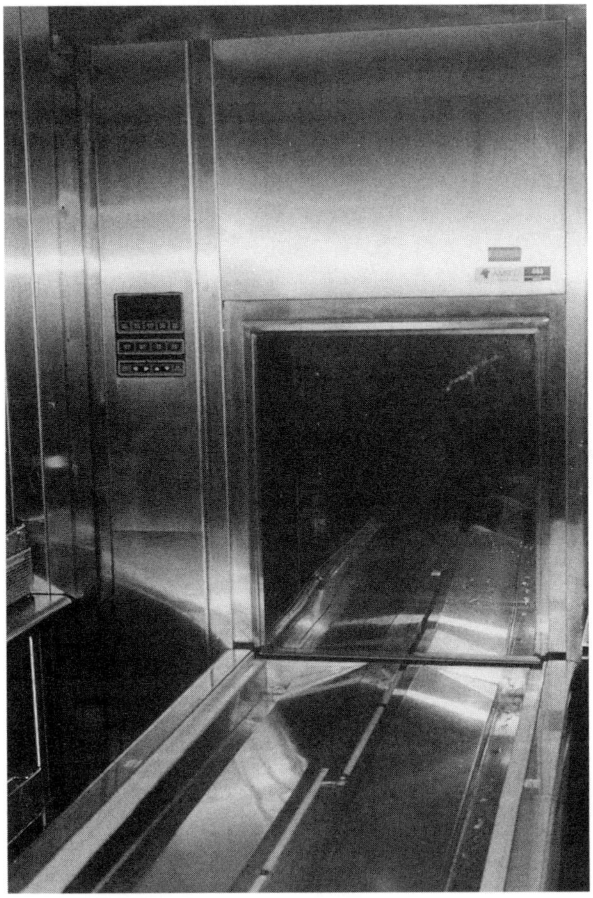

Figure 4.5. A Washer/Decontaminator.

Wire-mesh or mesh-bottom trays must be used to decontaminate utensils and instrument-container systems. Some have the capability of decontaminating respiratory therapy equipment. These units provide high-level disinfection, depending on the temperature and exposure time in the rinse phase of the cycle.

An advantage to using a washer/decontaminator is that very little handling or rearranging of instruments is needed before they are put in the unit. It is important for staff to handle items as little as possible before they are decontaminated as a protection against microbial contact. Another advantage is that delicate instruments can be decontaminated in some models of this type of equipment.

Ultrasonic Washers

The ultrasonic washer is used to remove *fine* soil from hard-to-reach places that other equipment and manual cleaning may not remove (Figure 4.6). Gross soil must be removed before putting items in the ultrasonic washer. If not done, the energy can be absorbed by the soil particles, making the process ineffective. The equipment works by converting high-frequency sound waves into mechanical vibrations in the solution. The high-frequency energy causes microscopic bubbles to form on the surfaces of the instruments, and as the bubbles become unstable and implode (collapse into themselves from the surrounding water pressure), minute vacuum areas are created, drawing out the tiniest particles of debris from the crevices of the instruments. This process is called cavitation (Figure 4.7).

The energy created in these machines is not designed to remove gross soil, and there is no evidence that it will kill microorganisms. Therefore, ultrasonic washing should not be considered a disinfecting process. Unless the solution is changed *frequently,* the bioburden in the solution will increase and eventually add bioburden to the instruments. It could also increase the risk of microorganism exposure to personnel operating or working in the vicinity of the ultrasonic washer. The ultrasonic process and subsequent rinses create fine aerosols containing microorganisms at the surface of the water. These aerosols may be harmful to personnel. Therefore, the covers on ultrasonic cleaners should always be closed when in operation. If the cover is not closed, or there is no cover, a face shield or goggles and a mask should be worn, along with other PPE, during operation of the washer.

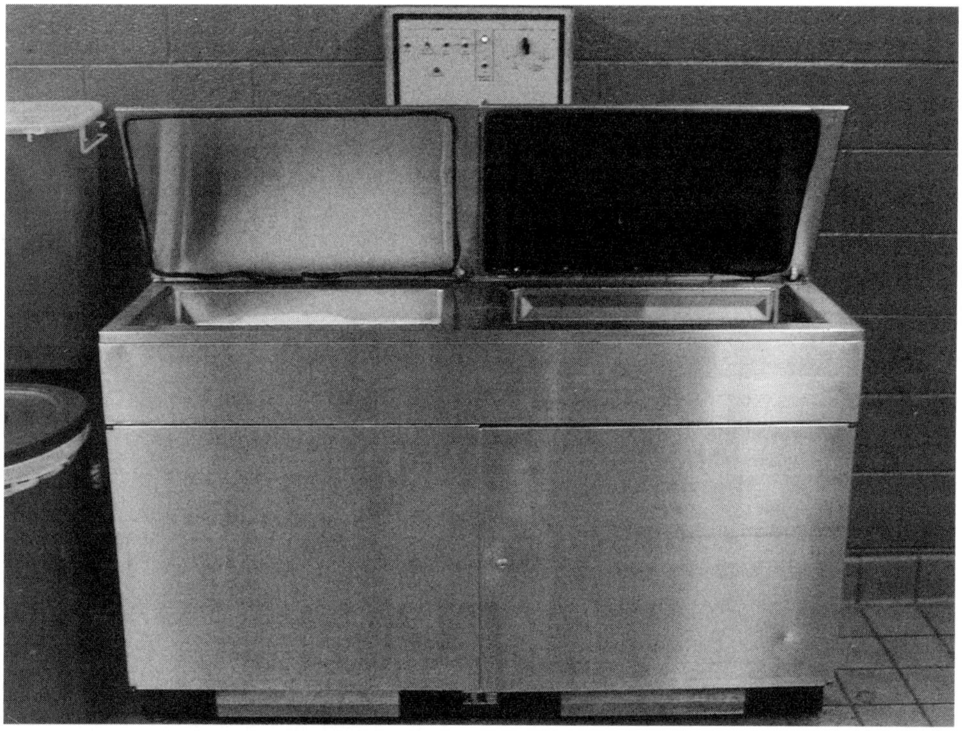

Figure 4.6. An Ultrasonic Washer.

A few ultrasonic washers automatically insert baskets of instruments through wash and rinse chambers; in others, the baskets must be moved manually from one chamber to the next. The wash chamber must contain a detergent that is specified for use in ultrasonic cleaners. If a detergent is selected that is not recommended for ultrasonics, the cleaning process can be adversely affected. The detergent label should specify that the product can be used in ultrasonic cleaners, not just mechanical washers. This solution should be changed frequently to keep the cleaning agents active. The rinse chamber sprays rinse water (preferably distilled or deionized) over the instruments. The time required for each process is usually 4 to 5 minutes. In some units, there is a chamber for hot-air drying. Of course, items that may be damaged by the heat should not be placed in this chamber, but should be air-dried on a rack instead. If a hot-air drying chamber is not available, instruments should be dried with absorbent materials so that no visible water drops remain, especially in hinges or box locks.

There are two theories on when in the reprocessing cycle the ultrasonic washer should be used. One theory is to clean and decontaminate the instruments, either by hand or by means of a washer/sterilizer, before placing them in the ultrasonic washer. Supporters of this sequence are concerned about the fine spray of microbe-laden particles from soiled instruments that can be caused by the ultrasonic washer and

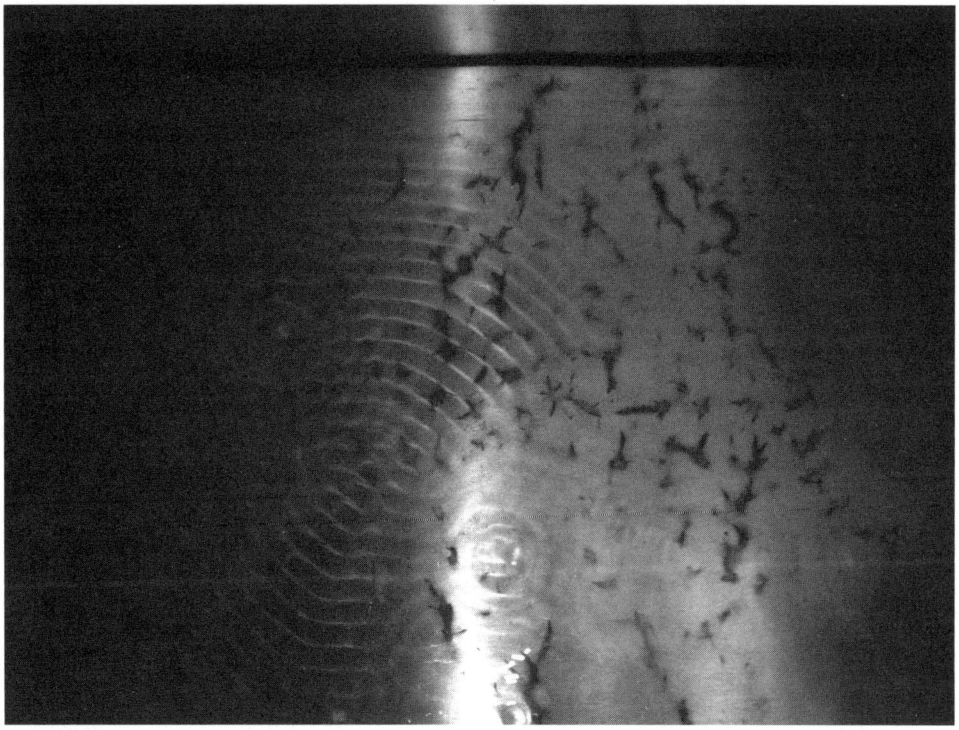

Figure 4.7. Cavitation.

the risk this may pose for workers. They also cite the cross-contamination that can occur if the ultrasonic washer chamber is not emptied and cleaned between loads. In the other approach, gross debris is rinsed off the instruments, and the ultrasonic cycle is used as the principal cleaning step. Supporters of this sequence say that instruments will be cleaner. Instruments may be incompletely cleaned in the wash cycle of a washer/sterilizer, and some debris may be baked on during the sterilization cycle that will be difficult to remove later.

Work practices must be adjusted to accommodate the approach used. If the first sequence (decontaminate, then apply the ultrasonic) is used, inspection procedures for instruments must be carefully maintained to detect any baked-on soil. If the second sequence (rinse, then ultrasonic, then decontaminate) is used, workers must wear adequate protective attire (a mask, eye protection, gloves, shoe covers, and impervious gown or jumpsuit) to minimize the risk of cross-contamination by aerosols. The wash chamber of the ultrasonic should be emptied and cleaned as needed.

Not all instruments can withstand ultrasonic cleaning. Hinges may be loosened in very delicate instruments. Chrome can be removed in chrome-plated instruments. Mixing different types of metals together in an ultrasonic cleaner load can cause one type of metal to plate with another type of metal. In general, the manufacturer's instructions should be checked before processing any instrument through an ultrasonic washer.

Instruments to be processed through an ultrasonic washer are placed loosely in a metal all-mesh basket. Plastic baskets cannot be used because they absorb the sonic energy. The basket is immersed in a solution of warm water (80° to 110°F) and a low-sudsing, free-rinsing detergent with a pH of 6 to 9 that is compatible with an ultrasonic cleaner. The solution in the cleaning chamber should be changed when it becomes cloudy or turbid and at least once during each work shift. After refilling the chamber with the water and detergent solution, one cycle should be run before it is used for instruments. This is necessary because the large gas bubbles formed during filling may absorb sonic energy, hence reducing the effectiveness of the machine. Running a cycle before actual use breaks down these air bubbles.

After the ultrasonic cleaning process, it is essential to rinse the loose, tiny debris from the instruments or it will be baked onto the instruments during final sterilization. Instruments should be final-rinsed in deionized or distilled water rather than in tap water. Tap water contains minerals that can stain instruments.

Glassware Washers (Dishwashers)

The glassware washer or laboratory dishwasher uses an automatically or manually fed detergent of high pH, which is very effective for cleaning glassware. The glassware is placed on special racks that securely hold it upside down. The items are washed with sprayer arms and then rinsed thoroughly. The rinse water must be distilled or deionized, because the minerals in tap water may interfere with some laboratory tests. Care must be taken during loading to be sure that items will not fall off the rack and break.

Glassware Dryers

Hot-air dryers are used for thorough drying of glassware and other such items. These items should be left inside the dryer only long enough to dry. When removing them, personnel should take measures to avoid burns.

Cartwashers

Carts and other transportation vehicles and containers must be cleaned routinely. Both automated and manual systems are available for cleaning carts. (See Figures 4.8 and 4.9.)

Automatic cartwashers have wash, rinse, and steam cycles. Some also have a drying cycle. Some models require the cart to be placed inside the washer in a tilted

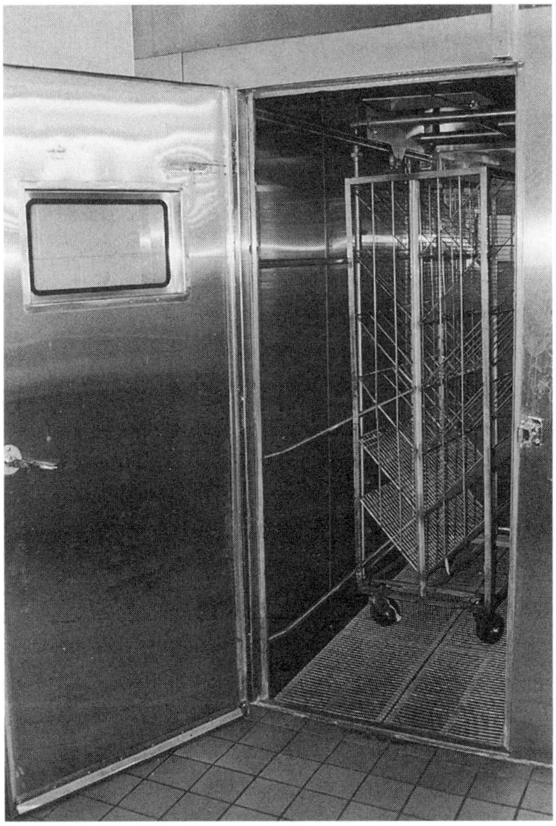

Figure 4.8. A Cartwasher.

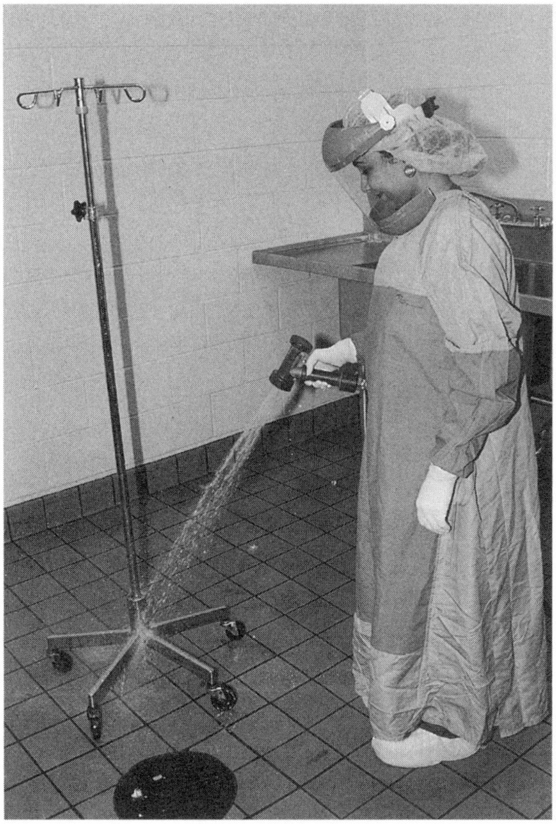

Figure 4.9. A Power Washer.

position to enable water to drain out and prevent restriction of any moving parts within the washer. Items removed from this type of washer are very hot and must be allowed to cool before they are handled. Carts must be inspected and usually need spot drying before supplies are placed in them.

Other means of cleaning carts and large equipment are the steam gun and power washer (Figure 4.9). These devices should be used in a confined area with a drain in the floor. The area should be well ventilated, and the floor drain must be cleaned periodically. Floors and walls must be cleaned frequently so that particles splashed off items being washed do not accumulate. The cart to be cleaned is tilted so that water will drain out. This equipment is then used to spray and sanitize all surfaces. A variety of cleaning and disinfecting procedures can be performed depending on the design of the equipment. These machines may also be filled with disinfectant and operated at very low temperatures, resulting in disinfection rather than sanitization with hot water. The steam gun and power washer must be handled with care. Insulated gloves, boots, aprons, and ear protection should be worn. Precautions should be taken to avoid slips and falls.

Utensil Washers

The utensil washer is used to clean and sanitize soiled utensils such as bedpans and wash basins. The utensils are placed on special racks to facilitate cleaning and rinsing. Some utensil washers have attachments to clean glassware and some instruments. The items are washed and rinsed with spraying action from various directions, depending on the headers used for various types of items.

Pasteurization Equipment

Pasteurization equipment consists of a wash chamber and pasteurization chamber or one chamber that can accomplish both processes. Respiratory therapy and anesthesia equipment can be processed in this manner. Items are placed in wire-mesh baskets that rotate in a water-and-detergent bath for a specified time. The solution drains and items are spray-rinsed. The baskets are then submerged in a water bath and rotated to get air out of all parts so that there is water contact on all surfaces, and the water bath is then heated to 150° to 170°F (65° to 77°C) and kept there for at least 30 minutes. This results in high-level disinfection. The equipment must be dried right after a cycle is completed by being placed in a drying cabinet. If items are not completely dried they will become contaminated with microorganisms (particularly pseudomonas) that will grow in the water droplets.

Drying Cabinets

Drying cabinets are beneficial for drying medical devices after they have been cleaned or disinfected to prevent growth of microorganisms. Drying cabinets are used to hang tubes lengthwise so that they can dry quickly and completely. Shelves may be available for drying other items.

Cleaning, Disinfection, and Preparation Procedures

Cleaning instructions, including disassembly, chemicals that the item can be exposed to, cleaning implements to be used, and the type of mechanical equipment the item can go into, must be obtained in writing from each device manufacturer. This information should be readily available to the CSD processing staff, to ensure that the device will be cleaned effectively. The instructions must be followed each time the item is reprocessed.

Upon arrival in the decontamination area, soiled items must be sorted according to the processing needed. Each type of medical device, patient care equipment, and supply item should be evaluated so that the most effective, most economical, and most appropriate cleaning and disinfecting methods are selected. Factors to be considered in this selection process are the type of contamination present and the desired use of the item for patient care (such as clean or sterile). Before using any disinfecting agent or method, the CSD technician must be knowledgeable about its toxicity, the pros and cons of its use, the expected results, and correct procedures.

All newly purchased instruments must be inspected for defects, proper function, and required specifications. New instruments have been handled many times during the manufacturing process in an uncontrolled environment. The instruments may also have a coating of oil to protect them during shipping. Therefore new instruments must be put through a decontamination process prior to sterilization. The same process must be used for repaired instruments returned to the facility.

Certain general considerations apply to instruments, patient care equipment, glassware, plastic or rubberized plastic surfaces, electronic devices, metal surfaces, and items with lumens. These considerations, with some examples, are discussed as follows.

Manual Cleaning and Decontamination

If a washer/sterilizer, washer/sanitizer, or washer/decontaminator is not available, instruments and other items can be cleaned manually. Hand cleaning and decontaminating are recommended for delicate instruments, items with long or small lumens, and items that cannot be immersed (e.g., some scopes and powered equipment).

The first step in the manual cleaning process is to immerse the instruments in a solution of water, detergent, or enzyme cleaner designed to remove blood and with a pH between 7 and 9. Each instrument is then individually cleaned with a soft-bristled brush (Figure 4.10) and friction, which loosens the soil. The brush and the instrument must be kept under the surface of the water to prevent contaminated droplets from being sprayed into the air (aerosolization). Never use abrasives because they scratch the surface and provide an area for microorganisms to hide. All surfaces of the instrument must be cleaned, with particular attention to any serrations on the ratchets, jaw, teeth, or spring lock, if present. Instruments with lumens or small holes (such as suction tubes and tips) can be cleaned using bottle or tube brushes of appropriate diameter, pipe cleaners, or handheld water pressure guns. Items that cannot be immersed are cleaned with a cloth or brush soakcd with detergent solution.

The cleaning solutions must be changed frequently. Each time contaminated instruments or the cleaning cloth are immersed, microorganisms and soil are added to the solution. There will be a point where microorganisms and soil will be added to the items rather than being removed. How frequently the solution needs to be changed depends on the amount of soil being removed. As discussed earlier, most disinfectants are inactivated by soil.

When soiled instruments will sit for any period of time before being cleaned, they should be immersed in an enzymatic solution or sprayed with an enzymatic

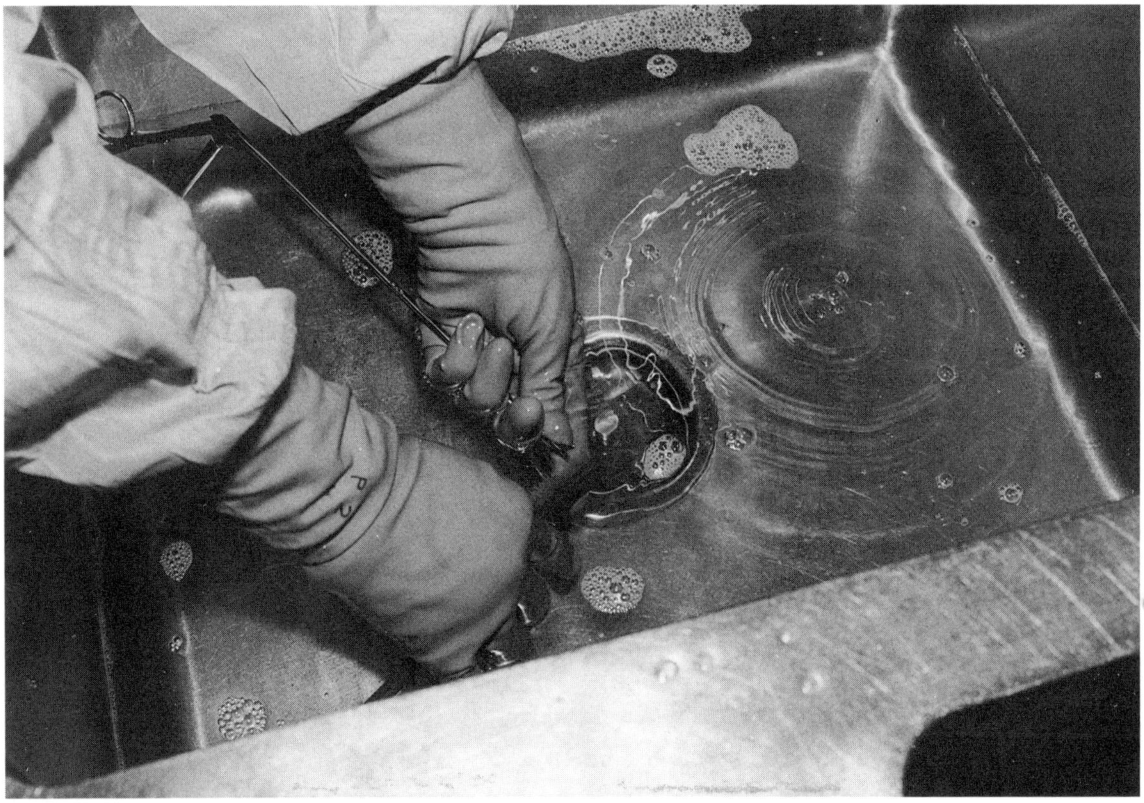

Figure 4.10. Manual Cleaning of a Surgical Instrument.

gel or foam. This is important because some microorganisms can form biofilms that are difficult to remove by ordinary cleaning methods. Biofilms are microscopic organisms that have the ability, when growing in water or water solutions or in vivo (i.e., bloodstream), to adhere to a surface and then exude over themselves a polysaccharide matrix. This prevents sterilants, disinfectants, and antibiotics from reaching the microbial cells. If biofilms have formed, friction and/or oxidizing chemicals are needed to remove them. Biofilms can form on many surfaces but are a problem mainly on devices with lumens. Therefore, it is extremely important to adhere to the guidelines outlined in this chapter for cleaning lumens.

This cleaning process lowers the bioburden. To disinfect devices, it is necessary to repeat the cleaning using a disinfectant solution designed for use on the particular material. The devices should have wet contact with the disinfectant for the length of time recommended by the disinfectant manufacturer.

The next step in the cleaning process is to rinse the instruments in deionized or distilled water. This type of water is recommended because the minerals present in tap water can cause staining or film formation on instruments as the tap water evaporates.

Items with Lumens

Items such as catheters, needles, tubes, and minimally invasive endoscopic instruments have internal passageways (lumens), which require special care for adequate cleaning. Blood or solutions can become dried and difficult to remove from lumens. It is necessary to reduce the surface tension to "lift" secretions from inner surfaces. Items should be soaked in an enzymatic solution. It is important to remember that to be effective, cleaning requires time, proper concentration of chemicals, and recommended temperature.

Some minimally invasive endoscopic instrumentation should be presoaked in a tall container allowing the instrument to be suspended from the top. Follow the manufacturer's recommendations for disassembly and cleaning of these devices. If recommended, place these instruments in a sonic cleaner, taking care to keep all parts for each instrument together. This will make it easier to reassemble after cleaning. Rinse thoroughly and allow to dry. There is also equipment available to flush lumens of endoscopic instrumentation.

Needle hubs may be cleaned by means of a small brush or cotton-tip applicator. Cleaning solution must be forced through the lumen with a syringe. The needles are then rinsed thoroughly with distilled water and inspected with a lighted magnifying glass for sharpness and burrs (see Figure 4.11). Burrs can also be detected by passing the needle tip over a gauze sponge or cotton ball. A dull or burred needle can cause trauma to the patient and should be removed from service and replaced.

All items with lumens must be thoroughly cleaned. Friction is essential to loosen the debris from inside lumens. Brushes in varying sizes (diameters) are needed to accommodate the different sized lumens to ensure proper cleaning. The brush should be large enough to rub against the inside of the lumen, yet not so large that the bristles fold back and do not apply friction. The brushes must be cleaned and disinfected daily. Hydrogen peroxide may be used for flushing to ensure that no blood remains. Any remaining blood will react with the hydrogen peroxide and bubbles will be seen; cleaning must be repeated until no more foaming is present. All hydrogen peroxide must then be thoroughly rinsed away.

Care and Handling of Handheld Surgical Instruments

For patient safety, it is vital that all instruments be maintained in proper working order. Instruments are usually contaminated with blood, tissue, and body fluids, and, therefore, present microbiological hazards to workers during the cleaning and decontamination portions of the reprocessing cycle.

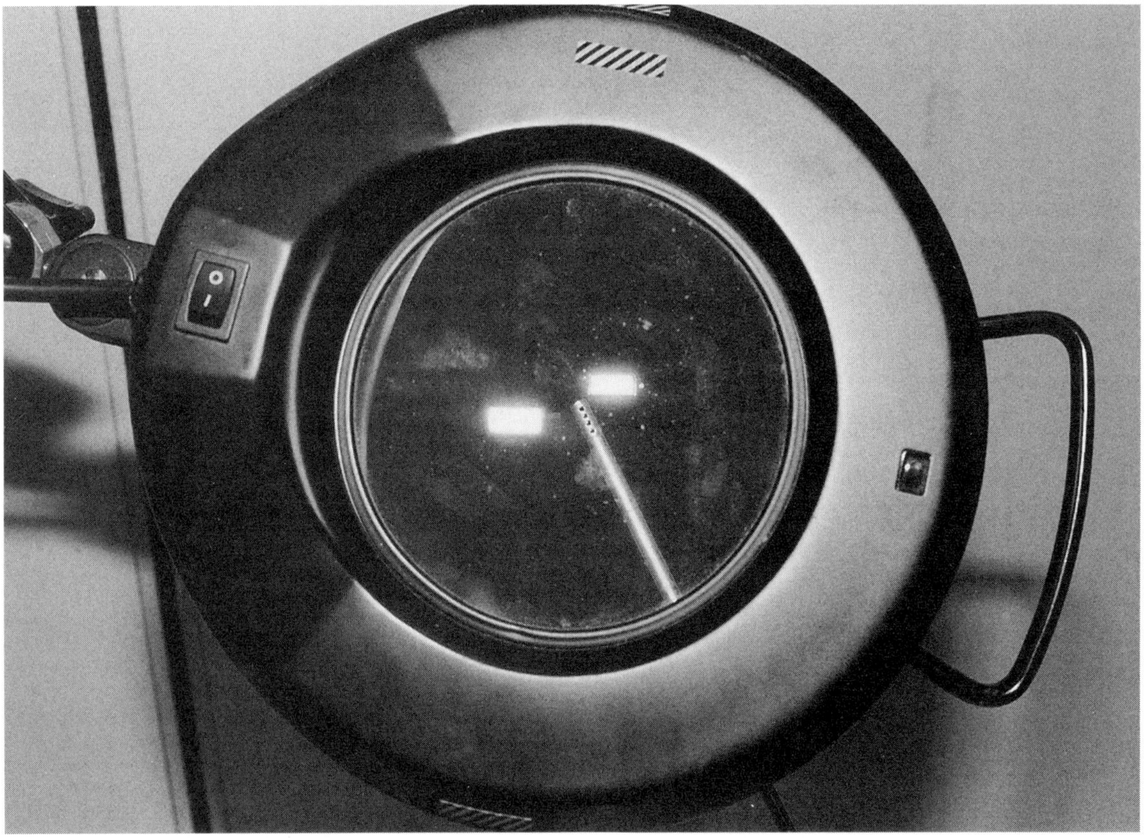

Figure 4.11. Inspect a Needle Under a Lighted Magnifying Glass for Sharpness and Burrs.

The complete reprocessing of surgical instruments involves the following steps:

- Safe transport from the point of use to the decontamination area
- Sorting
- Disassembly, soaking, and cleaning
- Inspection, reassembly, and set assembly
- Packaging and preparation for sterilization
- Sterilization
- Sterile storage
- Transport back to the point of use

SAFE TRANSPORT To prevent contamination of personnel or the environment, instruments should be contained during transport from point of use to the area where they will be cleaned and decontaminated. Plastic bags, totes with lids, carts with covered containers, or other methods may be used for this purpose. Sharp instruments must be transported in puncture-resistant containers.

CLEANING AND DECONTAMINATION Cleaning of the instrument to remove blood and other visible debris should occur as soon after use as possible. Such foreign material, if left on the instrument, serves as a reservoir for microbial growth and may damage the finish of the instrument. There are corrosive agents in blood and body tissue that can penetrate the passivation layer and cause rusting or pitting of the stainless steel. Initial cleaning at the point of use may consist of wiping off the gross debris with a damp gauze sponge.

If it is not possible to transport soiled instruments immediately after use, the instruments should be covered with a moist towel and placed in a plastic bag. In some areas instruments are placed in plain water or enzymatic solution in a closed container. There are also enzymatic gels or foams that can be sprayed on the instruments. These instruments are periodically transported to the CSD. Instruments should never be soaked in saline solution, for it is very corrosive. When transporting containers of liquid, care should be taken to prevent spillage. Any method used should be started by the personnel of the unit or department where the instruments were used.

During the initial cleaning procedure and all subsequent processing steps, instruments should be handled carefully to avoid damage to the instruments or injury to the worker. Workers should wear heavy-duty latex-free or plastic gloves when handling contaminated instruments. Instruments should be handled individually or in small groups to prevent them from becoming tangled. Never reach into a solution where instruments cannot be easily identified. The technician should be careful to avoid sharp cutting surfaces and should be especially alert for scalpels that still have the blade attached and for needles, either free or attached to syringes or needle holders. If found, knife blades and disposable needles should be removed and discarded in an impervious, rigid, hazard-labeled container. Reusable needles should be segregated and processed separately.

After instruments are cleansed of gross soil, delicate instruments (microsurgery needle holders, eye instruments, and any instruments with very fine tips) that require special handling should be separated from general instruments. Delicate instruments are usually washed by hand in a detergent specifically recommended for use on stainless steel surgical instruments. The instruments should be thoroughly rinsed and then dried. Most instrument manufacturers suggest that deionized or distilled water be used for the final rinse. This will reduce minerals that may remain on the instrument surface and cause staining or malfunctioning. Use of mechanical washers or washer/sterilizers is generally not recommended for delicate microsurgery instruments.

When used medical devices need to be returned to the manufacturer for repair or investigation of a potential malfunction, the manufacturer must be consulted for decontamination and shipping instructions. Devices should be decontaminated by the user facility before being sent to the manufacturer. There may be instances when the manufacturer requests the device not be decontaminated because it may obscure the problem with the device. The manufacturer must give written instructions for labeling, containing (sealed and leakproof), and shipping each device. U.S. Department of Transportation and postal regulations must be followed. This decontamination process also holds true for devices being sent for repair to a department within the facility.

Powered Instruments

Many surgical procedures require the use of powered instruments, such as saws and drills. Powered instruments should never be immersed in solution or come into contact with saline solution, detergents with very high or very low pH, or chemical disinfectants. They should never be cleaned in an ultrasonic washer.

The first step in cleaning an air-powered instrument is to disassemble it according to the manufacturer's instructions. If an air hose is part of the equipment, it is inspected for damage and washed with lukewarm running water, using a mild detergent and a cloth or soft-bristled brush. The hose should be held coiled with both ends hanging down to prevent water from entering the open ends. If the equipment has an electrical cord, the cord should be inspected for cracks in the insulation and wiped with a cloth soaked with mild detergent solution. Other components are also cleaned with lukewarm water, a mild detergent, and a soft brush, or as recommended by the manufacturer (i.e., Blitzcleaner for 3-M drills). All components are then rinsed with distilled or deionized water and wiped dry.

Endoscopic Equipment

There are two major types of endoscopic instruments: rigid and flexible. Each has its own care and handling recommendations.

Rigid endoscopes have channels, holes, hinges, and joints that must be thoroughly washed and rinsed to remove residual mucus, blood, and other body fluids. Endoscopic instruments and accessories that can be disassembled for cleaning should be, according to the manufacturer's recommendations. Soaking the endoscope in an enzymatic product is recommended to facilitate the cleaning process. Use of a water-cleaning pistol for washing and compressed air for drying will expedite this otherwise very time-consuming job. Care must be taken, however, to avoid the contaminated aerosols that may result from the use of a water-cleaning pistol. If such a device is not available, a soft cotton material should be used. The type of detergent used should be that recommended by the instrument manufacturer. After the instrument has been cleaned, it must be dried before it is stored, since moisture enhances bacterial growth. Lumens should be flushed with alcohol and forced-air dried. Eyepieces can be easily scratched and other components of these instruments are very delicate; consequently, they should be handled with extreme care throughout the rinsing, cleaning, and drying procedure.

Most flexible endoscopes are not disassembled for cleaning. There may be several accessory tools, such as biopsy forceps, biopsy brushes, and snares, that are cleaned separately. When cleaning a flexible endoscope, it is essential to follow the manufacturer's directions. Soaking in an enzymatic solution will enhance the cleaning process, ensuring all suction ports are open. Thorough rinsing will also help dislodge any debris. The exterior of the scope should be cleaned with a detergent recommended by the manufacturer and a soft brush or cloth. The suction, biopsy, air or water, CO_2, and elevator wire channels of the instrument must be cleaned. After cleaning, the scope should be dried. Lumens should be flushed with alcohol and forced-air dried.

Because most of the accessories are long and flexible and have small springs, adequate cleaning may require immersion in a blood-dissolving detergent solution to remove tiny particles trapped in the springs. Whatever the decision regarding disinfection versus sterilization of the scope itself, the accessories should be thoroughly cleaned (most manufacturers recommend ultrasonic cleaning) and then the items should be sterilized by the method recommended by the manufacturer (usually steam). Because it is so difficult to clean these items, some hospitals purchase disposable, single-use, springhandled accessories.

Patient Care Equipment

Many types of reusable electrical and mechanical equipment are used in patient care. In the CSD, each piece of equipment must be cleaned, disinfected if needed, inspected and tested, reassembled per department policy, and stored until requested. There are so many varieties of patient care equipment that it is difficult to generalize about cleaning, disinfection, and testing procedures. The manufacturer should be consulted about specific cleaning and testing procedures for each type of equipment. These instructions should be incorporated into the CSD's procedures.

Electrical patient care equipment must be routinely tested by the biomedical engineering staff for electrical safety. A label should be attached to each piece of equipment to indicate the results of testing and the date when the next check is due. The CSD technician should check these labels and ensure that equipment due for electrical inspection is not returned to service until it has been tested. Also, electrical cords and plugs should be routinely inspected. Any piece of equipment with a frayed or cracked cord must be removed from service and sent to the biomedical engineering department for repair.

Some examples of frequently used patient care equipment and its uses are listed below:

- Wagenstein suction pump: intermittent gastrointestinal suction
- Oral suction machine: continuous suction for nose, throat, and bronchial tubes
- PCA (patient-controlled analgesia) pump: allows patients to control, within certain parameters, the amount of pain medication they receive and when they receive it
- IV infusion pump: controls delivery of intravenous solutions and medications
- Feeding pump: controls delivery of food through a gastric tube
- Sequential compression machine: pumps air to sleeves, which expand and contract, that are placed around postoperative patient's leg(s) to aid circulation and prevent blood-clot formation
- Hypo/hyperthermia machine: increases or decreases body temperature using pads that have warm or cold water running through them

Electronic Devices

Cables, probes, and other electronic devices are used in conjunction with electrical patient care equipment and must be cleaned between uses. When cleaning such devices, the manufacturer's instructions must be followed carefully. Care must be taken to avoid damaging the electronics. The surfaces, which may be metal or plastic, should be cleaned with a mild detergent solution and then rinsed and dried thoroughly. Electronic equipment must never be immersed in cleaning agents or disinfectants, unless otherwise stated by the manufacturer. If sterilization is required, ethylene oxide (EtO) gas is usually recommended by the device manufacturer, whose written instructions must be followed carefully. Figure 4.12 illustrates some common types of electronic devices.

Plastic Items

A variety of plastic compounds or components can be easily damaged. Harsh detergents, elevated temperatures, disinfectants, or combinations of these may cause crazing, cracking, or discoloration of surfaces. In particular, alcohols or phenolics should never be used.

Anesthesia and respiratory therapy items should be disassembled, washed manually or mechanically, and rinsed thoroughly. If a pasteurization system is used, this process occurs immediately after rinsing. After pasteurization the items are dried. Items not pasteurized may be chemically disinfected or sterilized by EtO. The items should be dried in a mechanical dryer, manually, or with compressed air before disinfection or sterilization.

Glassware

Glass syringes require special attention for thorough cleaning. Syringe plungers and barrels must be separated and immersed in an enzyme product to facilitate the removal of blood or body fluids. Syringe components may then be handwashed,

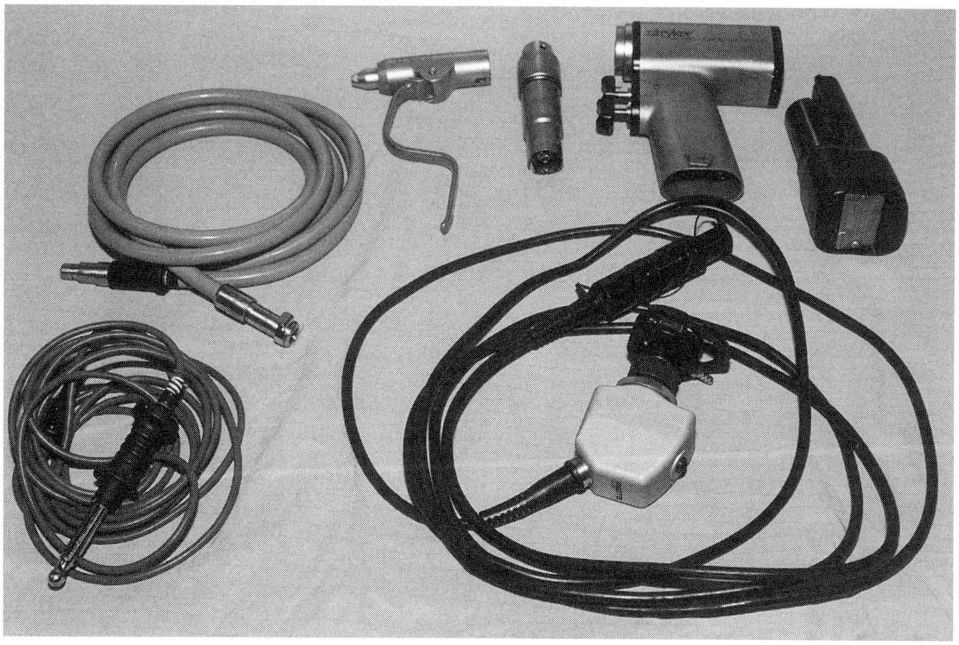

Figure 4.12. Common Types of Electronic Devices.

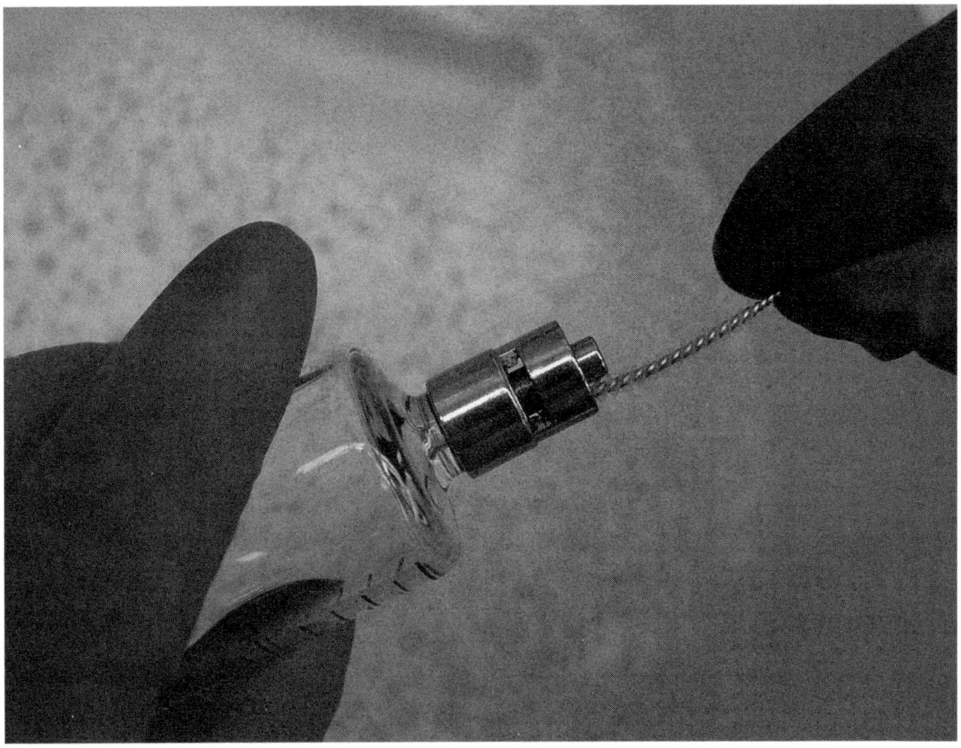

Figure 4.13. Handwashing a Syringe.

with special attention to the tip (a soft-bristled brush, pipe cleaner, or cotton-tipped applicator should be used—see Figure 4.13), or placed in a glassware washer or ultrasonic washer.

The cleaned syringes should then be rinsed with distilled water and may be mechanically dried or allowed to air dry. Careful rinsing, drying, and handling will remove all mineral and soap residue from the syringe and will help prevent the barrel and plunger from sticking together. Some syringes have a dedicated barrel and plunger, which have the same number on both the parts. Barrels and plungers are kept separate when being sterilized. If they are numbered, make sure matching numbered parts are placed in one package.

Items such as glass bottles, beakers, and flasks should be cleaned with the same detergent and in the same manner as syringes. Distilled water should be used for the final rinse, and the bottles should be inspected for chips or cracks.

Traction Equipment

Traction equipment parts should be cleaned with a mild detergent solution and disinfected with the chemicals recommended by the manufacturer. Pulleys and sliding parts must be checked for easy movement, and clamps must be checked to make sure they tighten all the way. Traction rope should never be reused.

Summary

Cross-contamination is one of the most serious infection-control problems in the health care facility. This chapter has presented what central service departments can do to prevent cross-contamination. Of particular importance are the containment of microorganisms in the decontamination area and the use of proper techniques for cleaning and disinfecting contaminated items. Ways for the CSD staff to protect themselves from pathogens and chemical disinfectants were discussed. How various types of chemical disinfectants are used, what microorganisms they are effective against, their damaging properties to some materials, and potential hazards to staff were also presented.

Technicians should be able to make informed decisions about the decontamination of various materials that are sent to them. The function of various mechanical equipment in the cleaning and disinfecting process was reviewed. Also discussed was the care in the cleaning of specific groups of items (i.e., instruments, items with lumens, powered and endoscopic equipment, electrical and mechanical patient care equipment, electronic devices, glassware, syringes, and plastic materials).

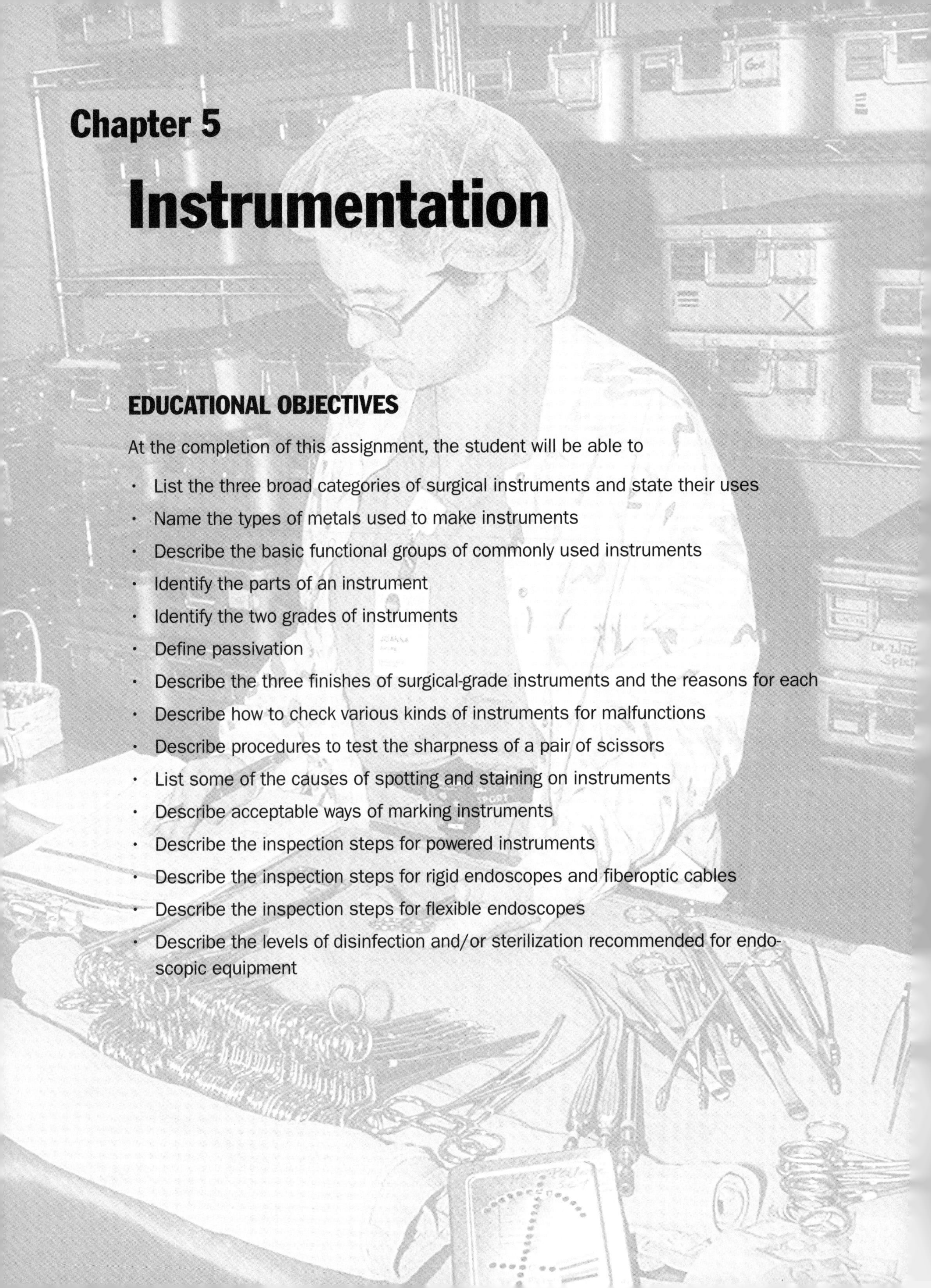

Chapter 5

Instrumentation

EDUCATIONAL OBJECTIVES

At the completion of this assignment, the student will be able to

- List the three broad categories of surgical instruments and state their uses
- Name the types of metals used to make instruments
- Describe the basic functional groups of commonly used instruments
- Identify the parts of an instrument
- Identify the two grades of instruments
- Define passivation
- Describe the three finishes of surgical-grade instruments and the reasons for each
- Describe how to check various kinds of instruments for malfunctions
- Describe procedures to test the sharpness of a pair of scissors
- List some of the causes of spotting and staining on instruments
- Describe acceptable ways of marking instruments
- Describe the inspection steps for powered instruments
- Describe the inspection steps for rigid endoscopes and fiberoptic cables
- Describe the inspection steps for flexible endoscopes
- Describe the levels of disinfection and/or sterilization recommended for endoscopic equipment

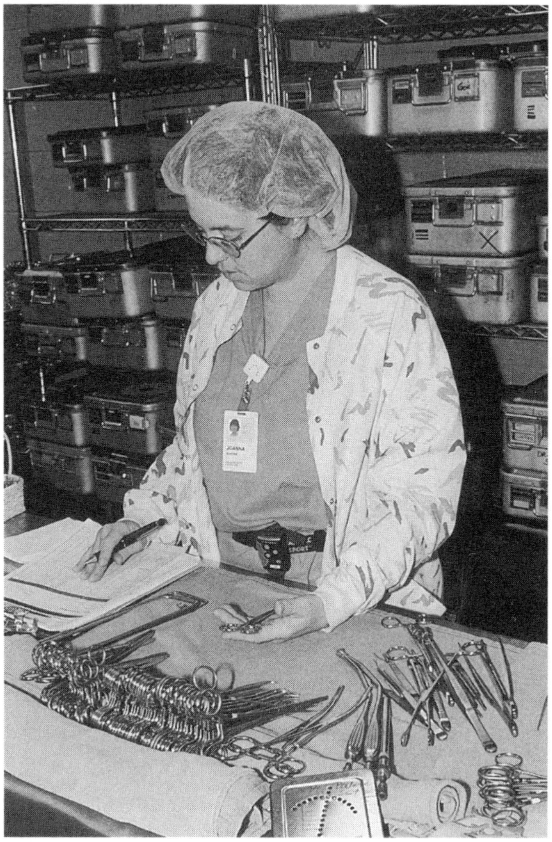

A VAST ARRAY OF INSTRUMENTS and medical devices are used in surgical procedures today. These instruments and devices range from delicate microsurgery needle holders to air- and battery-powered drills and complex endoscopic equipment with sophisticated lens systems and fiberoptics. The surgery department uses the greatest number and variety of instruments. Instruments are also used in other areas of the health care facility, such as the Emergency Department, endoscopy, delivery area of obstetrics, outpatient surgery areas, surgicenters, and critical care units.

The retrieval, reprocessing, storage, and distribution of surgical instrumentation make up the major portion of the work load in many CSDs. Central service department technicians must be able to identify many types of instruments, medical devices, and equipment, depending on the types of surgeries performed in the facility. They must clean and disinfect or sterilize each item. They must assemble instrument packs and trays for use in specific surgical, obstetrical, and specialty procedures.

Included in this chapter will be an overview of the care, handling, and *general* description of types of instruments and devices. With this basic knowledge, CSD technicians should be able to properly care for the majority of instruments in their work setting. The identification of specific instruments and devices can be learned by comparing them with pictures in the manufacturer's catalog (many instruments have identifying numbers on them), consulting with surgery staff (especially when nicknames are used), and working alongside experienced technicians. Some facilities have a computer system that can put a picture of a specific instrument on the screen.

The three broad categories of surgical instruments are as follows:

- Handheld, nonpowered surgical instruments used for cutting, clamping, retracting, chiseling, holding, and manipulating tissue or bone
- Tools powered by electricity, compressed gas, batteries, and light sources (i.e., laser) used for drilling or cutting bone or cauterizing tissue
- Endoscopic equipment and instrumentation used to biopsy or perform minimally invasive surgery or examine internal organs through natural openings or very small incisions

Together, these three categories represent a substantial financial investment and resource for every health care facility. The CSD technician is part of the team that ensures proper care and handling, which is essential in maintaining the value of this investment.

Surgical instruments are essentially extensions of the surgeon's hands. There are numerous advantages to their use. Instruments can be cleaned and sterilized for use in incision sites. Instruments grasp tissue more effectively than fingers can. Instruments hold other instruments; for example, needle holders hold the suturing needles. Instruments can conduct electrical impulses, as in electrocoagulation of bleeding vessels, or transmit a high-frequency light, as in laser fiberoptics. Other instruments cut tissue, sutures, and dressing.

Handheld Surgical Instruments

Handheld surgical instruments are usually made of stainless steel. Other metals, such as titanium alloy, sterling silver, chrome, copper, and brass, are also used. Surgical instruments are finely crafted tools designed by or for surgeons to accomplish particular functions in specific surgical procedures. There are thousands of different patterns and designs, although the only difference between some is size.

Instrument Names and Structure

The names or descriptions for instruments generally include a proper name, functional name, and size. In many facilities the CSD technicians may have to become familiar with instrument nicknames. Proper names often refer to the name of the facility or person who designed the instrument (e.g., Kelly forceps, Mayo scissors). The functional name designates the purpose of the instrument. The basic functional groups of commonly used instruments are

- Forceps—Grasp tissue, sponges, dressing
- Scissors—Cut tissue, suture, dressings
- Hemostats—Occlude arteries
- Needle holders—Hold suturing needles
- Retractors—Displace tissue or body organs
- Miscellaneous—Do not fall into above groups

Some of the common nicknames used are sharp, stat, Dr. X's [instrument], pickups, and clamp. In some instances using a surgeon's name is appropriate. A surgeon at a particular facility may have modified an instrument for his or her particular use. In this case, there would be no way of identifying the instrument other than using that surgeon's name along with the functional name.

The structure of many handheld instruments (e.g., forceps, hemostats, needle holders) includes a jaw, box lock, shank, ratchet, and finger rings (see Figure 5.1). The jaw is the working part (clamps, holds, grasps). The jaws may be smooth, have various designs of serrations (crosswise, lengthwise along jaws, or fine criss-cross), and have a tooth or teeth at the tip or teeth spaced along the jaws. The jaws also differ in length. The various lengths and designs on the jaw help identify its function and proper name. Jaws of instruments can be difficult to get clean because of the serrations and teeth.

The box lock is the hinge point of the instrument. This is the most difficult part of the instrument to clean. The box lock is the weakest part of the instrument. When the instrument is misused or when there is a buildup of debris within the box lock, a crack can occur in the joint around the pin. When this occurs, the instrument can fail at any time and must be removed from the set. Cracked box locks cannot be repaired.

The shanks provide the closing force on the jaws.

The ratchets lock the instrument in a closed position. This part of the instrument is also difficult to get clean. To release the lock, put outside sideways pressure on the finger rings.

The finger rings are usually a complete oval circle. The user controls the action of the jaws with the finger rings.

Some forceps do not have finger rings or box locks, and they are known as "tissue" or "dressing" forceps. This tweezer-designed instrument cracks at the proximal end, and the teeth can break off at the distal end. Finger pressure is the method to open and close this type of forcep.

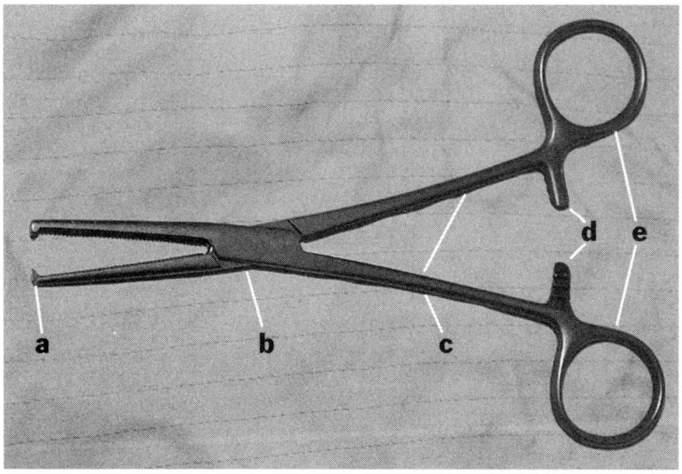

Figure 5.1. Structure of a Typical Surgical Instrument.

Note: a = jaws, b = box lock, c = shanks, d = ratchets, e = finger rings.

Other identifying features for instruments include straight or curved jaws and the length of the instrument. The length is determined by measuring from the tip of the jaw to the bottom edge of the finger ring.

Grades of Handheld Surgical Instruments

The overall quality or grade of a surgical instrument is determined by the quality of the materials used in its construction, the precision of features such as ratchets, cutting edges, and box locks, and its finish, particularly the degree of corrosion-resistance. The two general grades of instruments are *surgical grade* and *floor grade.*

Surgical instruments are made from uniform quality forgings, most often of German origin. The raw materials for the steel are carefully controlled, so that the alloy is consistent from one batch to another.

Stainless steel is rust-resistant, but not totally immune to corrosion. To strengthen their resistance to damage by chemicals and water, surgical instruments undergo a process known as passivation as one of the final manufacturing steps. Passivation removes all foreign debris from the surface of an instrument and begins the formation of a layer of nonreactive chromium oxide. As the instrument ages, this layer increases and the instrument surface becomes highly resistant to corrosion. The passivation layer can be damaged by engraving, using abrasive cleaning equipment, and exposing the instrument to damaging chemicals. Ultrasonic cleaning can remove the passivation layer, therefore lubrication of surgical instruments should be performed after every cleaning.

The ring handles, ratchets, shanks, and jaws of surgical instruments are finely machined, so that there are no rough edges on which gloves might be torn or that may interfere with comfortable handling and use. The box lock is secured with a rivet made of the same material as the rest of the instrument so that reaction between metals will not weaken this union. The box lock is then polished so that the rivet is not visible on the surface.

Cutting edges can be sharpened to a fine degree. Some surgical instruments have cutting edges or grasping surfaces made of tungsten carbide. Tungsten carbide is a very hard metal that holds a cutting edge well and resists wear. Instruments with tungsten carbide inserts (see Figure 5.2) can usually be identified by their gold-plated handles. Some scissors are identified with a black handle indicating that they have "super sharp" edges. These are not as strong as tungsten carbide but will stay sharp significantly longer than regular stainless steel scissors.

Shiny or mirror, satin or patina, and dull or matte are three types of finishes commonly available for surgical instruments. Satin and matte instruments reflect less light and help to minimize glare. Glare created by the deflection of the surgical lights contributes to visual fatigue and interferes with visual acuity. On the other hand, dull finishes show stains more than shiny ones. Staining can be caused by the chemical impurities in water and steam, by some other chemicals, and by detergent residues. An additional finish is available for instruments used in laser surgery.

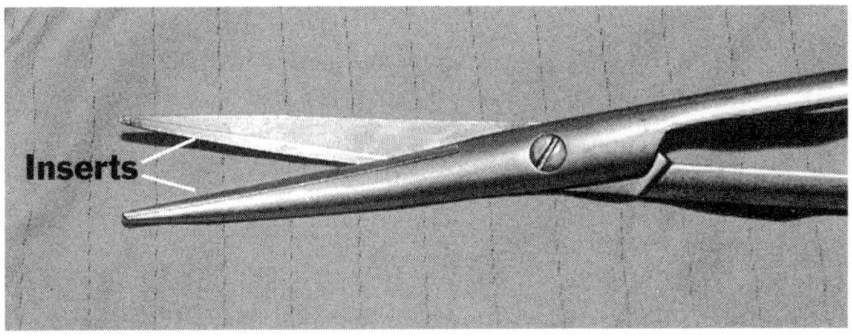

Figure 5.2. A Surgical Instrument with Tungsten Carbide Inserts.

This finish has a black, microscopically irregular surface to scatter and absorb light and minimize the energy generated by lasers from bouncing onto and destroying tissue surrounding the intended target.

Some instrument companies offer different tiers of surgical instruments. The difference in the tiers is mainly aesthetics, for example the finish and some less refined, nonessential features such as the thickness of the instrument. The overall function and quality is the same, though some tiers are lower cost.

Some common instruments—the so-called "soft tissue" instruments—are available in floor grade. Floor-grade instruments are made from forgings of lower quality and consistency. They may bend or break easily, and the precision of key features such as ratchets and box locks are less exact. These instruments are usually not passivated and may rust and pit after being steam-sterilized a few times. Plated instruments can become scratched or chipped and must then be refurbished or replaced. The trade-off is, of course, that floor-grade instruments cost substantially less than surgical instruments. They are appropriate for use in noncritical trays such as a dressing kit where the lower quality does not markedly interfere with effective use. They are also often used when security measures to prevent loss or theft of instruments are inadequate. Although not considered disposable items, these instruments will need much more frequent replacement than instruments of surgical grade.

Lubrication of Instruments

Clean instruments with box locks may be immersed in a water-soluble lubricant solution, a process referred to as "milking." Immersion may be either mechanical or manual. Manual lubrication requires following the manufacturer's instructions for dilution and expiration dating. It also requires that instruments be dry before immersion to avoid further dilution of the lubrication. This lubrication protects the hinges and box locks as metal moves on metal and coats the surface of the instrument to reduce spotting. This can be particularly useful in regions with hard water. This lubricating process is often considered an optional step in processing. The Association for the Advancement of Medical Instrumentation (AAMI) recommends that instruments with moving parts be lubricated with a lubricant compatible with sterilization.

After the instruments are removed from the lubricant bath, they should not be hand-dried. The preferred method is to allow the machine to dry them or use room air. Not all instrument lubricants are suitable for use in steam, gas plasma, and EtO sterilization. It is important to read the label before use.

Care must be taken to not increase the bioburden in the lubricant solution. Only decontaminated instruments should be immersed in the solution. If manual submersion is the method, a perforated inside container must be used so that no one reaches into the solution to retrieve the instruments.

Silicone- or oil-based lubricants should only be used for specific applications recommended by the device manufacturer (i.e., lubricants used for powered drills). The solution chosen must be water-soluble so as not to interfere with steam contact during sterilization. Lubrication of surgical instruments is recommended to prevent spotting and to help repassivate the instruments. Ultrasonic cleaning removes instrument "milk," so the lubrication should be performed after ultrasonic cleaning and before sterilization. The label on the lubricant should clearly indicate that the solution is designed for use on stainless steel surgical instruments. The use of instrument-lubricating solutions will sometimes mask incomplete cleaning of hinges and box locks by allowing them to move even with some debris present. If an instrument is found to be "stiff" (that is, the hinge or box lock is stiff), it should be inspected for debris and not just "milked."

All instruments with hinged or moving parts must be lubricated after every use. A spray-on or machine-applied neutral pH lubricant should be used. Silicone- or oil-based lubricants should not be used.

Instrument Inspection

Before decontaminated instruments are stored or prepared for sterilization, they must be carefully checked for cleanliness and proper working function. A lighted magnifying glass facilitates the inspection process. Each instrument should be visually inspected for cleanliness, any corrosion or pitting, any burrs or nicks, and cracks. Areas to inspect closely for cleanliness include ratchets, serrations, box locks, hinges, and lumens. Common areas where cracks may be found are the box locks, hinges, and near the base of the jaws.

Instruments must be checked for properly aligned jaws (Figure 5.3) and a freely moving box lock. If the instrument has teeth, they must all be there and mesh properly.

Instruments with box locks and ratchets should be tested to see if the proper tension is being maintained. The tips of a clamp should meet just before the ratchet is engaged. As the ratchets are engaged, the entire jaw of the instrument should approximate or mesh. To test further, the clamp should be set on the first ratchet and gently tapped on a flat surface such as a worktable. This test will determine if the instrument is "sprung." If the instrument is sprung, the ratchets open when tapped on a flat surface.

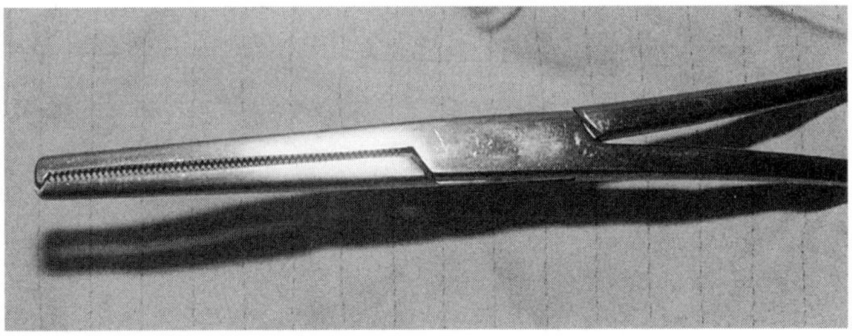

Figure 5.3. The Instrument's Jaws Must be Aligned When Closed.

Self-retaining retractors should be checked to make sure the ratchets hold well in the open position. One way to check this is to open the retractor and put pressure on both shanks. The ratchet should unlock with minimal opposing pressure on finger rings.

Multipart instruments must be checked to make sure all pieces are there and they fit together properly. Sliding parts must move smoothly and always be cleaned and lubricated. Screw-on retractors must function easily—check for misthreading. Check for bends on instruments with lumens (e.g., trocars and needles).

Needleholder jaws are designed to wear out. To inspect a needleholder correctly, separate the rings and inspect the tread wear on both needleholder jaw tips. If tread wear is visible, schedule the needleholder for repair. Cardiovascular needle holders often need to be demagnetized. To test if this step needs to be done, put a needle next to the instrument. If it is magnetized, it will draw the needle to it. A demagnetizer must be available, either in the area of the facility in which the instrument is used or in the area where instruments are processed and checked.

The hinges on scissors should not be stiff, but must retain the proper tension to bring cutting surfaces smoothly together. Check cutting edges for gouges or burrs. To test the sharpness of scissors larger than 4½", use (Theraband) red scissors test material. The scissors should cut through completely, all the way to the tip of the scissors. The final test of scissors is the opening and closing, which should be smooth. To test micro scissors 4½" and smaller, use (Theraband) yellow scissors test material. The scissors should be able to go through completely, all the way to the tip of the scissors. The scissors opening and closing should be a smooth action. Paper should never be used to test the cutting edge of surgical scissors, because cutting paper is not a true test for sharpness and it dulls the instrument.

When an instrument is found to need repair, it should be set aside in a designated location. Surgical instruments are finely crafted precision devices and should only be repaired or sharpened by those with specific training in this type of work. An improperly repaired instrument may not work the next time it is used or, of greater consequence, may cause injury to a patient.

Instrument Spotting or Staining

There are several causes for spotting, staining, corrosion, and pitting on instruments. A checklist of causes can be established and each cause checked off as eliminated during the investigative process. Some of the causes include cleaning or sterilizing dissimilar metals at the same time, detergent residue on textile towels (used to line trays or protect instruments) or reusable textile wrappers, condensation after sterilization, inadequate cleaning, water impurities, chemicals from the boilers or steam piping, chemical residue from improper rinsing of sterilizer chamber walls after cleaning, and use of abrasives on instrument surfaces. Saline and bleach are highly corrosive to surgical instruments, and exposure to these chemicals should be avoided. Sometimes the color of the stain may indicate the cause. Major instrument manufacturers have troubleshooting sheets that can help in the investigative process.

New Instruments

All *new* instruments must be cleaned and inspected for proper function before being put to use. The manufacturer puts a protective coating that is not water soluble on the instruments. Instruments are inspected by the manufacturer, but may be handled numerous times before reaching the facility. Damage can occur along this chain of events.

Insulated Instruments

Insulated instruments require careful inspection to make sure there is no breach in the insulation. There are insulation testers available, and these should be used to verify the integrity of the insulation each time the instruments are processed.

Marking Instruments

Instruments should never be engraved. Engraving destroys the passivation layer in that area and will cause corrosion. There are etching processes that are acceptable. Preferably, markings should be done by the manufacturer.

Placing colored tapes on instruments must be done carefully. The tape must overlap, but not be multilayered, and be smooth. There must not be irregular areas for soil and microorganisms to adhere. These areas potentially cannot be cleaned in the routine cleaning process. Tape should not be placed on areas of the instrument that will be handled. Rough edges may put holes in gloves. The tape must be changed whenever the edges curl or start to come off the instrument. The tape must be sterilant permeable.

Some instrument manufacturers can mark instruments by using a coating process on parts of the instruments, such as the finger rings. The various colors used could represent the surgical specialty (e.g., emergency room, OB, clinics), or specific trays the instruments belong to in the facility. The coating should be inspected for breakage after each use, and if breakage is noted the instrument should be removed from service and sent back to the manufacturer for recoating.

Instrument Storage

Instruments must be thoroughly dried before being put in the storage area. The storage area must remain dry and humidity controlled. Instruments with ratchets should be stored in the open position. Locking the ratchets puts constant tension on the jaw, shanks, and box lock, which could cause damage.

Misuse of Instruments

Surgical instruments must be used only for their intended use. Do not grasp material or solid objects with forceps. Prying objects with the jaw of an instrument can crack it or put the jaw out of alignment. If instruments are dropped, they must be checked carefully for burrs, misalignment, cracks, and bends. If an endoscopic instrument is dropped, it must be checked by a qualified repair person.

Sterilization

Most handheld surgical instruments are sterilized by exposure to saturated steam under pressure (see Chapter Seven for description). However, some manufacturers may recommend low-temperature sterilization (i.e., EtO sterilization and aeration or gas plasma sterilization) for delicate microsurgery instruments (although most of these instruments will tolerate steam sterilization). It is thought that low-temperature sterilization protects delicate, high-carbon-content cutting edges and instruments made of several different metals from the rigors of rapid heating and cooling present in steam sterilization. No published scientific evidence demonstrates whether low-temperature sterilized instruments last longer, so the issue calls for a judgment in each health care facility, in consultation with surgical instrument manufacturers. Sterilization with EtO will affect the processing turnaround time and may result in greater inventories of instruments. Other low-temperature sterilization methods have shorter turnaround times.

Manufacturers' instructions for correct sterilization method and parameters (time at a certain temperature) must be obtained in writing for manufactured sets of instruments, both facility-owned and loaner sets. Some manufacturers give instructions for particular sets of instruments (especially orthopedic) that include extended time exposures.

Powered Instruments

Some surgical instruments are designed to be connected to a power source during use to cut or drill. The power source may be electricity, either battery or line current, or compressed medical gases, such as nitrogen, compressed air, or carbon dioxide. In common usage, these are all referred to as powered instruments. Examples include reamers, drills, powered screwdrivers, and the saws used by orthopedic surgeons, the craniotomes and perforators used by neurosurgeons, the dermatomes that plastic surgeons use to take skin grafts, and the sternal saws used by thoracic surgeons.

Because their designs vary, each type of powered instrument should be cared for and sterilized in accordance with the manufacturer's instructions. Powered instruments should be lubricated as recommended by the manufacturer. This usually requires connecting the equipment to the proper power source and running it for several seconds (see Figure 5.4). This procedure also tests the function of the equipment before sterilization. Lubricants should be used as specified. Because the inner spaces of these instruments are complex, and the lubricants are oil-based, extended sterilization exposure times are often recommended by the manufacturer.

Endoscopic Instruments

Endoscopic instruments are used to look at the body's organs, either through natural openings such as the mouth or anus, or through small incisions (over joints or in the abdomen, for instance). These instruments are complex, often consisting of several lenses carefully aligned along the instrument, one or more lumens, and, frequently, fiberoptic glass bundles. There are two major types of endoscopic instruments: rigid and flexible (see Figure 5.5).

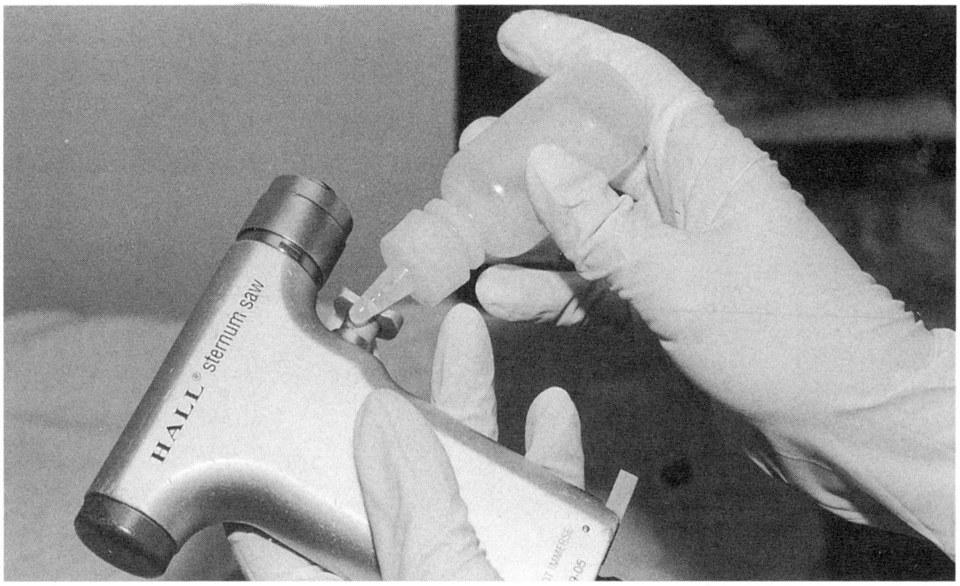

Figure 5.4. Lubricating and Checking an Air-Powered Drill.

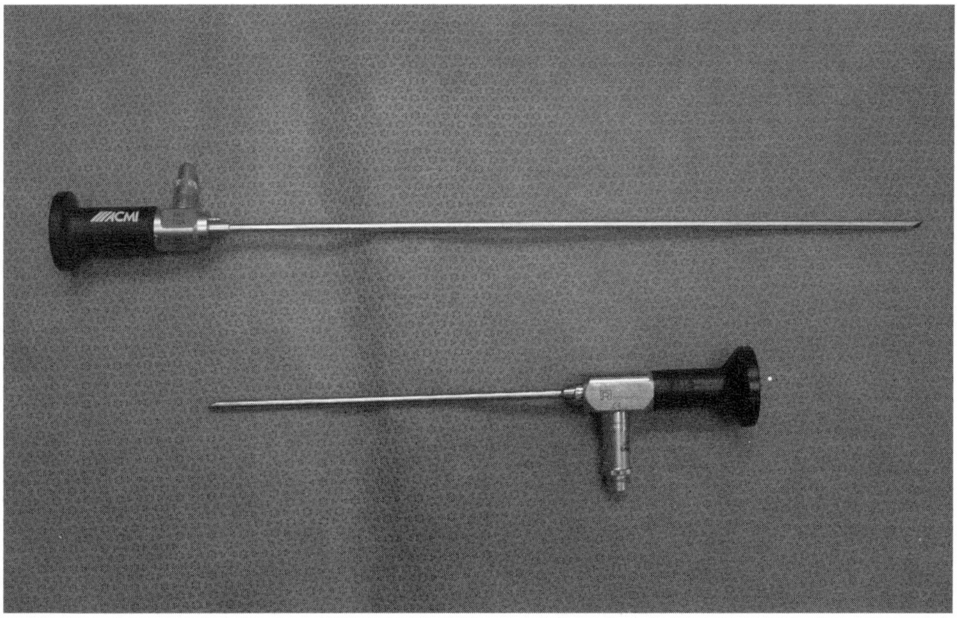

Figure 5.5. Flexible (above) and Rigid (below) Endoscopes.

Rigid Endoscopes

Examples of rigid endoscopes include cytoscopes, resectoscopes, laparoscopes, arthroscopes, and hysteroscopes. Some endoscopes are available in both rigid and flexible designs (bronchoscopes, gastroscopes, and sigmoidoscopes).

After the endoscopic instrument is clean and dry, it should be inspected to ensure that it is functioning properly. There is now a tester to facilitate identification of defects in rigid scopes before processing. The telescope should be checked to verify that the field of vision is clear. If the field is not clear, the telescope should be washed and dried again, then reexamined. If spots still remain, a magnifying glass may be used to inspect the cover glass on the working end for any cracks or chips. A "half-moon" but otherwise clear view could indicate that the telescope has a dent on the outside sheath. If the cover glass appears "foggy," that means that leakage has occurred at the sealed ends or that there are residual surfactants from disinfectants on the lens. If surfactant is the cause, wiping the lens with alcohol should correct this problem.

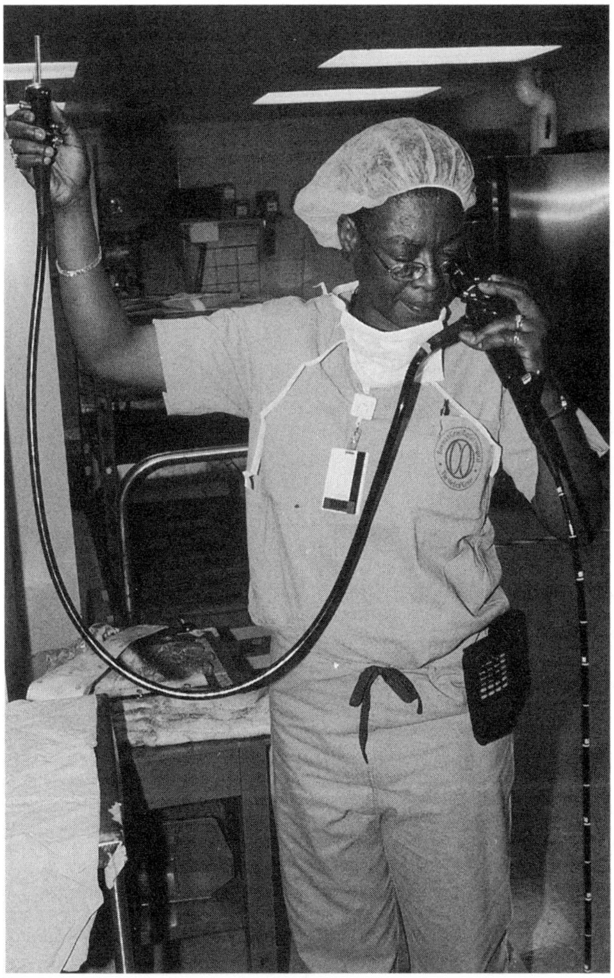

Figure 5.6. Checking a Fiberoptic Cable.

To see inside the body, light must be brought to the end of the endoscope. This is done by bundles of special glass rods that conduct light very well. The rigid instrument is connected to a powerful light source by a flexible cable made of hundreds of these very thin glass rods. Care must be taken not to break these fibers by bending the cable at sharp angles or dropping it.

The fiberoptic cable should be inspected after each use by holding one end toward the ceiling light and observing the other end (see Figure 5.6). Numerous black dots indicate that many fibers are broken and the light transmission will be reduced. Repair or replacement will be necessary if the light transmission has been reduced sufficiently to impair the physician's visualization of internal structures.

Not all rigid endoscopes are subjected to a sterilization process before reuse. Some are high-level disinfected by immersion in a chemical disinfectant. This disinfection may be done in the department where the scope will be used (the operating room, emergency room, or endoscopy clinic). The decision concerning which scopes require sterilization and which only need high-level disinfection is made by the using department, in consultation with the CSD and the Infection Control Department.

Regardless of how the telescope portion of an endoscope is processed, all completely metal components of endoscopic instruments can and should be steam sterilized. Because of the complexity of the instrumentation, each piece must be carefully inspected for cleanliness before being packaged and sterilized. If the rest of the scope will not be steam sterilized, these components should be wrapped separately. There are some insulated components, such as resectoscope sheaths, and some accessory instruments that consist of both metal and plastic. These also can be steam sterilized, but it is important to recognize that the expansion during heating and contraction during cooling are completely different for plastic and metal. This may cause changes in the plastic materials during and after steam sterilization. Therefore, the manufacturer's instructions should be followed for how these components should be sterilized. The number of times a device is sterilized and the specific cycle time and temperature that plastic or metal components can withstand before cracking, becoming brittle, or shedding particles may be limited, and the manufacturer's recommendations must be followed.

Manufacturers of some telescope components of endoscopes claim that they can be steam sterilized, but the wide variety of materials that make up telescopes complicates the steam sterilization process considerably. A telescope is made up of tiny lenses or glass rods inserted into a thin metal tube. This tube is in turn surrounded by fiberglass threads and another metal tube. The system is enclosed at one end with the eyepiece for viewing and at the other end (the objective) with a cover glass. When steam sterilizing telescopes, the manufacturer's instructions must be followed carefully.

Even if the instructions for steam sterilization are followed meticulously, the life of a steam-sterilized telescope is usually shorter than that of an EtO-sterilized one. Because the cost of the telescope is almost 50 percent of the total cost of an endoscopic instrument set, EtO, ozone, and glutaraldehyde sterilization or other low-temperature systems are considered the methods of choice by many health care facilities. EtO sterilization of endoscopic equipment offers distinct advantages over steam sterilization, because the instruments are less likely to be damaged. The only real disadvantage is the delay in availability of the instruments caused by the need for aeration after sterilization. Aeration is essential to remove toxic EtO residuals, and an endoscope should never be removed from the aerator until the process is complete.

The fiberoptic light cable can usually be steam-sterilized. It should be loosely coiled, to avoid any sharp bends that might break the glass fibers, and packaged for sterilization.

Flexible Endoscopes

Flexible endoscopes consist of fiberoptic glass bundles arranged around a lumen or lumens, a series of lenses and mirrors, coils or springs, and cables running the entire length of the instrument to control the movement of the tip, and an impervious covering. These are all put together to produce an instrument that can bend gently (not sharply at right angles) and maneuver through the lumens of the gastrointestinal and respiratory tracts, with less discomfort to the patient than rigid scopes and the ability to reach deeper into the body.

The manufacturer's instructions must be followed for checking the function of these endoscopes. Check for proper movement of the scope tip and the covering for flaking and cracking. Usually the light source must be checked. Testing for leaks is done after each use and before immersion in the cleaning solution.

As with rigid endoscopes, not all authorities agree on the necessary level of terminal sterile processing. In some health care facilities, flexible scopes are routinely sterilized by EtO or other low-temperature methods. In others, high-level disinfection is considered adequate. This is a decision that must be made at each health care facility, in consultation with the CSD and the Infection Control Department.

Summary

Health care facilities have a large financial investment in medical instrumentation and devices. The CSD technician is part of the team that cares for that investment by the proper handling and preparing of these items for use. The instruments and devices must function as intended so users do no harm to the patient or themselves.

An orientation to the general types of surgical instrumentation (handheld, powered, and endoscopic) was presented in this chapter. Being able to identify general functions and structure of this instrumentation prepares the CSD technician to carry out the physical steps and visual observations (discussed in this chapter) needed to identify when various kinds of instruments need repair.

Hard-to-clean areas on instruments were discussed. The CSD technician is responsible for the thorough cleanliness of instruments before they are put through the sterilization process.

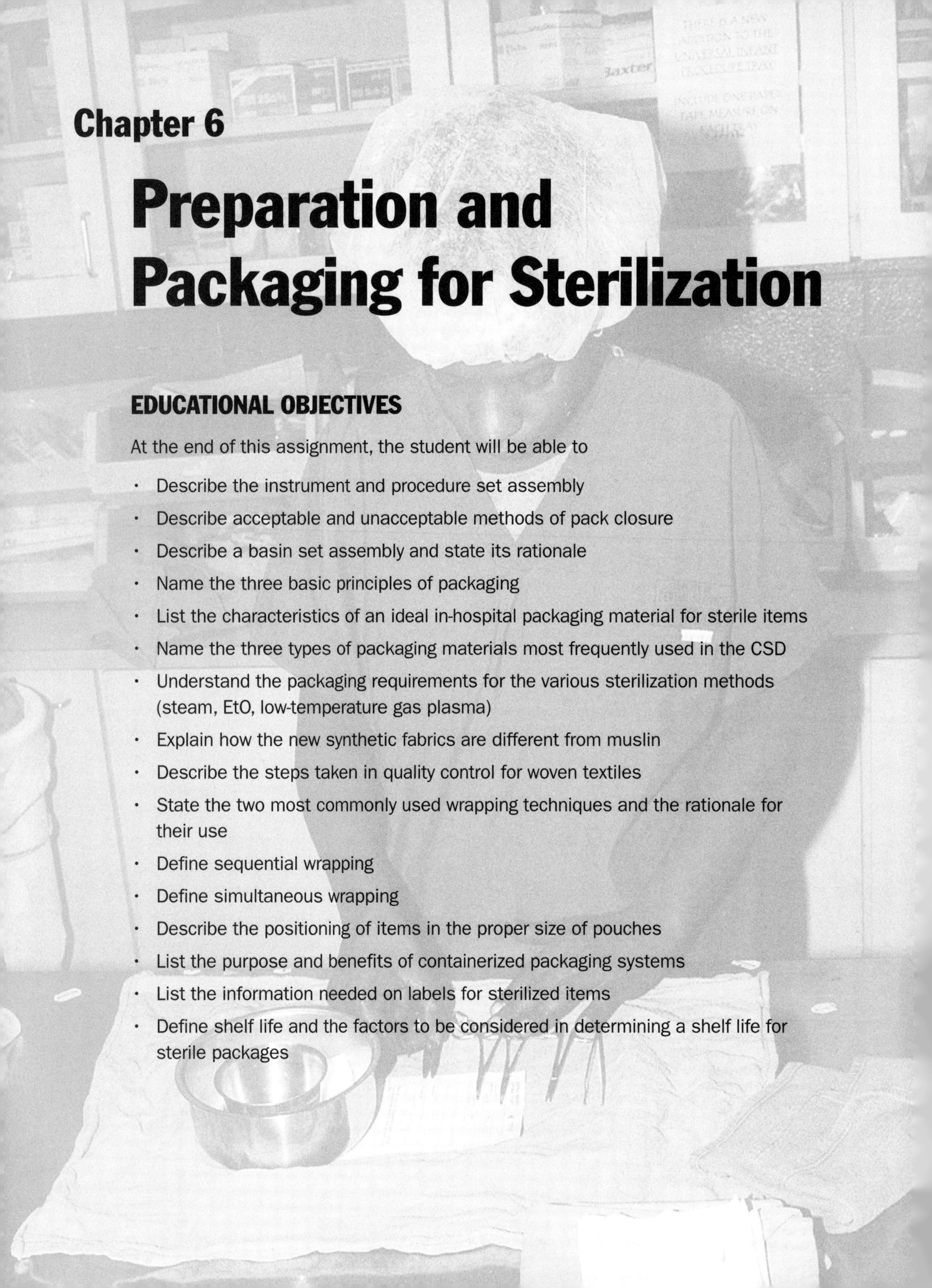

Chapter 6

Preparation and Packaging for Sterilization

EDUCATIONAL OBJECTIVES

At the end of this assignment, the student will be able to

- Describe the instrument and procedure set assembly
- Describe acceptable and unacceptable methods of pack closure
- Describe a basin set assembly and state its rationale
- Name the three basic principles of packaging
- List the characteristics of an ideal in-hospital packaging material for sterile items
- Name the three types of packaging materials most frequently used in the CSD
- Understand the packaging requirements for the various sterilization methods (steam, EtO, low-temperature gas plasma)
- Explain how the new synthetic fabrics are different from muslin
- Describe the steps taken in quality control for woven textiles
- State the two most commonly used wrapping techniques and the rationale for their use
- Define sequential wrapping
- Define simultaneous wrapping
- Describe the positioning of items in the proper size of pouches
- List the purpose and benefits of containerized packaging systems
- List the information needed on labels for sterilized items
- Define shelf life and the factors to be considered in determining a shelf life for sterile packages

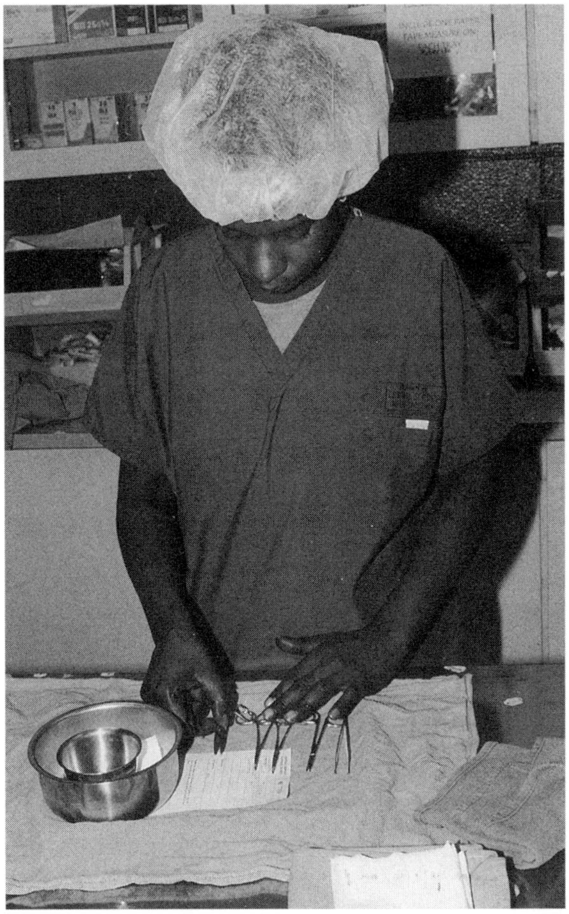

SURGICAL INSTRUMENTS, supplies, and most other medical devices must be prepared and packaged so that their sterility can be maintained to the point of use. Preparation involves inspecting items for cleanliness, ensuring that all parts are present and functional, and assembling multiple component sets or packs. The materials and techniques used for packaging must permit air removal, allow the sterilant to contact the device, protect the device from contamination during storage and handling before it is used, and let the item be aseptically removed. In this chapter, preparation of devices for sterilization and the properties, types, and methods of packaging will be explored.

Preparation of Instruments

Some instruments are packaged by themselves or in groups of two or three, either because the instruments are the only ones needed to perform a procedure or because they are specialty instruments used only in certain circumstances by certain surgeons. These instruments can be placed in paper-plastic pouches (see Figure 6.1) or wrapped in envelope fashion using a flat wrapper (see Figure 6.2). Pouches are often preferred when visibility of an item is important. However, pouches are primarily used for single lightweight devices and instruments. If the instrument has sharp points, these should be protected by means of commercially available tip guards, commercially made holders, or foam sleeves. The manufacturer's instructions should be checked to ensure that the protectors are permeable to the sterilant (steam or EtO). This is especially critical if using tip guards. Latex tubing should never be used to protect instrument tips because it will inhibit sterilant penetration. The presence of latex tubing can also compromise the setup for a latex-sensitive patient. Gauze squares should never be used because the additional gauze might affect sponge counts.

Instruments for small sets (often called *procedure trays*) may be packaged along with a few needed towels, gauze sponges, and other supplies (see Figure 6.3). These may be placed in an autoclavable mesh or perforated-bottom basket or arranged on a perforated autoclavable tray. The use of a cuffed towel will help keep instruments open and in place (one finger ring placed under cuff and the other on top of the cuff).

Most handheld instruments are prepared in sets (also called trays or kits in some health care facilities). A set may consist of the few instruments needed for procedures, such as suturing lacerations or performing a venous cut-down (opening the skin and dissecting muscle and fascia to reach a deep vein so that intravenous fluids may be given). Or, the set may contain a hundred or more instruments, as in the

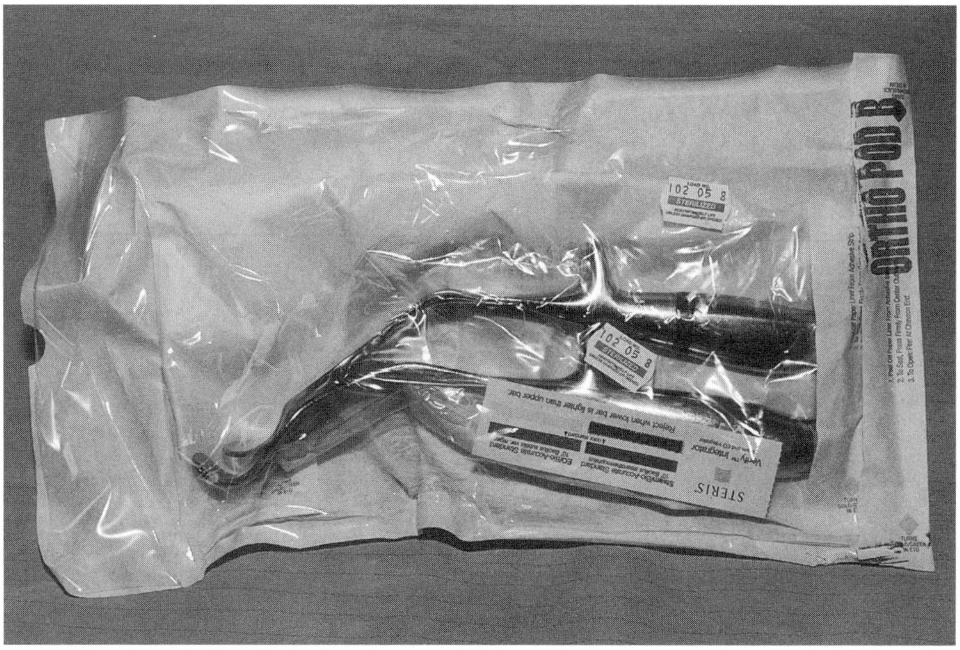

Figure 6.1. Packaging a Surgical Instrument in a Paper-Plastic Pouch.

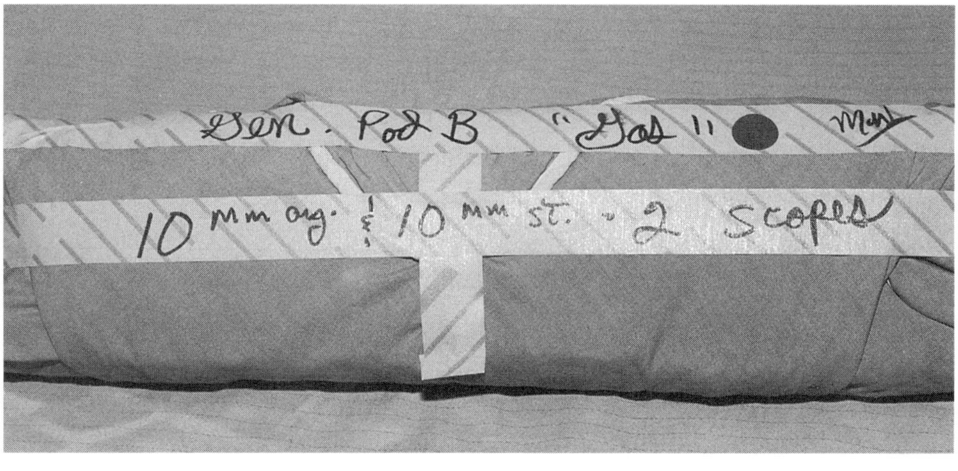

Figure 6.2. Packaging a Surgical Instrument in a Flat Wrapper.

case of the sets needed to perform a laparotomy (opening the abdominal cavity) or thoracotomy (opening the chest cavity).

The contents of each set are usually determined by the staff of the department in which the set will be used. Whenever practical, the contents of each set should be standardized so that the same instruments are packaged no matter which physician is performing the procedure. Also, when possible, sets should be standardized for use in several different, but related, procedures. For example, a basic laparotomy set could include instruments used in opening the abdomen or pelvic cavity in general surgery or in gynecological or urological procedures. Ancillary sets of specialty instruments could be prepared for specific operations in each of these categories. For example, "stomach and bowel instruments" might be one specialty set, "abdominal hysterectomy instruments" another.

Whatever the scheme for determining the contents of each set, the procedure should be specified in writing on a tray list or count sheet, similar to a recipe (Figure 6.4). This tray list should be used every time the set is put together to make sure it is complete and that the instruments are in the proper order. Incomplete sets may create delays in performing surgical procedures, and such delays may harm patients. In most health care facilities, the person who prepared the set signs his or her name or initials along with the date of preparation on the tray list and somewhere on the label after the set is packaged. This accountability allows for problem identification and correction.

Instruments for large sets are placed in a stainless steel, anodized aluminum, or heat-tolerant plastic basket of appropriate size and with a wire-mesh or perforated bottom. The container manufacturer should provide written documentation as to

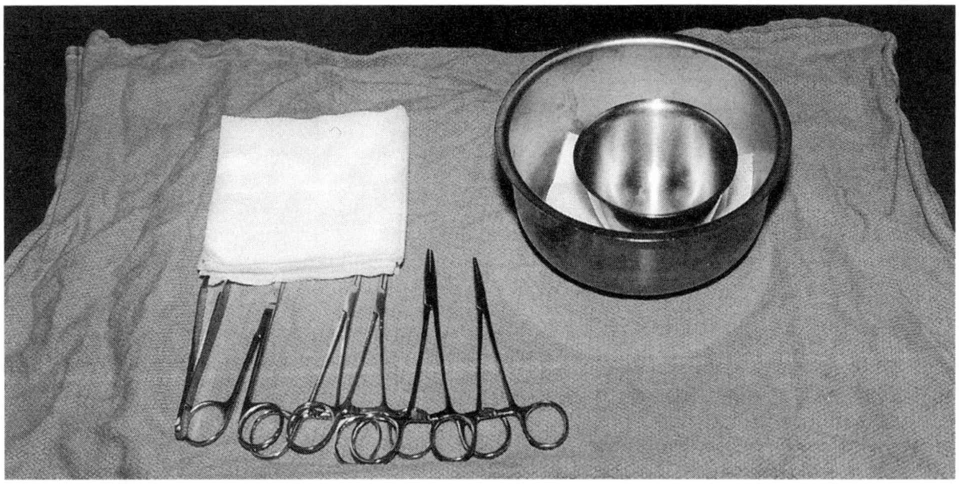

Figure 6.3. Instruments for a Small Set Packaged Along with Other Necessary Supplies.

MAJOR TRAY						
Count	**Quantity**	**Description**	**Vendor**	**Catalog #**	**OR Pre-count**	**OR Post-Count**
	1	Large Tray	Mueller	SU-2987-003		
	2	Tray Tags				
	1	Prep Forcep 7 in.	Mueller	MO-1760		
		Needle Holders				
	2	7 in. Mayo Needle Holder	Mueller	SU-16061		
	2	8 in. Mayo Needle Holder	Mueller	SU-16062		
		Scissor Set				
	1	6 3/4 in. Straight Mayo	Mueller	SU-1801		
	1	6 3/4 in. Curved Mayo	Mueller	SU-1802		
	1	7 in. Curved Metzenbaum	Mueller	MO-1600		
		Ring Handled/Clamps				
	2	5 in. Straight Mosquitos	Mueller	SU-2700		
	6	5 in. Curved Mosquitos	Mueller	SU-2702		
	2	5 1/4 in. Straight (6 1/4) Criles	Mueller	SU-2732		
	24	5 1/4 in. Curved (6 1/4) Criles	Mueller	SU-2737		
	6	6 in. Allis	Mueller	SU-4055		
	6	6 in. Kocher (Oschner)	Mueller	SU-2800		
	6	6 in. Babcock	Mueller	SU-5000		
	6	5 in. Large Towel Clip	Mueller	SU-2905		
	4	9 in. Sponge Sticks Straight	Mueller	GL-650		
	6	8 in. Curved Peans	Mueller	SU-2764		
	6	8 in. Mixters	Mueller	SU-10524		
		Long Needle Holders				
	1	10 in. Mayo (9 in.)	Mueller	SU-16063		
		Long Scissors				
	1	9 in. Curved Metz	Mueller	CH-2032		
	1	11 in. Curved Metz	Mueller	CH-2030		
		Long Clamps				
	2	9 in. Allis (10 in.)	Mueller	CH-1560		
	2	9 in. Kocher (Oschner) Straight	Codman	30-4066		
	2	9 in. Babcock	Codman	34-7030		
	2	10 in. Mixter	Mueller	CH-1726		
		Knife Handles				
	2	#3 Knife Handles	Mueller	SU-1403-001		
	1	#7 Knife Handles	Mueller	SU-1407		
		Thumb Tissue Forceps/Misc.				
	2	Adson W	Mueller	NL-1400		
	2	6 in. Tissue W	Mueller	SU-2333		
	2	6 in. Tissue W/O	Mueller	SU-2303		
	2	6 in. Martins	Mueller	SU-2490		
	2	7 in. DeBakeys	Mueller	CH-5902		
	2	9 1/2 in. DeBakeys	Mueller	CH-5904		
	1	10 in. Tissue W	Mueller	SU-2337		
	2	10 in. Tissue W/O	Mueller	SU-2307		
	2	9 in. Nelson Tissue	Mueller	CH-1500		
	1	10 in. Russian	Mueller	SU-2454		
	1	5 1/2 in. Short Probe	Mueller	SU-10810-600		
	1	8 in. Long Probe	Mueller	SU-10810-800		
	1	Pool Suction	Mueller	SU-13000		
	2	Log Large Applier (Syringe Envelope)	Weck	52-3180L		
	2	Log Med. Applier (Syringe Envelope)	Weck	52-3111M		
	2	45'		E.H. - O.R. #25		
Signature: ______________________			Date: ______________________			

Figure 6.4. An Instrument Tray List.

the devices the manufacturer has validated for use inside their container (e.g., power equipment, lumens, etc.). The instruments are arranged so that like instruments are together. All hinged instruments must be open to permit sterilant contact on all surfaces. All multipart devices must be disassembled for sterilization unless otherwise specified in writing by the device manufacturer. Ring-handled instruments can be placed on racks, pins, or stringers (with their box locks open), so that they will be easier to handle at the point of use (see Figure 6.5). Malleable (bendable or flexible) retractors or probes are straightened. Heavy instruments are placed on the bottom or at one end of the basket to avoid damage to other instruments. Placing instruments in the general order of use will facilitate case setups and may save vital time in emergency operations. Microsurgery instruments may have their own special trays or containers designed to secure the instruments and protect them from damage. The CSD management and the staff of the departments using the sets should agree on how the sets should be arranged.

To enhance drying of surgical instrument sets, it might be necessary to wrap heavier items (e.g., a weighted vaginal speculum) in an absorbent material (e.g., a huck towel). If instruments need to be separated inside a set they may be wrapped in single-ply packaging material. A chemical indicator should be placed inside each separately wrapped item. Peel pouches should not be used inside wrapped or containerized trays since they cannot be kept on their side for sterilization. The weight limit of an instrument set is based on the ability of personnel to lift and carry the set without injury, the configuration of the set (how the instruments are placed on the tray), and the total metal mass of the instruments. For rigid containers, consult with the container manufacturer regarding the weight and density of sets. It is the responsibility of the sterile processing department to determine that sets can be effectively sterilized and dried.

Pack Construction

Packs vary in size, shape, and composition, but the size, density, and metal mass (if applicable) of any pack must be limited to proportions that will be compatible with the sterilant, temperature, and exposure time used during the sterilization cycle. Packs containing woven materials should not exceed the accepted maximum size of 12 by 12 by 20 inches, nor should they weigh more than 12 pounds. The density of linen packs should not exceed 7.2 pounds. Larger or denser packs require longer sterilization cycles and prolonged drying times, and exposure times must be tested in each health care facility.

Drapes and sheets should be fan-folded to enhance air removal and steam penetration. All reusable linen should be inspected on a light table. Lint should be removed using a lint roller. Holes should be patched on both sides of the wrapper

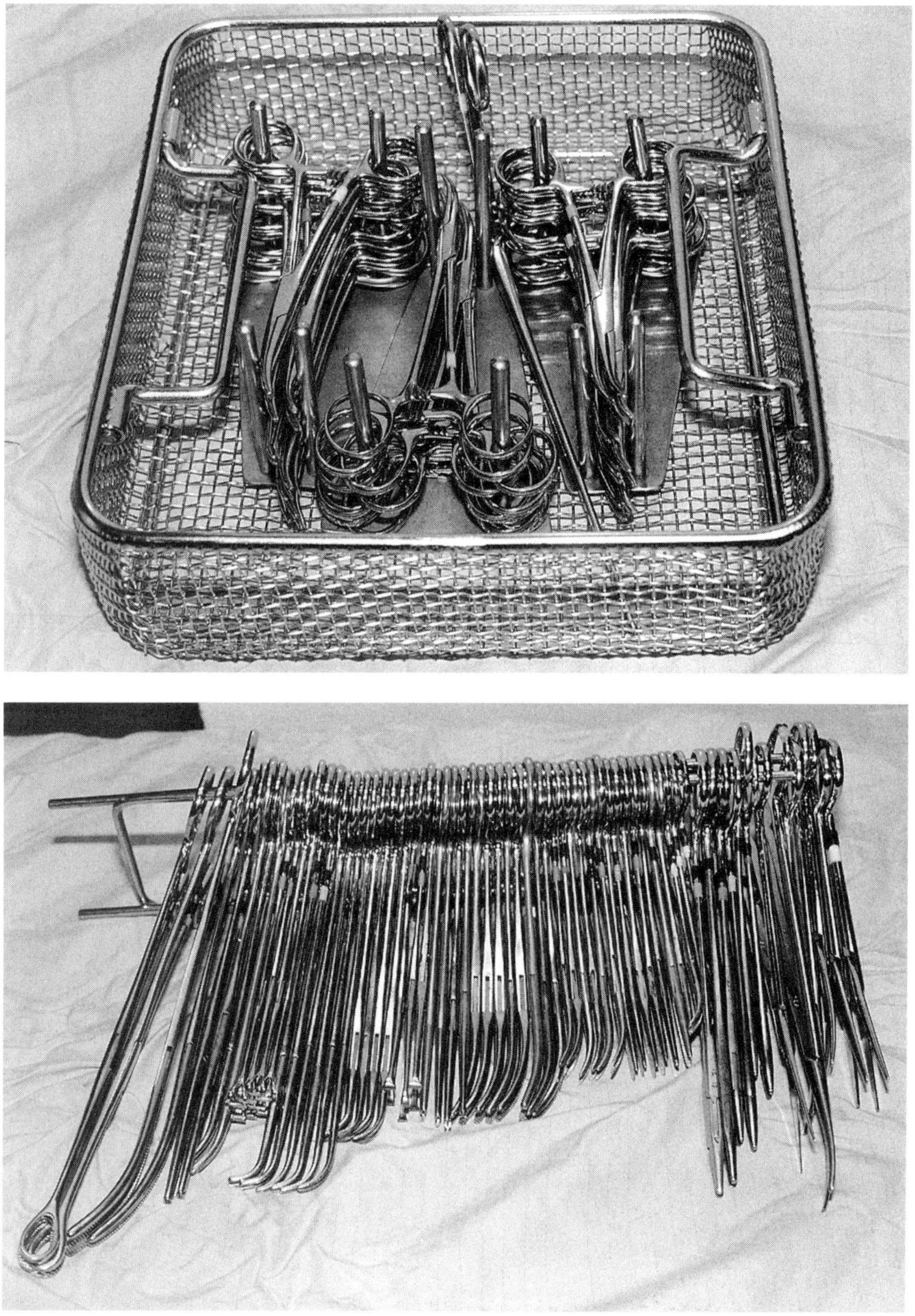

Figure 6.5. Ring-Handled Instruments Are Placed on Racks (Above), Pins, or Stringers (Below), with Their Box Locks Open.

using a heat patch machine. Drapes and sheets should not be cross-stitched because this presents additional openings for bacteria to enter.

The exact procedures used to fold specific reusable surgical items are sometimes difficult to comprehend when written. This is truly a case of actions speaking more clearly than words, for it is much easier to learn by watching than by reading. Maintaining aseptic presentation and minimizing handling at the point of use are the two goals in folding any linen that will be used as part of a sterile procedure.

Special care must also be taken in preparing and folding the items so that they can be handled aseptically. For example, gowns are folded with the inside surface of the body of the gown toward the outside. The gown can then be grasped just below the neckline and it will hang open ready to put on without touching the outer surface, which must remain sterile. Drape sheets are folded so that minimal handling will be necessary to open and place them around the operative site on the patient. Special sheets, such as those with apertures or openings for the wound site (e.g., laparotomy drapes, lithotomy drapes), are folded so that they can be fully opened in one direction (usually toward the head or feet of the patient) and then in the opposite direction, so that the patient ends up fully covered with a sterile surface.

Reusable textile pack contents are arranged generally in the order of use. For example, a towel is always placed on top of each gown (for drying the hands and forearms after a surgical scrub or handwashing). Gowns are placed on top of the Mayo stand cover, which is on top of the draping towels, which are on top of drape sheets, and so on. The order of placement is mutually agreed on by the user department and the CSD management. During pack assembly, the layers should be alternated so that the folds do not all go in the same direction. This will aid air evacuation and steam penetration. Generally, metal items (e.g., basins, bowls) should not be placed inside linen packs.

Basin Set Preparation

Basin sets should be constructed so that smaller basins nest inside the largest basin (see Figure 6.6). Nested basins should differ in size by at least 1 inch. All basins should face in the same direction, and a material that will absorb and wick moisture should be placed between basins to facilitate steam getting to all surfaces and revaporization (see Figure 6.7). The weight of wrapped basin sets should not exceed 7 pounds. Excessive metal mass can cause excessive condensation, slower heat-up time, and inefficient drying.

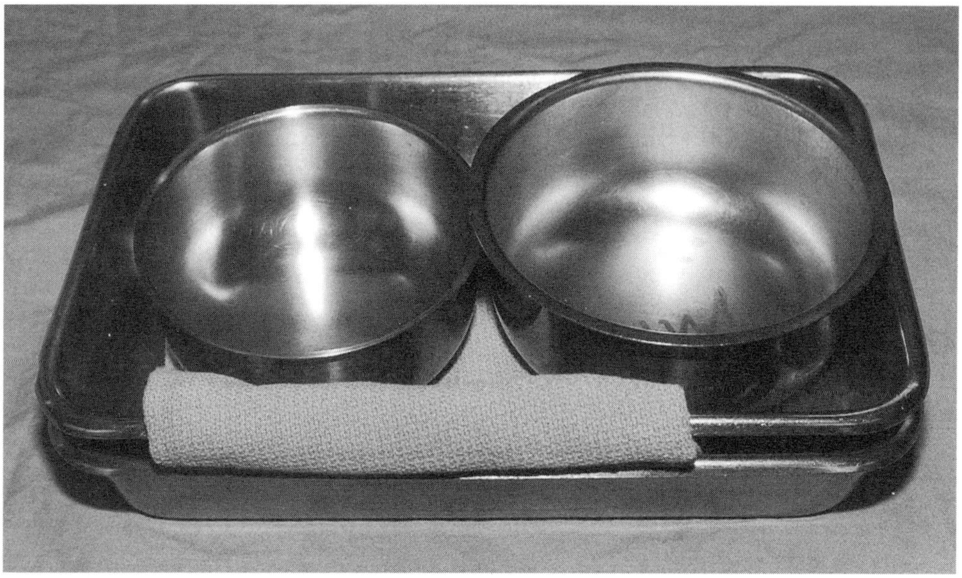

Figure 6.6. Smaller Basins Should Nest Inside Larger Basins.

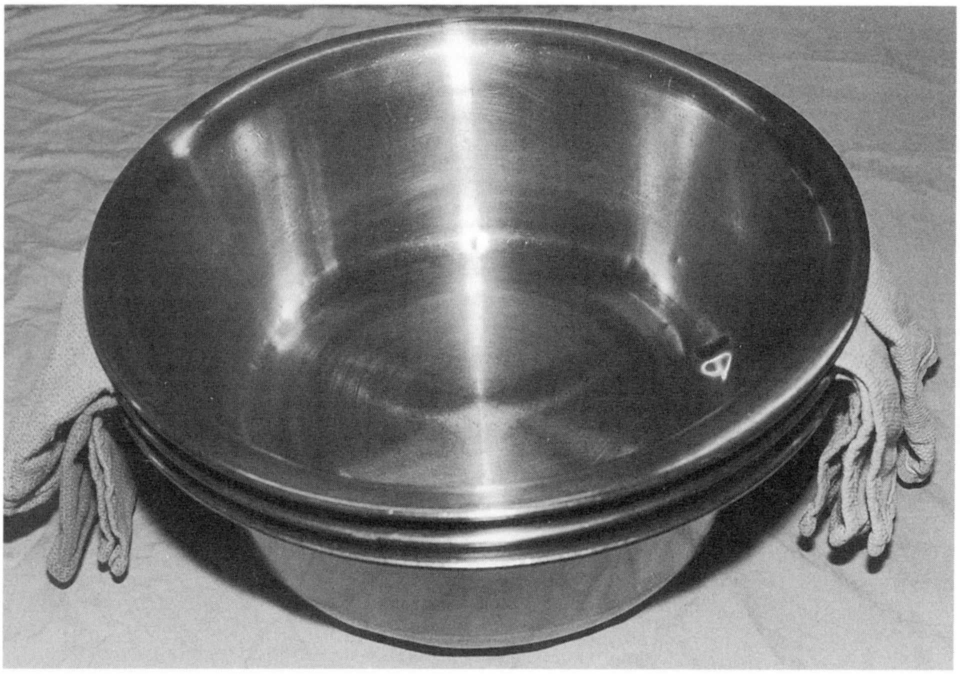

Figure 6.7. Material to Absorb Moisture Should Be Placed Between Basins.

Miscellaneous Preparation

Syringes should be inspected for any chips or cracks and for proper fit of plunger and barrel. When the plunger and barrel are fitted properly, liquid should not flow between them when drawn up in the syringe. For sterilization, the barrel and plunger should be disassembled, but packaged together and protected with a soft material such as 4x4 gauze (see Figure 6.8). To aid in steam contact, items with lumens must be flushed with sterile, distilled water immediately before sterilization.

Principles of Packaging

The packaging chosen for sterile products must conform with three basic principles: it must allow sterilant contact, provide a barrier to microorganisms, and allow sterile presentation of the package contents. It is important that CSD technicians understand these basic principles and the specific properties of packaging materials that relate to these principles. With this knowledge, they can appreciate the rationale for the procedures they must follow in choosing the appropriate material and packaging techniques and in handling sterile products.

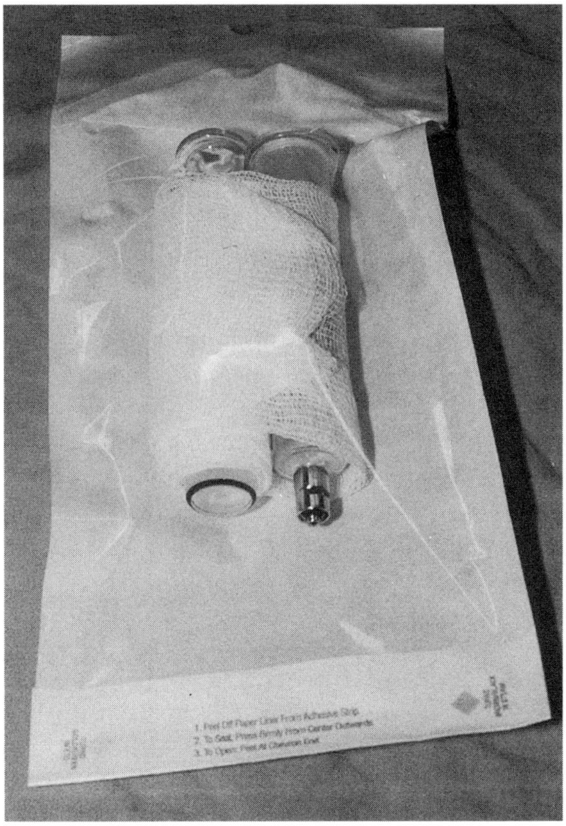

Figure 6.8. Before Sterilizing, the Barrel and Plunger Should Be Disassembled, Packaged Together, and Protected with a Soft Material.

The ideal in-hospital packaging material would have the following characteristics:

- It withstands the physical conditions of the sterilization process chosen for the device (e.g., high temperature, moisture, and steam-sterilization pressure).
- It allows for adequate air removal.
- It is easily penetrated by the sterilant, enabling sterilization of the package contents.
- It allows adequate removal of the sterilant.
- It is a reliable barrier to microorganisms.
- It repels water and other liquids.
- It is sealed in such a way that tampering will be evident.
- It adapts to the size, shape, and nature of the item to be packaged.

- It resists tearing and puncturing under ordinary conditions of use.
- It protects the package contents from physical damage.
- It allows aseptic removal of the contents.

Unfortunately, the perfect packaging material has not been developed. Therefore, many CSDs will have two or more different types of packaging materials (for example, textiles, nonwoven materials, and pouches). Depending on the nature of the particular product to be packaged, how it is used, the method of sterilization used, and where it is stored, some of these characteristics may be more important than others. For example, some devices require more physical protection than others. Or, it may be important to be able to see the device through the packaging.

The physical conditions of the sterilization process depend on the method chosen. However, whatever the method, these conditions differ from normal room conditions. The chamber pressure and temperature in steam sterilization rapidly rise to levels well above ambient. The first step in a prevacuum steam process is the creation of a vacuum. With EtO sterilization, a vacuum may also be created and the chamber temperatures may be somewhat above normal room temperature. Packaging materials must be able to tolerate these changes in pressure and temperature without melting, burning, rupturing, or otherwise being altered or destroyed.

Adequate air removal is essential in steam sterilization, because air will inhibit direct contact with the steam necessary for sterilization to occur. In some EtO sterilizers, a vacuum is created because it is necessary to reduce the amount of air in the chamber in order to allow for more rapid diffusion of the sterilant gas. Packaging materials must therefore allow the rapid removal of air without compromising the integrity of the package.

The packaging material must be permeable to the sterilant agent used, because the sterilant must contact all surfaces of the item being sterilized. Some packaging materials resist penetration by steam (for example, plastic films), and are therefore unsuitable for packaging items to be steam-sterilized. Other packaging materials are not permeable to EtO (for example, nylon or aluminum foil), and are therefore unsuitable for packaging items to be sterilized with EtO. Textile products are unsuitable for packaging and protecting items to be sterilized with gas plasma (one of the sterilants used for low-temperature sterilization). Follow the manufacturer's recommended practice for these systems.

The process of steam sterilization causes water to condense on the item being sterilized. In order for the item to dry, the water must be revaporated. Ethylene oxide is a toxic chemical that must be removed from the package before the sterilized item is used. Therefore, packaging materials must not only allow penetration of the sterilant, but also allow *removal* of the sterilant within the time allowed for that phase of the sterilization cycle.

In order to move from place to place, microorganisms must have a vehicle or medium. They can travel in a liquid, on hands, or on dust particles smaller than the eye can see. Therefore, packaging materials must provide a reliable barrier. This barrier is created by establishing a *tortuous path.* The tortuous path (i.e., a series of turns or bends) forces dust particles to turn at right angles many times before reaching the package contents, making penetration difficult.

Microorganisms can readily move in any direction in fluids. Moisture can "wick" along fibers and move through the spaces between fibers, carrying microorganisms with it. Packaging materials can *resist moisture penetration* either by retarding wicking action or by being treated with a process that will render the material repellant to water.

Packaging materials must ensure that the contents remain within the package. It should not be possible to open and reseal the package without it being evident that the seal has been breached and the sterility of the contents compromised. The term for this property is *tamper proof.*

Another consideration is the *adaptability* of the packaging material to the size, shape, and nature of the item to be packaged. The package should not extend beyond the actual size of the contents, because excessive packaging material can inhibit sterilant penetration and create the potential for contamination.

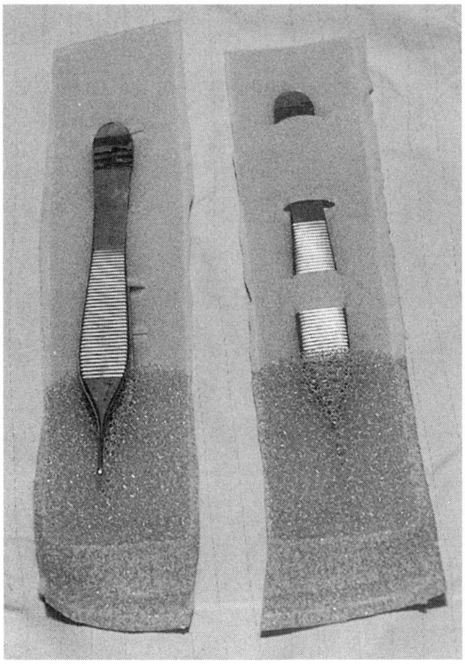

Figure 6.9. Foam Inserts Help to Protect Delicate Instruments from Damage.

A packaging material must be durable so that it withstands, without tearing or puncturing, the impacts and pressures of normal handling. Also, a packaging material must not degrade over the usual storage time—folds must not become holes, the materials must not become brittle and crack, and the seals must not deteriorate and break open with age.

Many medical devices and instruments are fragile and may require physical protection from damage, even during routine handling. For such items, rigid plastic and metal containers are sometimes chosen. Clips, pins, foam inserts, commercially made folders, and sleeves may also be used in the standard mesh bottom trays to protect instruments (Figure 6.9).

The packaging material must allow the package to be opened, either in the hand or on a flat surface, in a manner that will permit *aseptic transfer* of the contents. In some cases, the packaging material may also serve as a drape to establish a sterile field. Consideration must be given to the size of the product being wrapped when selecting the packaging material.

Lint can act as a carrier for microorganisms. Therefore, although lint cannot be completely eliminated, the packaging material should generate as little as possible when the package is opened.

Types of Packaging Materials

Several materials and combinations of materials are available for in-hospital packaging, including woven textiles, papers, cellophanes, plastics, nonwoven synthetics, and sterilization containers. The particular type or combination of types chosen for use at a given health care facility depends on the resources and specific needs of that institution.

Woven Textiles

The types of woven textiles that are used for sterilization packaging are 100 percent cotton, cotton-polyester blends, and synthetic blends. Unbleached, double-thickness muslin of 140 threads per square inch was for many years the standard sterilization wrap. This type of wrapper has been replaced at many facilities with cotton-synthetic blends, synthetic blends, and nonwoven materials.

In a single layer, the spaces between the threads of any woven material are large enough to allow microorganisms and even dust particles to pass through. In order to minimize this transfer, two approaches have been taken in the design of textile packaging materials: using multiple layers or increasing the number of threads per square inch (the "thread count"), thus making the spaces between threads smaller. In addition, because the cotton fibers in these textiles will wick moisture into a package, the fibers may be treated with chemicals that make them water-repellant. This combination of multiple layers, tighter weave, and chemical treatment has made modern woven textiles suitable for use in sterilization packaging. Woven textiles are reusable, of course, and require laundering, inspection with a lighted table, delinting, and folding between uses.

Nonwoven Materials

Nonwoven packaging materials are made of plastic polymers, cellulose fibers, or washed paper pulp bonded under pressure into sheets (not woven on a loom). The nonwoven materials commonly used in health care facilities are designed for single use and thus must be disposed of after use.

The spaces between fibers in nonwoven material are very small and randomly placed, and significantly reduce the possibility of microorganisms or dust particles being transferred. Whether or not the material resists wicking and thus moisture penetration depends on the fiber used. Plastic polymers, for example, are impervious to droplet moisture, whereas packaging materials made of untreated, washed paper pulp can be easily wetted.

Durability varies widely within this group. Washed paper pulp products can be easily torn or punctured by sharp objects, whereas polymers such as spun-bonded olefin are more resistant to tears and punctures.

Wrapping Techniques

Surgical instruments, medical/surgical supplies, and other items to be sterilized must be wrapped or otherwise packaged to ensure that they will stay sterile during storage and until they are used. As explained above, the properties of the packaging material are important in ensuring and maintaining sterility. Even the best material is of little value if the package is not correctly prepared. Specific procedures must be followed when preparing any package to ensure its intended purpose.

Some heavier sets may need additional protection on the corners of the tray to prevent tears. This can be accomplished by placing a towel under the tray or using commercially made corner protectors.

After a pack is prepared, it must be wrapped in suitable packaging material. Two wrappers, sequentially applied, are used to ensure adequate protection of the package contents. These wrappers may be two double-thickness woven wrappers, two nonwoven wrappers, or a combination. This double-wrapping procedure essentially creates a package within a package. Items are first wrapped with one wrapper, then with the second. The second or outside wrapper is taped to secure the closure and the tape is labeled to identify the contents. There is also a newer method called simultaneous wrap, which is explained later in this chapter.

Choosing the correct size wrapper is very important. The wrapper must be large enough to completely enclose the items being packaged and to allow all edges and corners of the wrapper to be tucked in securely. However, excessive packaging material can inhibit sterilant penetration and release. Wrappers should be folded tight enough to secure the contents but not so tight as to hinder air removal and sterilant penetration.

When the wrappers will also be used to create a sterile field (e.g., back table in surgery), they must be large enough to extend at least 6 inches—below the edge on all four sides of the table.

The wrapper must be properly folded to secure the package content and allow the contents to be aseptically presented at the point of use. The folds must always be in the same sequence (as described on the following pages) to allow person(s) opening the packages to establish a standard pattern of movements and conserve time. The two most common methods are the "square fold" or "straight method," which is used to wrap large packs and instrument trays, especially when the wrappers will be used to create the sterile field. The "envelope fold" or "diagonal method"

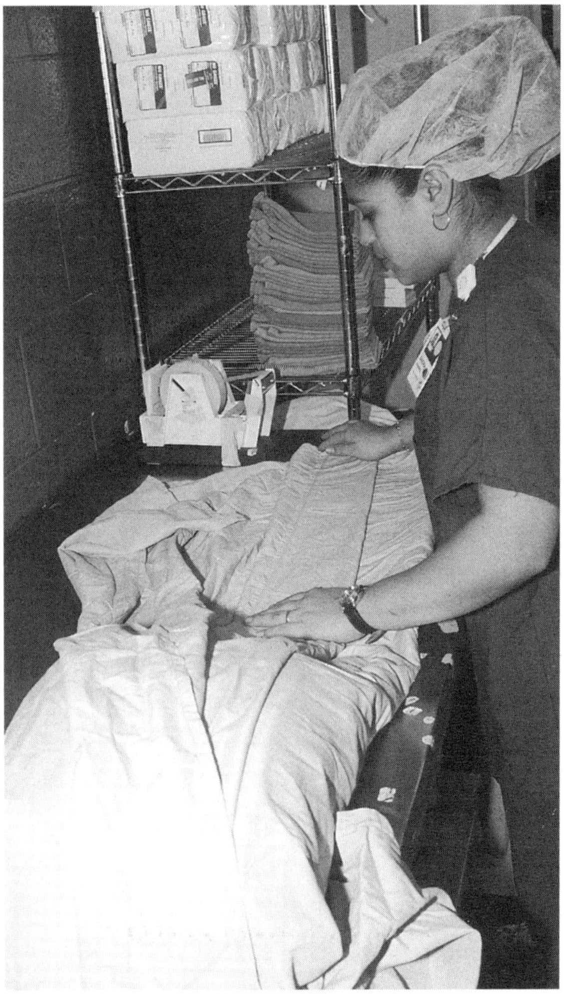

Figure 6.10. Square Fold (Straight Method).

is used for small packs, most instrument sets, and individual items. The specific procedures used are as follows:

Square Fold (Straight Method)
See Figures 6.10 and 6.11.

1. The wrapper is placed lengthwise across the table. The linen pack or instrument tray is placed in the center of the wrapper square or parallel with the edges.
2. The edge of the wrapper at the front of the table is folded over the top of the pack or tray to cover the lower half of the pack or tray and then folded back to form a cuff.
3. The opposite edge of the wrapper is folded over the upper half of the pack or tray, then folded back to form a cuff overlapping the previous cuff.
4. The left edge of the wrapper is folded snugly over the pack and then folded back to form a cuff.
5. The right side of the wrapper is folded over the pack, overlapping the previous fold to make a snug pack, and then folded back to form a cuff.

6–9. The procedure for applying the second wrapper used with large packs and instrument trays is the same as that for the first wrapper.

10. The package is usually secured with sterilization-indicator tape.

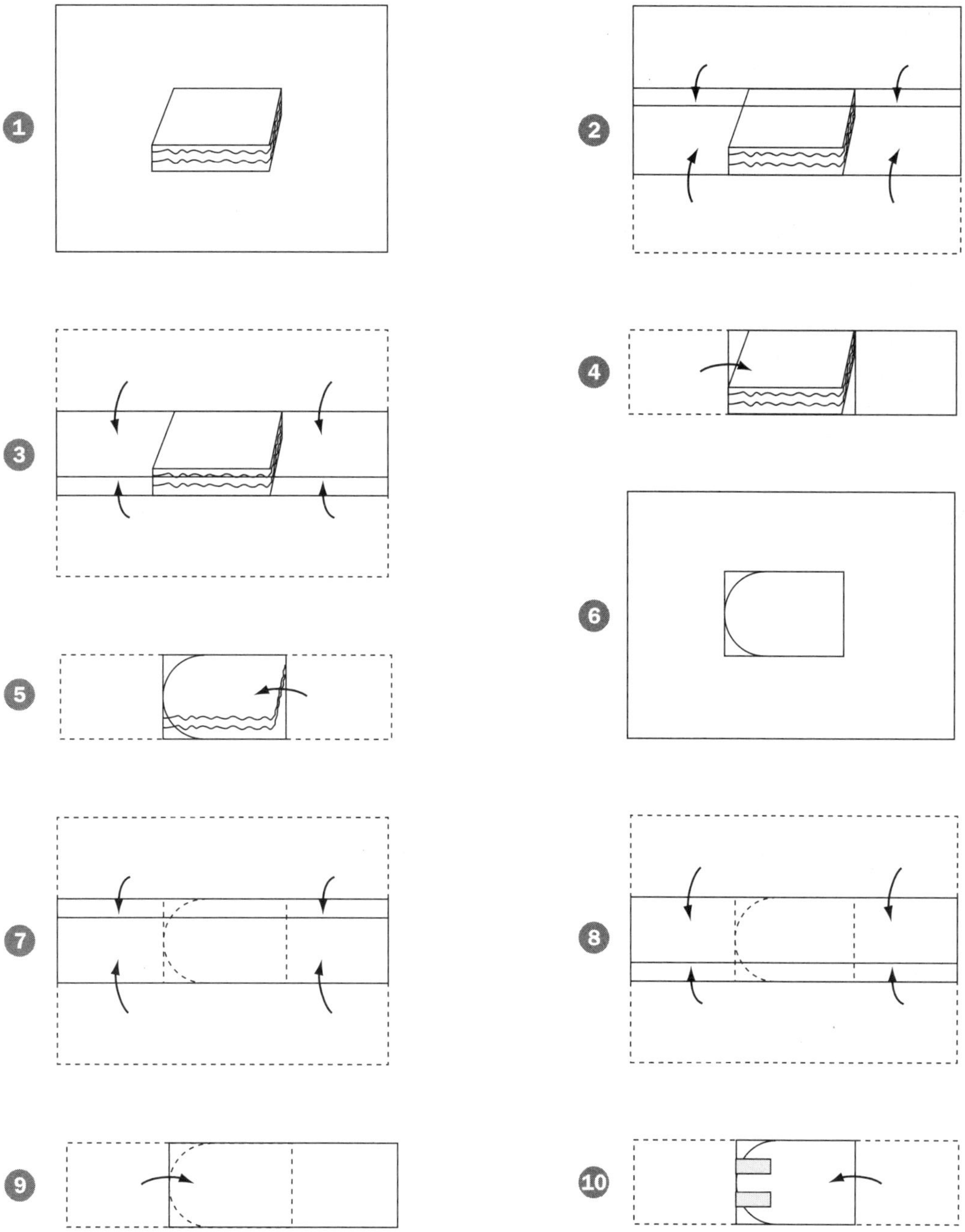

Figure 6.11. Illustration of the Square Fold or Straight Method of Wrapping Packs.

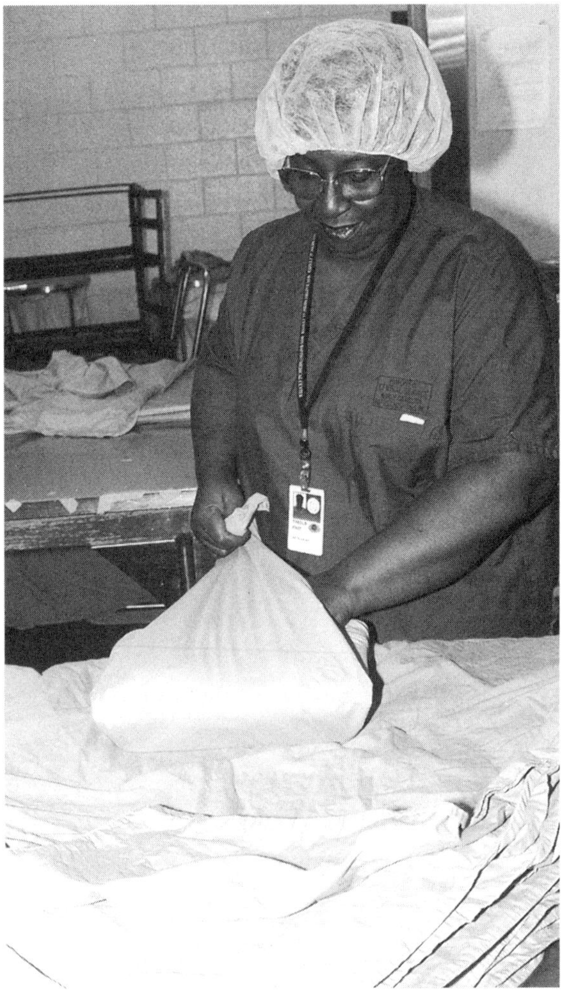

Figure 6.12. Envelope Fold (Diagonal Method).

Envelope Fold (Diagonal Method)

See Figures 6.12 and 6.13.

1. The square wrapper is placed diagonally on the work table, with one corner pointing toward the front of the table. The item to be wrapped is placed in the center of the wrapper at right angles to a line between the top and bottom corners of the wrapper.
2. The bottom corner is folded over the item and then folded back to form a tab or flap, which will be used, like a cuff, to open the package at the time of use.
3. The left corner of the wrapper is folded over the item and then folded back to form a flap.
4. The right corner of the wrapper is folded over the item, overlapping the previous fold, and then folded back to form a flap.
5. The top corner of the wrapper is folded over the item, and the flap is tucked under the previous left and right folds, leaving a small tab visible for easy opening in the sterile environment.

6–8. The second wrapper is applied in the same manner.

9. The package is usually secured with sterilization-indicator tape.

Simultaneous Wrapping Method

Some facilities are using a new method for wrapping items, which involves the use of *two* wrappers made of nonwoven material that have been *attached* on the edges by the manufacturer. This simultaneous method serves the same purpose as the

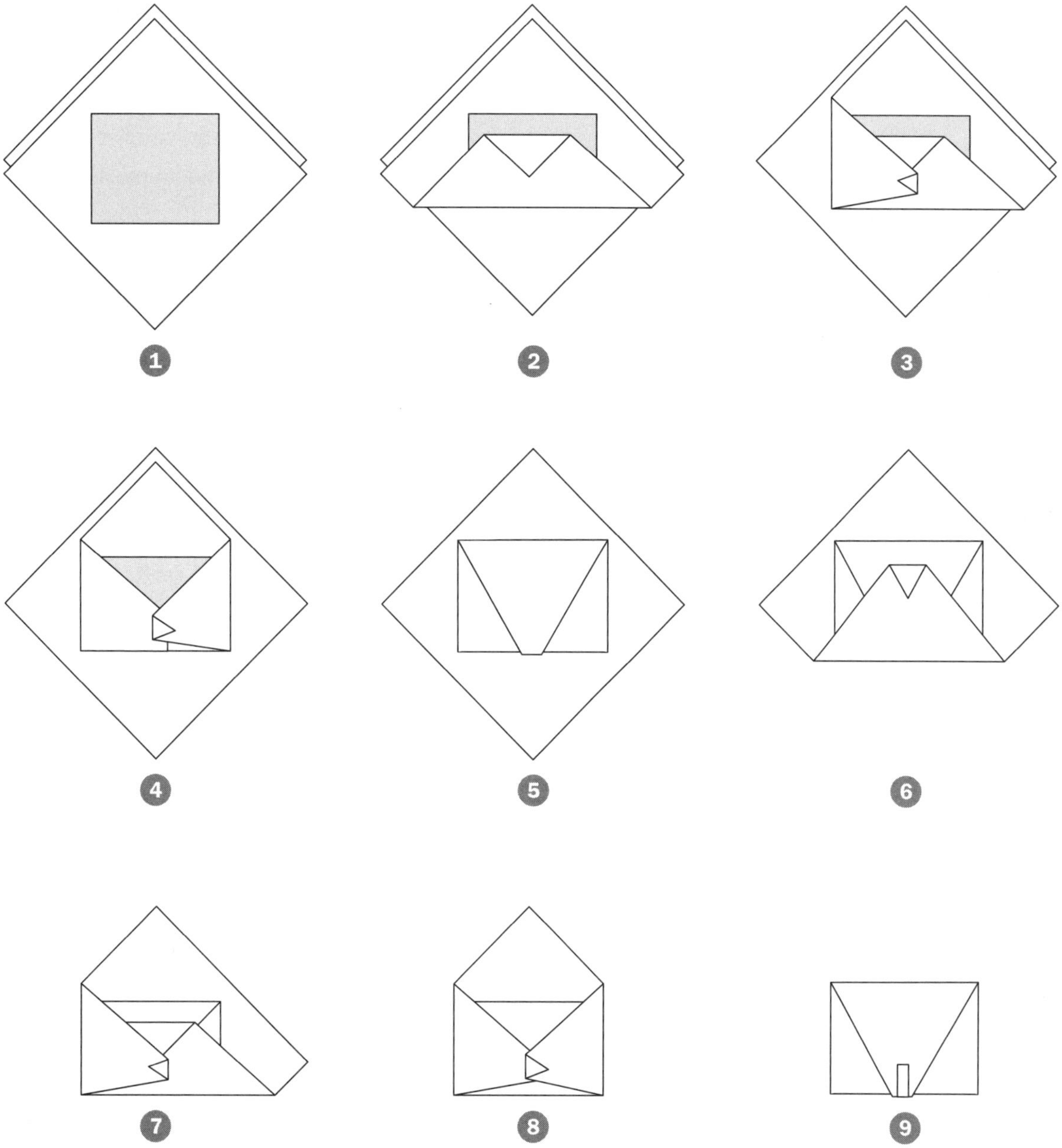

Figure 6.13. Illustration of the Envelope Fold (Diagonal Method) of Wrapping Packs.
Copyright © 1980 by the Association for the Advancement of Medical Instrumentation.

sequential double wrap to protect instruments from contamination. The square fold (Figure 6.11, steps 1 to 5 and 10 only) and the envelope fold (Figure 6.13, steps 1 to 5 and 9 only) wrapping methods are used with this type of wrapping material. Make sure the first fold covers all the contents. The advantage of using this wrapping method is the time saved when wrapping items and aseptically opening the package.

After the pack is wrapped, the closure must be properly secured. Sterilization indicator tape is the recommended method. The use of indicator tape serves several purposes. It securely seals the closure of the wrapper and provides external visual indication, by changing color, that the package has been subjected to sterilization conditions. It is also a label for identifying the pack contents and can be removed easily at the time of use.

Wrapped packs should not be secured with pins, staples, or any other sharp objects. Sharp objects can penetrate the wrapping material, break the fibers, and leave an opening through which microorganisms can enter and contaminate the package contents. Paper clips should not be used because they can be accidentally removed in handling or storage.

Pouches

Pouches are often used to package lightweight individual items, especially when visibility of the item is important. Pouches should not be used for heavy or bulky items because the seals will be stressed and might break open. These preformed pouches are fabricated from a variety of materials, including paper, polyethylene, cellophane, TyvekR (spun-bonded olefin), and various paper-plastic combinations. Items are placed in pouches so that the end of the item to be grasped (such as the finger rings of an instrument) will be presented first when the package is opened at the point of use.

Care must be taken to choose the correct-size pouch. It is important to leave a minimum of 1 inch of space between the item and the seals of the pouch. The pouch or seals may rupture if the item is too close to the seals. Pouches that are too large may allow excessive movement of the contents, which in turn may break the seals.

Heat sealing is the most widely used method of sealing. Special machines are available for this purpose. Heat sealers must be used according to the manufacturer's instructions. When using these machines, personnel should take care to avoid burning themselves on the extremely hot sealer jaws. There are a variety of heat sealing machines available.

For paper-plastic pouches, the general sealing procedure is to place the open end of the pouch between the sealer's jaws, apply pressure with the jaws while they are hot, then release the jaws, and allow the seal to cool. This process bonds the plastic to the paper. After the seal is made, it should be inspected to ensure that it is complete (with no wrinkles) and secure. For plastic-plastic pouches, the procedure is the same, except that the jaws of the sealer are not released until the seal has cooled. In this process, the two plastics are melted together. Cooling the seal under pressure prevents stretching of the hot plastic and weakening of the pouch and seal. When using heat sealers, CSD personnel should take care to avoid burns. The proper temperature (heat setting) should be verified before use to ensure proper sealing.

Some paper-plastic and plastic-plastic pouches are self-sealing. The seal is made with a sticky strip at the end of the pouch, which is folded over the opening. These seals must be folded carefully to avoid gaps or wrinkles, which will allow microorganisms to enter and contaminate the package contents.

Paper-plastic and plastic-plastic pouches should not be secured with paper clips, pins, staples, or any other sharp objects. These methods of closure may damage the integrity of the packaging material.

In addition to being used in nonwoven synthetics, some plastic polymers can be extruded into sheets of varying thicknesses. During this process, it is possible for small pinholes to form in very thin sheets (those less than 1 millimeter [$^{1}/_{1,000}$ inch] thick). Therefore, for packaging applications, it is recommended that plastic films be at least 2 millimeters thick (whether a single sheet or two sheets bonded together).

Water cannot penetrate plastic films in either the liquid or vapor phase; thus plastic film cannot be used as a packaging material for steam sterilization. Pouches have been designed with paper on one side of the pouch to allow steam to penetrate. If items are "double peel pouched" (i.e., the item is placed in a peel pouch and the pouch is placed in a second, larger pouch), it must be paper against paper, plastic against plastic, to allow sterilant penetration. The inner package must not be folded. Double packaging is not required except for very small items, which may need to be contained. Plastic films absorb EtO and allow its passage, but not humidity, which is necessary for sterilization. For this reason, plastic pouches designed for EtO may be either paper on one side or contain a Tyvek port. Polyvinyl chloride (PVC) is not used because it is penetrated poorly by EtO and retains the gas for a prolonged period after the sterilization cycle.

Plastic films (i.e., sterility maintenance covers) are often used after sterilization to provide a moisture- and dust-impervious barrier.

Containerized Packaging

Specially designed metal or plastic containers are also used to package items for sterilization, usually surgical instrument sets. These containerized packaging systems (Figure 6.14) have the following components:

- A top that can be removed for aseptic presentation of the contents
- Perforations in the top and bottom or valves that allow air removal and sterilant penetration and removal
- A microbial filter system or secured valve closure to maintain the sterility of the contents
- A means of securing the top to the bottom
- A means of identifying the contents
- A means of distinguishing processed containers from unprocessed containers

Containerized packaging systems must be disassembled and cleaned after each use. Single-use filters should be removed and discarded. The container may be washed with a mild detergent. Most container manufacturers recommend a neutral pH detergent. The container manufacturer should be consulted on the types of detergents and filters that can be used. The container should be rinsed thoroughly with clear water because soap residues will cause spotting. Containers can also be cleaned in an automatic system (e.g., washer/decontaminator, washer/sterilizer).

When the containerized packaging system is being reassembled for reuse, gaskets should be inspected and replaced if torn, cracked, or no longer soft and pliable. Most systems use filter paper and a retainer frame. The filter is usually a precut sheet of nonwoven wrap that is held securely to the container by the retainer frame (Figure 6.15). Care must be taken to ensure that the retainer frame is secure. If it is not, the filter plate may become dislodged and the supplies within the container will be contaminated. This problem is usually not found until the set is opened in

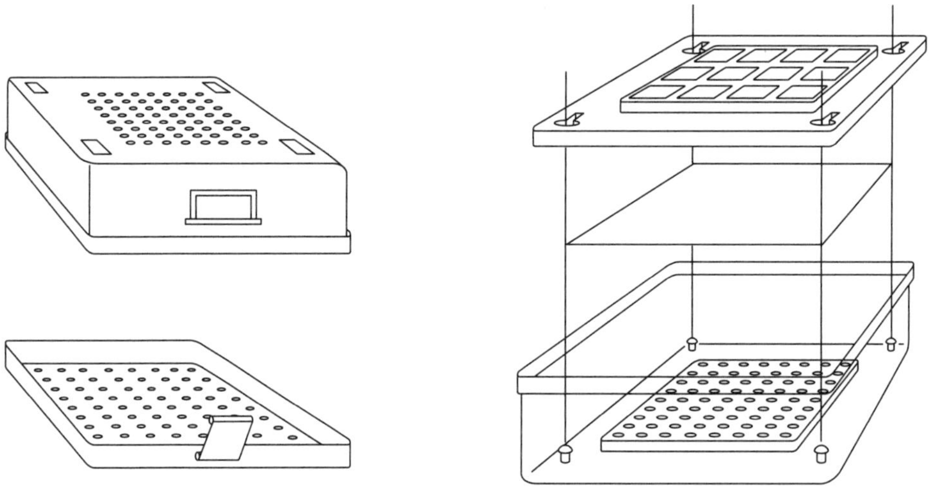

Figure 6.14. A Containerized Packaging System.

the operating room. In one type of containerized packaging system, a valve is used instead of filter paper and a retaining frame. This valve must be checked for proper working order in accordance with the manufacturer's instructions. If the valve is not working correctly, the sterilization process may be inhibited.

The prepared instrument set in a mesh basket is then placed in the bottom of the container and the lid is attached. The container manufacturer should provide written documentation as to the devices the manufacturer has validated for use inside their container (e.g., power equipment, lumens, etc.). Several types of locking mechanisms are available. The locking mechanism serves two purposes: it prevents accidental opening and contamination of the contents, and it serves as a tamper-evident seal (see Figure 6.16). The lid should never be forced onto the bottom of the container, as this may damage the instruments or the container. If the lid cannot be secured without force, it should be removed and the instruments inspected to ensure that they are not out of place.

Once the container is locked, the contents must be identified on the outside. There is usually a space where the label can be attached. This indicator will distinguish which sets have been processed and which have not. The processing indicator is usually a customized one available from the manufacturer of the container. A piece of indicator tape may also be used. Careful removal of the tape and adhesive is necessary each time to avoid buildup (see Figure 6.17).

Unless otherwise specified by the container manufacturer, containerized packaging should only be used in prevacuum steam sterilizers. Gravity displacement

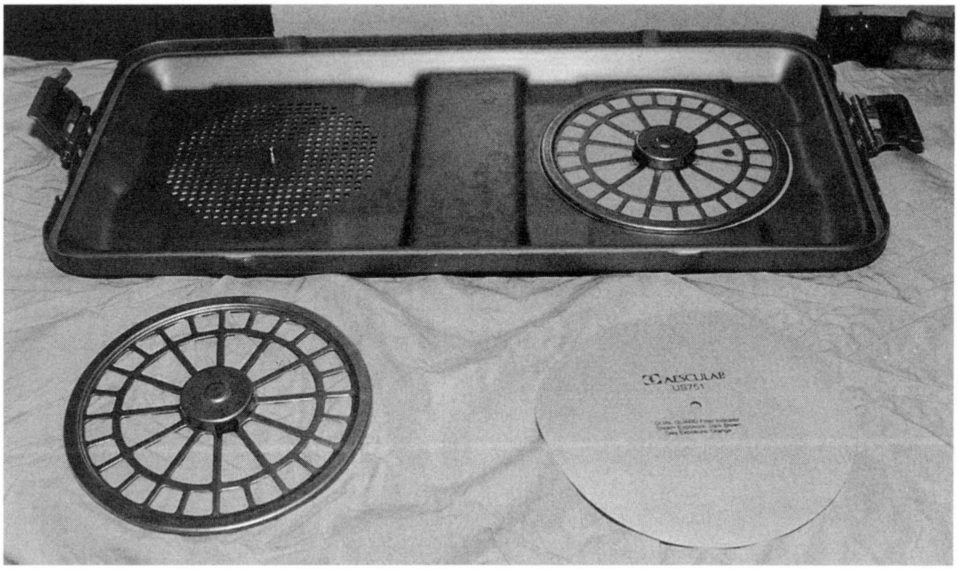

Figure 6.15. Most Containerized Packaging Systems Use Filter Paper and a Retainer Frame.

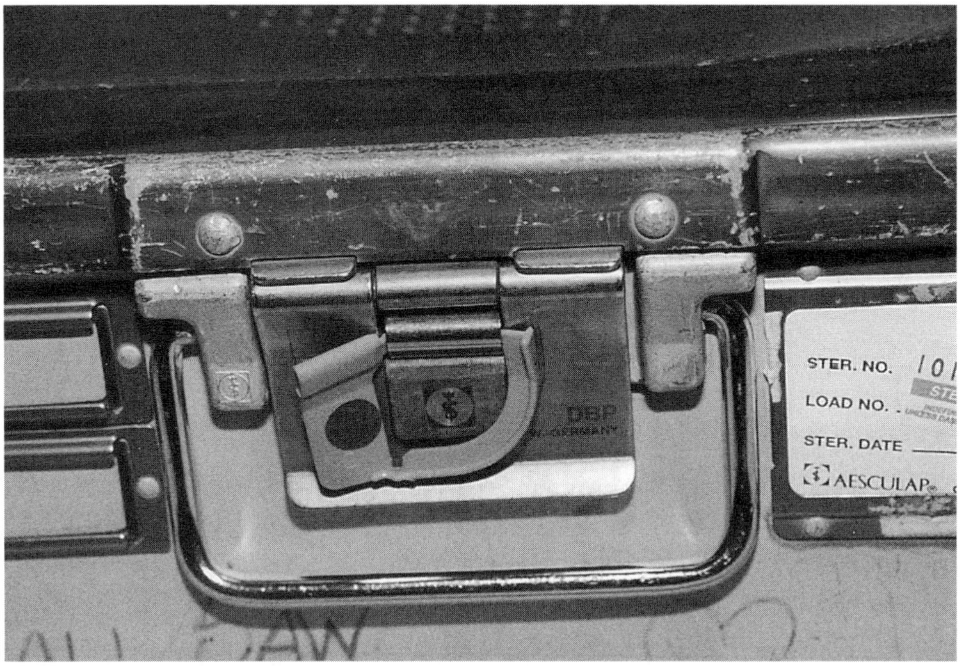

Figure 6.16. A Locking Mechanism on a Container.

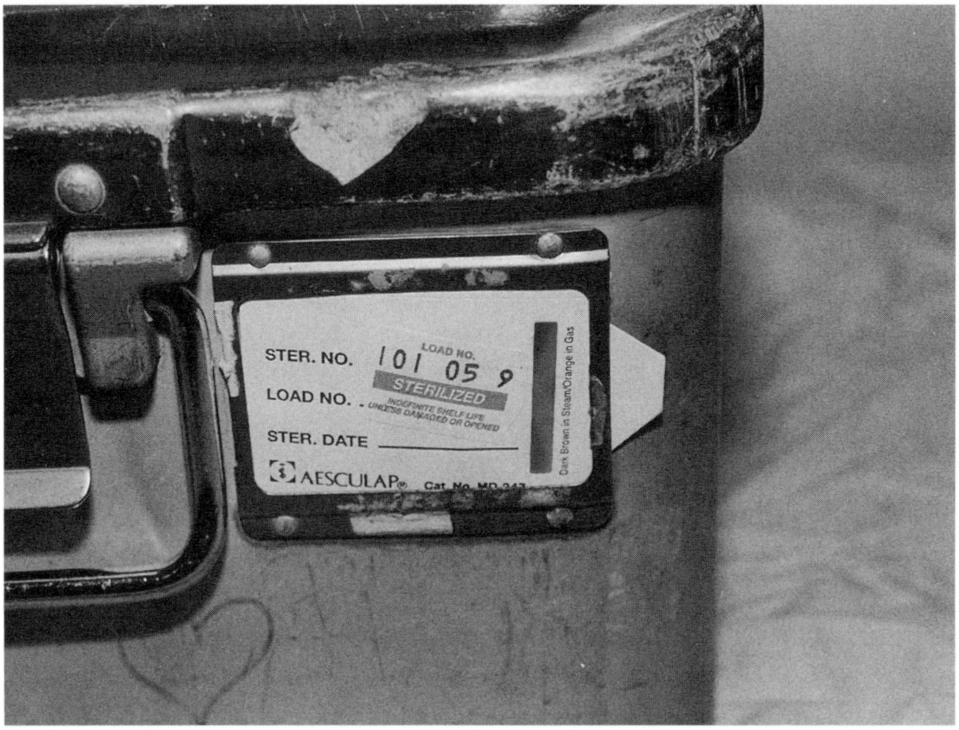

Figure 6.17. A Label Attached to a Container.

steam sterilization is not usually recommended because of the difficulty of air removal. Manufacturers of the containers must provide recommended processing instructions for exposure and dry times if containers are used in a displacement steam sterilizer. If containers are used in a gravity displacement steam sterilizer, they must have filters in the top and bottom to facilitate air removal and steam penetration inside the container. *Some* containerized packaging can be used in EtO, gas plasma, or ozone sterilizers. Check with the container manufacturer for acceptable types of sterilants that can be used with their containers and whether special aeration times will be needed for removal of ethylene oxide residuals.

Containers should be processed for the length of time and temperature recommended by the manufacturer. However, if you are processing a specialty instrument or device that requires a nonstandard exposure time, the difference between the manufacturer's standard and the irregular exposure time must be reconciled. Metal containers cannot absorb condensate like fabric wrappers do. During sterilization, condensate collects on both the exterior and interior surfaces of the containers. These beads of condensate are difficult to revaporize. Therefore, an extended drying time may be necessary. If condensate is present after a 20-minute drying time, usually there are too many instruments in the set or they are too heavy and dense (for example, automatic retractor systems). Wet packs are discussed in Chapter Seven.

The shelves of the sterilizer cart should be arranged so that there is space above and below the containers to allow maximum air removal and steam penetration. Containers should be placed flat on the shelf. Containers should not be stacked unless specifically recommended by the manufacturer. After sterilization, however, containers can be stacked for storage without danger of contamination due to puncturing or tearing.

It is essential for SPD workers to know if their sets are dry at the completion of the sterilization cycle. This is difficult, because one cannot see inside the container. Therefore it is recommended that verification of drying be performed and documented. Sterilize as usual the largest (heaviest) sets (e.g., Laminectomy, total hip). Allow to cool on the autoclave shelf after sterilization. Open the set and inspect for moisture on the instruments, moist towel or foam (if used inside the inner basket), or visible water in the corners of the baskets. If any moisture or water is noted, the set needs additional drying time. Sometimes the drying of sets can be helped by "preconditioning" the load. Place the load inside the steam sterilizer, close the door, and allow the set to "heat up" for 15 minutes. Then start the cycle. The instruments will be heated up from the heat inside the chamber, resulting in less condensate formation. Drying verification should also be performed on wrapped sets as well. All drying verification studies should be documented. The tests only have to be repeated if a change is made to the tray (more instruments added).

Some instruments are from outside manufacturers (loaner instruments) and may be provided in organizing cases. These organizing cases can be made of plastic, metal, or a combination of both. Always open and completely decontaminate loaner instrumentation, even if it is brought into your facility wrapped. You have no information as to how the tray was cleaned and sterilized; therefore, you should completely process it according to your facility's policies.

Labeling Packages

Because the contents of a package must be identified before the package is opened, it is important that the package be labeled completely and correctly. Also, proper labeling is necessary for quality assurance, inventory control, and stock-rotating purposes. Packages should always be labeled before sterilization.

A method of labeling that will not damage the packaging material should be selected. Generally, a felt-tip, quick-dry alcohol-based nontoxic marker may be used to record the necessary information on the tape. Never write on the wrapper material—use the tape for this purpose. Indelible ink is necessary so that the marking will not run or fade. Felt-tip, indelible-ink markers may also be used on pouches. For paper-plastic pouches, the labeling must be on the clear plastic side. Writing on the paper side may damage the material and the ink may bleed through and contaminate the package contents. Preprinted indicator tape can be purchased for standard high-volume items.

The label information should include a description of the package contents, the expiration date or other shelf-life indication, the CSD technician's initials, identification of the sterilizer and cycle number to be used, and the date of sterilization. Usually the contents are hand-labeled on the tape with the preparation employee's initials. The sterilization information is usually contained on a printed label that is affixed during load preparation. Standardized terms and abbreviations should be used. The department to which the package is to be sent after sterilization may also be identified on the label.

Shelf Life

Sterility is event-related. Shelf life is the period during which an item is considered safe for use. This can be a specific period or may be indefinite. If packages are handled and stored properly, many packaging materials will maintain sterility without regard to time. The longer an item remains in storage, however, the greater the chance of contamination.

Some packaging materials are better than others. Also, some packaging materials may deteriorate over time. Decisions about which packaging materials to use should be based on the frequency of events (i.e., the number of times a package is handled before use).

Many commercially sterilized items have an indefinite shelf life. The manufacturer indicates on the label that the contents are sterile unless the package integrity has been compromised (that is, unless the package is torn, cut, wet, cracked, dirty, or open). Some commercially prepared products carry a specific expiration date, which is usually indicated by an hourglass symbol followed by a date. See Appendix C for an example of this symbol as well as other commonly used symbols that the International Standards Organization (ISO) has designated for use on medical-device packaging. When indefinite shelf-life dating is used for health care–produced products, a control date should be established. This date is usually six months.

Shelf life should be thought of as event-related rather than time-related. Contamination does not suddenly occur on the last day of the labeled shelf life. It occurs because of some event that allows penetration of the package and introduction of microorganisms (for example, the package is dropped on the floor or the wrapper is wet or punctured). The less impervious and durable the packaging material and the more the package is handled or subjected to an environment loaded with microorganisms, the shorter the length of time assigned as the shelf life. In many hospitals every package is labeled with an exact *outdate,* the last day the item may be used. Of course, a package can become contaminated at any time after leaving the sterilizer if it becomes wet or the package is punctured or torn.

Assigned shelf-life dates may also be used as part of an inventory control system. Expiration dating is used to help keep active stock rotated, to reduce outdates, and to allow periodic review of rarely used items. Items that frequently outdate should be evaluated to determine if they are obsolete and should be removed from inventory. Infrequently used items should be stored separately from frequently used items to prevent contact, preferably in closed cabinets that are not often opened.

The expiration date does not indicate whether an item is sterile. Limited handling, correct storage, and package integrity are the keys to maintaining sterility.

Summary

Chapter Six has presented the types of materials and systems used for packaging items for sterilization, including methods used for preparing packages and the importance of proper labeling. The next major step in the reprocessing cycle is the sterilization process itself.

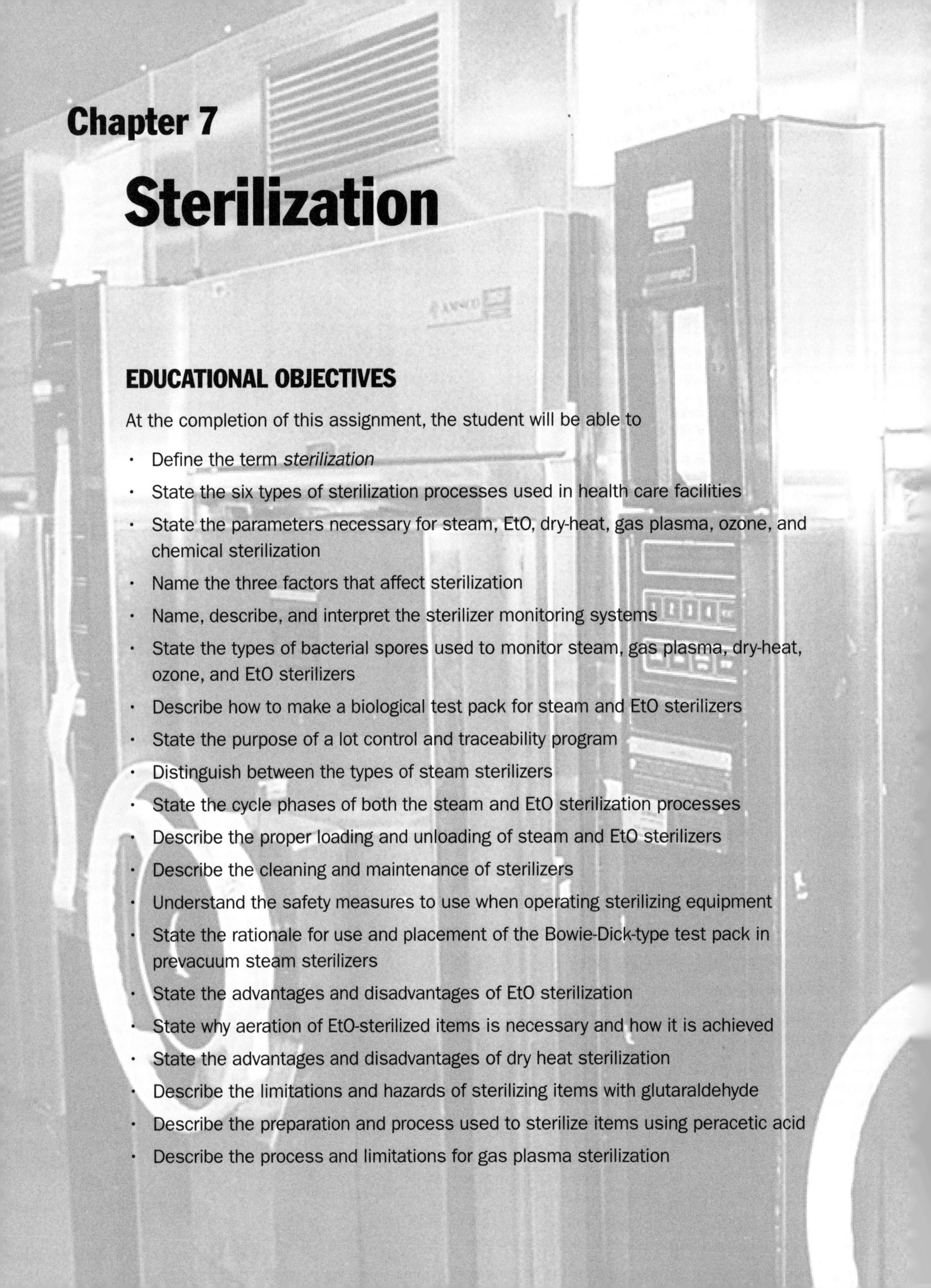

Chapter 7

Sterilization

EDUCATIONAL OBJECTIVES

At the completion of this assignment, the student will be able to

- Define the term *sterilization*
- State the six types of sterilization processes used in health care facilities
- State the parameters necessary for steam, EtO, dry-heat, gas plasma, ozone, and chemical sterilization
- Name the three factors that affect sterilization
- Name, describe, and interpret the sterilizer monitoring systems
- State the types of bacterial spores used to monitor steam, gas plasma, dry-heat, ozone, and EtO sterilizers
- Describe how to make a biological test pack for steam and EtO sterilizers
- State the purpose of a lot control and traceability program
- Distinguish between the types of steam sterilizers
- State the cycle phases of both the steam and EtO sterilization processes
- Describe the proper loading and unloading of steam and EtO sterilizers
- Describe the cleaning and maintenance of sterilizers
- Understand the safety measures to use when operating sterilizing equipment
- State the rationale for use and placement of the Bowie-Dick-type test pack in prevacuum steam sterilizers
- State the advantages and disadvantages of EtO sterilization
- State why aeration of EtO-sterilized items is necessary and how it is achieved
- State the advantages and disadvantages of dry heat sterilization
- Describe the limitations and hazards of sterilizing items with glutaraldehyde
- Describe the preparation and process used to sterilize items using peracetic acid
- Describe the process and limitations for gas plasma sterilization

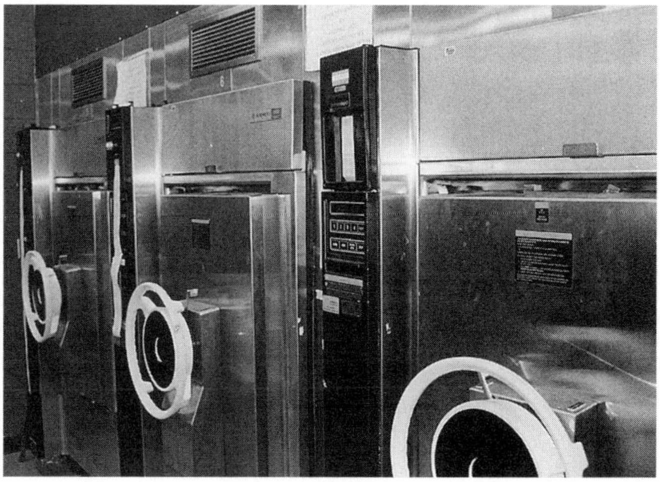

TYPES OF STERILIZATION processes used in health care facilities are steam sterilization, EtO sterilization, dry-heat sterilization, gas plasma sterilization, ozone sterilization, and liquid chemical sterilization. Most items sterilized in U.S. health care facilities are processed by steam. Technicians must know the factors that affect the process of sterilization and the maintenance of sterility, as well as the specific procedures that should be followed for all types of health care sterilization processes.

Because all forms of sterilization are intended to kill microorganisms, sterilizing agents and equipment can be hazardous to personnel. Therefore, CSD technicians should observe the safety precautions described in this chapter, in the sterilizer manufacturer's user manuals, and in their department procedure manuals.

Factors Affecting Sterilization

Sterilizing an item involves the following three essential factors:

- Conditions lethal to microorganisms must be present. In practice, this means that the sterilizer or other sterilizing system must be properly designed and used to achieve the correct combination of temperature and sterilant concentration.
- The amount of bioburden must be low enough to ensure the effectiveness of the sterilization process. The higher the bioburden, the more difficult it is to kill all microorganisms. Therefore, it is very important that items to be sterilized are as clean as possible before sterilization is attempted.
- There must be adequate contact of the sterilant, for sufficient time, with all surfaces of the item.

Achieving these conditions depends not only on the proper design and operation of the sterilizer, but also on how items are assembled, packaged, and loaded into the sterilizer. Maintaining product sterility, once it is achieved, requires that items be handled and stored properly after the sterilization process has been completed.

Even under ideal processing and handling conditions, a "sterile" product is one that has only a high probability of being sterile. Sterilization is a complex process, and there is no practical way of proving that an individual item is actually sterile without contaminating it. It is possible, however, to verify that an item has been exposed to a processing cycle in a sterilizer that provided the conditions necessary for sterilization. Therefore, procedures have been developed for monitoring and documenting the effectiveness of sterilization processes. However, these procedures are only one element of sterility assurance. All CSD technicians must clearly understand that many variables affect the achievement and maintenance of product sterility, not just the exposure of items to a sterilization process. They must strictly adhere to established policies and procedures concerning personal hygiene, attire, and handwashing; cleaning, decontaminating, assembling, and packaging items to be sterilized; and handling, storing, and transporting sterile items.

Monitoring the Sterilization Process

Because so many variables affect the achievement of sterility, monitoring the sterilization process is essential. Mechanical, chemical, and biological monitoring methods are used, as well as procedures for lot control and traceability. In addition, administrative monitoring processes must be in place.

Administrative Monitoring Processes

Quality assurance steps and policies and procedures for cleaning, packaging, operating sterilizers, and loading and unloading sterilizers must be written and reviewed annually due to changes in technology and/or updated. CSD technicians must follow all manufacturers' instructions for use and care of CSD equipment and patient care equipment and devices. There should be scheduled preventive maintenance processes for all sterilizers and other department equipment, and CSD personnel should be aware of what the processes involve (e.g., filters changed, valves replaced, temperature checked, seals changed) and make sure they are being consistently followed.

Environmental conditions (humidity and temperature) in packaging, sterilization, and sterile storage areas should be checked and documented using a schedule determined by the facility. The CSD supervisor or peer review group must monitor CSD employees by observing their techniques for loading, unloading, handling sterile items, and following procedures.

Mechanical Monitoring

Effective sterilization processes depend on the exposure of items to an adequate amount of sterilant for a specified period of time under specific environmental conditions. Sterilizers are equipped with recorders and gauges that enable the operator to verify that all important *cycle parameters* have been met (Figure 7.1). These parameters vary with the type of sterilization process. They must be monitored and documented either manually or by means of an automated recording device. If an automated device is used, the operator must check that the cycle parameters were maintained and initial the recording at the end of every cycle (Figure 7.2). If an automated device is not available, the operator must look at the gauges at critical points in the cycle to verify that the parameters are being met and then record the readings on a sterilizer record sheet or card.

Chemical Monitoring

A chemical indicator is used inside or outside a package, or both, to verify that an item has been *exposed* to one or more sterilizing conditions. Chemical indicators are also used to test, in an otherwise empty chamber, the air-removal characteristics of prevacuum steam sterilizers. This test, which is called a Bowie-Dick

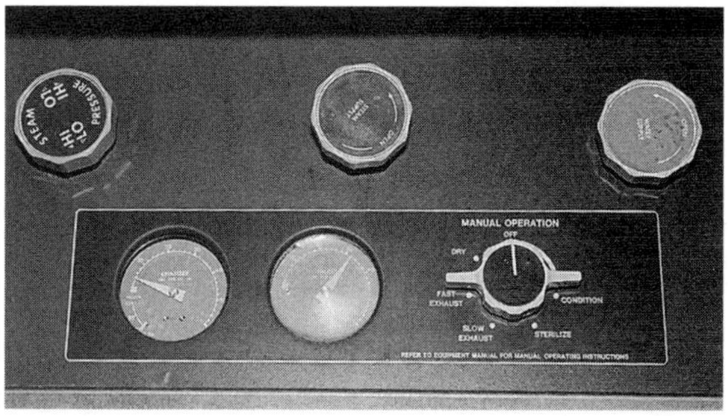

A

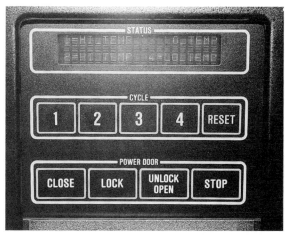

B

Figure 7.1. Several Examples of Sterilizer Recorders and Gauges for Monitoring Cycle Parameters: Gauges (A), Digital Display (B), and Recorder (C).

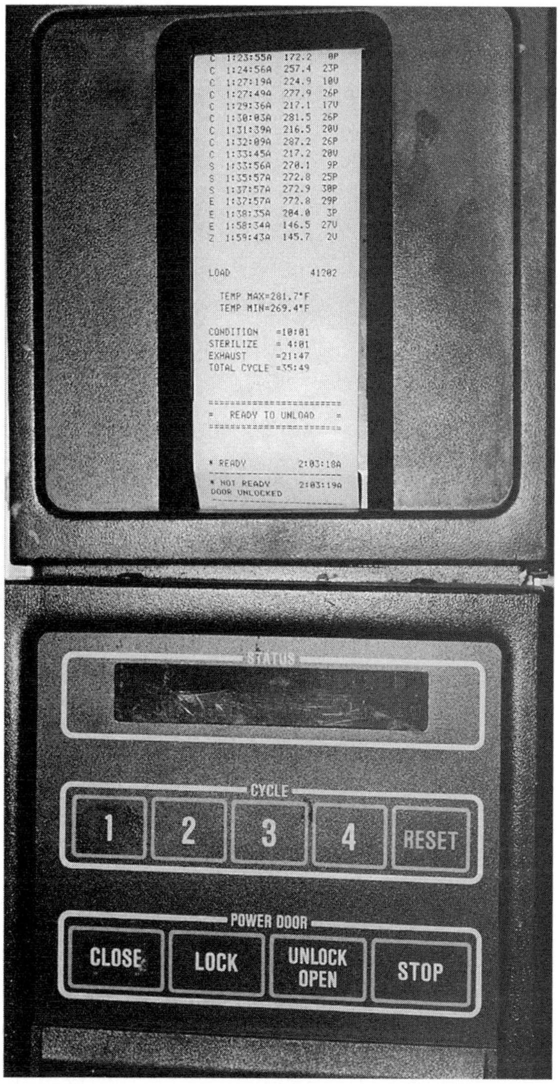

C

test, is described later in this chapter. Some chemical indicators consist of paper that has been chemically treated to change color if exposed to a specific temperature. Others are designed to melt a chemical inside the indicator when subjected to the correct sterilizing temperature, humidity, or sterilant for a specified time. These are called chemical integrators. Integrators measure multiple parameters of the sterilization process. Follow manufacturers' instructions for storage conditions (temperature and humidity levels), factors affecting use (such as exposure to sterilant or to fluorescent light), sterility assurance level of test, and expiration date information.

There are five classifications of chemical indicators. Each class is designed to provide specific information regarding a response to one or more physical conditions inside the sterilizer. *Class I,* or process indicators, respond to only one parameter of the sterilization process. An example would be autoclave tape. *Class II* indicators are designed for a specific use, such as the Bowie-Dick test (also known as the Dynamic Air Removal test). *Class III* indicators are single-parameter indicators that respond to only one of the critical parameters of the sterilization process. *Class IV* indicators are multiparameter indicators designed to react to two or

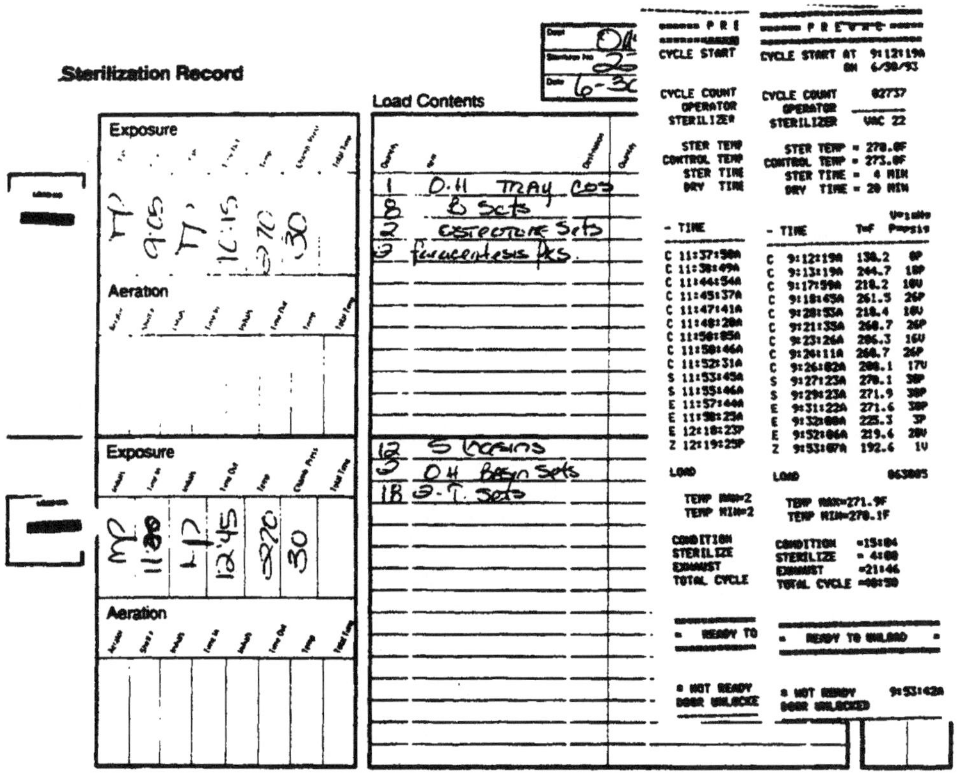

Figure 7.2. Documentation of Cycle Parameters.

more critical parameters of the sterilization process. *Class V* indicators are designed to react to all the critical parameters of the sterilization cycle. In many cases, the response of an integrator corresponds to the performance of a biological monitor. However, integrators do not contain spores and are not considered a biological monitor test.

External chemical indicators are placed on the outside of packaged items to be sterilized and are often used as package closures (for example, autoclave tape). Essentially, an external chemical indicator only illustrates whether the packaged item to which it is affixed has been in the sterilizer and exposed to the sterilization process. If the external chemical indicator has "turned" (changed color), sterilization conditions were not necessarily met inside the package. The use of external chemical indicators is an important quality control tool, because it is a safeguard against the distribution of items that are intended to be sterile but that have not actually been processed in a sterilizer.

Internal chemical indicators or process integrators are placed inside packages to indicate whether the contents have been exposed to one or more of the conditions necessary for sterilization. The placement of the chemical indicator/integrator is in the center of the pack or tray. An exception is the placement of chemical indicators/integrators in two opposite corners of the inside basket of rigid containers. This is done because air can be trapped in the corners of rigid containers. The sterilant must penetrate the packaging long enough to change the color on the indicator or change the color a certain distance along the bar on the integrator. These indicator/integrators are read when the package is opened at the time of use. Internal indicator/integrators do not establish whether or not an item is sterile. If the indicator/integrator has not reacted appropriately, however, the contents of the package may not have been subjected to the correct temperature or other sterilizing conditions. In this event, the item should be considered nonsterile.

CSD staff must keep current on internal chemical monitoring recommendations that may change from time to time. Question what class of indicators should be used for the type of items being sterilized. Some instrument set manufacturers are recommending longer than usual exposure times. Questions regarding appropriate reaction of the monitor being used for each of the extended exposure times (e.g., 8 minutes, 18 minutes, etc.) must be answered by the chemical monitor manufacturer.

Biological Monitoring

A biological indicator (BI) is a device that has been impregnated with a known number and type of microorganism and is used to verify that all the conditions necessary for sterilization have been met. Most biological indicators contain from 100,000 to 1,000,000 bacterial spores, *Geobacillus stearothermophilus* (formerly called *Bacillus stearothermophilus*) for steam, ozone, and peracetic sterilization, and *Bacillus atrophaeus* (formerly called *Bacillus subtilis*) for EtO, gas plasma, and dry-heat sterilization. The number and resistance to sterilization of these populations far exceed the number and resistance of the microorganisms (bioburden) *expected* to be present on items to be sterilized.

In an earlier chapter the importance of thorough cleaning of items before sterilization was stressed because the assurance of the bioburden being below what the sterilization process can destroy is one of the variables that affect the achievement of product sterility. The sterilization cycles used in health care facilities are designed to destroy the microorganisms on the BIs and therefore provide an "overkill" relative to product bioburden, building a margin of safety into the sterilization process.

Biological monitoring involves placing a specifically constructed test pack containing one or more BIs in an otherwise routinely loaded sterilizer, processing the load through a routine cycle, and verifying that the microorganisms on the biological indicator are killed. Because the BI itself provides an "overkill," and because the test procedure is designed to make it more difficult to sterilize the BI than other items in the load, biological monitoring challenges sterilizer performance and validates the entire sterilization process. Follow manufacturers' instructions for storage conditions needed for biological indicators.

A control BI test, with the same lot number as BI test packs being used, must be processed once a day and whenever a different lot numbered pack will be used during the day. The control BI test is processed without having been through sterilization. The results of the test should be positive according to the color change in the vial or fluorescence detection. The control BI test confirms the same lot number as the BI test packs containing the live bacillus.

The general procedure is to place the BI inside a *standard* test pack, either in-house manufactured or commercially available. Different test packs are used for each type of sterilization process, because different types of items are sterilized by these methods and because different sterilizing conditions are being challenged. *Ethylene Oxide Use in Hospitals: A Manual for Health Care Personnel* (third edition, published by the American Hospital Association), describes commonly used test packs for biological monitoring of EtO sterilization cycles. Organizations such as the Association for the Advancement of Medical Instrumentation (AAMI) have defined standard test packs for both steam and EtO sterilization processing. There are BI tests specific to peracetic acid, gas plasma, ozone, and dry-heat sterilizers. The specific composition of the test packs used in any given health care facility is determined by the manager of the CSD and defined in the department procedure manual. Test packs manufactured within the facility must be consistent from pack to pack. The components, arrangement of items, placement of the BI, and size of the pack must be the same each time a pack is manufactured.

The test pack is placed in the portion of the sterilizer where it is most difficult to sterilize items. For steam sterilizers, this *cold point* is usually on the bottom shelf of the sterilizer, directly above the chamber drain. For EtO sterilizers, this point is usually the approximate center of the load. For gas plasma sterilizers, this point is on the first shelf at the back of the chamber. Follow the sterilizer manufacturer's instructions for placement of the test pack for the newer sterilization technologies (i.e., peracetic acid and gas plasma). The test pack is removed from the sterilized load and the BI is taken out. The BI is then incubated according to the manufacturer's instructions. Rigid containers must be validated prior to evaluation and at least once a year during use with biological indicators. Refer to the *AAMI Guidelines for the Selection and Use of Reusable Rigid Container Systems for Ethylene Oxide Sterilization and Steam Sterilization in Healthcare Facilities,* AAMI ST 33 1996, for the specific process.

If on examination of the culture it is determined that no microorganisms have survived, the BI test is negative. If microorganisms have grown in the culture, the BI is considered positive and the performance of the sterilizer is considered suspect, as is the sterility of the load from which the BI was taken. Some types of BIs must be incubated and interpreted in a laboratory by conventional microbiological techniques. *Self-contained* BIs can be incubated and read within the CSD. It is important to place the biological indicator in the correct incubator or "block" to ensure it is incubated at the correct temperature. *Geobacillus stearothermophilus* requires a temperature of 132°F (55°C) to grow. *Bacillus atrophaeus* requires a temperature of 98.6°F (35°C) to grow.

After sterilization, self-contained BIs are crushed and nutrient broth covers the spore-impregnated disk. After completion of incubation (24 to 48 hours), if bacteria live through the sterilization process, the nutrient broth turns yellow as a result of a chemical byproduct that the bacteria produce. Final reading of the test is in 48 hours. Other types of self-contained BIs, which are called rapid readout BI tests, are based on the fluorimetric detection of a spore-bound enzyme. The growth media contain a nonfluorescent substrate, which is converted to a fluorescent substrate by reactions with the spore-bound enzyme. A machine the BI is put into detects the fluorescence. This type of BI provides test results after a short incubation time (1 hour for unwrapped rapid readout, 3 hours for wrapped). There are separate BIs for flash sterilizers (1-hour readout) and prevacuum sterilizers (3-hour readout). It is recommended that at least once a week one of the rapid readout BIs should be incubated for 48 hours and checked for any color change, or a regular self-containing BI could be used for the 48-hour test.

There are a variety of causes for positive BIs. Sterilizer malfunction may cause improper vacuum, temperature, sterilant concentration, or exposure time. Failure of the operator to properly load the sterilizer, set the correct parameters, or follow procedures can also cause positive BIs.

When a positive BI occurs, it is important to immediately determine whether the cause was sterilizer malfunction, operator error, a BI incubation problem, or if the BI was incubated at the wrong temperature. If the sterilizer has malfunctioned, it is necessary to recall and reprocess all unused items in loads run in that sterilizer since the last satisfactory BI test, to quarantine and repair the sterilizer, and to retest it until the BI results are acceptable before resuming routine use of that sterilizer. If items from those loads were used, there must be a process for notifying those who may be able to identify which patient the items were used for and can notify his or her physician. BIs and controls must be documented in a manner approved by your facility's infection control department.

A recall policy must be established in each health care facility, and must be followed. The facility's infection control staff should be notified of any positive BI results. They are an important part of the team that assesses the cause of a positive BI and assists in carrying out the steps of the policy. In the case of operator error, which can often be identified by examining the results of mechanical monitoring for the cycle in question, it may only be necessary to recall and reprocess the particular load in which the positive BI was found.

So-called *false positives* sometimes occur. The usual reason for a false positive is that the BI was contaminated during the process of removing it from the test pack and transferring it to the culture medium or during the incubation procedure. Because of the possibility of false positives, a positive BI culture may be further analyzed to determine what type of microorganism is present. If it is not *Geobacillus stearothermophilus* or *Bacillus atrophaeus* (depending on the BI being used), then the positive was false and due to accidental contamination.

The frequency with which sterilizer loads are monitored varies with the sterilization process used, the type of item being sterilized, and the policies of individual health care facilities. Every load containing implantable items should be monitored, regardless of the sterilization method used, because of the grave consequences of implanting a nonsterile item into a patient and because biological monitoring gives better assurance of sterility than do mechanical and chemical monitoring. Implanting a nonsterile device carries a greater risk than does the transient or temporary introduction of a nonsterile item into the body. During implantation of a device, the tissues immediately adjacent to the implant are often injured. Microorganisms that might have posed no threat to healthy tissue can rapidly multiply in injured tissue. Also, the implanted device itself can interfere with the body's ability to fight infection. Thus, there is more concern about the sterility of implantables.

Ethylene oxide sterilization is a more complex process than steam sterilization. Consequently, EtO-sterilized loads are, in general, monitored more often than steam-sterilized loads. Every EtO-sterilized load should be monitored. For steam-sterilization processing, the frequency of biological monitoring varies from every load to one load per week. At a minimum, steam sterilizers should be monitored weekly. Steam sterilizers that need frequent maintenance may need to be BI monitored daily or with each load. Whenever there is a new sterilizer installed, a sterilizer is relocated, or there are major repairs to a sterilizer, it is recommended that three consecutive BI tests be performed back to back in the empty sterilizer. All tests must be negative before the sterilizer is put into service. As explained earlier, if the sterilizer malfunctions, items must be recalled from all loads back to the last negative BI monitored load. Infection control staff should review and monitor all patients that had items from the bad sterilization load used on them, going back to the last negative BI monitored. This should be considered when deciding the frequency of running biologicals. Peracetic acid, ozone, and gas plasma should be monitored frequently because they are newer sterilization technologies. Each facility must evaluate the manufacturer's recommendations, consult with the facility's infection control department, and establish policies on the frequency of BI monitoring for each method of sterilization in the facility.

The time factor involved in microbiological culturing and analysis of biological indicators varies, depending on the system used. In some health care facilities, loads containing implantable items are quarantined (not released for distribution) until the results of biological testing are available. At some health care facilities, all sterilizer loads that are biologically monitored are quarantined pending the test results. While this may be the ideal procedure, quarantining all sterilizer loads is not possible at many facilities because of time constraints, the cost of maintaining extra inventory, and other factors. Consequently, sterilized items may be released to sterile storage or for distribution on the basis of mechanical and chemical monitoring results only. This is why lot control and traceability are so important. If a BI test is positive, it is essential that items from that load be retrieved as quickly as possible for reprocessing.

Lot Control and Traceability

Each package to be sterilized should be labeled with a lot control number designating the sterilizer used, the date of sterilization, and the cycle number. This is commonly done by placing a lot-control sticker stamped with this information on each package, preferably prior to sterilization (except with gas plasma, unless the sticker is made specifically for gas plasma use) to help prevent errors. In addition, detailed records kept for each sterilizer should identify the sterilizer operator for each load processed and document the load contents, the lot number, and the results of mechanical, biological, and chemical monitoring (see Figure 7.2). All this information is written on the record form or, where available, attached to the form (such as printouts and chemical monitors).

The purpose of labeling each package with a lot number and maintaining detailed sterilization records is to enable items processed in a particular load to be retrieved if their sterility becomes suspect. Often, results of biological testing are not available until after the items in a load have been stored or distributed. If the items from a suspect load can be easily traced, it is possible to retrieve or recall them quickly or to attempt to identify the patients for whom they have been used. Newer bar coding systems can help with this process.

Steam Sterilization

Saturated steam under pressure is the most economical and reliable method of sterilization. Steam sterilization is based on direct steam contact with all surfaces as well as with each thread, fiber, or particle of porous material subjected to the sterilization process.

Steam permeates and heats through the process of condensation. In the sterilization of soft goods or fabrics, the steam first contacts the outer layers of fabric. The coolness of the fabric causes a film of steam to condense, leaving a small amount of water in the fabric. Heat is then absorbed into the fabric until it reaches the temperature of the surrounding steam. The steam passes through each layer, condensing and heating until the entire mass of fabric has been heated. This same process of condensing and heating applies to devices undergoing surface sterilization only, such as instruments, metalware, and glassware. Steam cannot permeate these devices, so the coolness of the metal or glass condenses the steam until the surfaces are heated to the temperature of the steam.

Steam Sterilization Cycle Parameters

The essential parameters (conditions) of steam sterilization are time, temperature, and the presence of saturated steam. The steam throughout the load must be hot enough to destroy all microorganisms in the time allotted for sterilization. In an open container, water will boil at 212°F at sea level and even lower temperatures at higher elevations. To increase the amount of thermal energy contained in the steam, the temperature of the steam must be increased. The temperature of the steam is increased by increasing the pressure in the closed chamber. Saturated steam is the condition in which all water present in the sterilizer chamber is in the vapor phase rather than the liquid phase. The reason that saturated steam must be used for steam sterilization is to ensure that the steam will quickly release its heat and change into water on contact with a cool object, resulting in the heating and condensation process described above. The condensation process releases the thermal energy contained in the steam and transfers that thermal energy to the item being sterilized. The steam entering the sterilizer must contain 2 to 3 percent liquid water; excessive liquid water will lead to wet loads and the need for longer drying times. Steam with less than 2 percent water can be superheated, causing a sterilization failure due to lack of heat transfer to the load contents. The sterilizer chamber must not contain any air, because air pockets prevent the steam from contacting all items in the load. Therefore, steam sterilizers are designed to eliminate air from the chamber at the beginning of the cycle. Sterilizers must be properly loaded to ensure free circulation of steam to all surfaces of items being sterilized, to avoid liquid buildup, and to avoid air entrapment. (This is explained later in the chapter.)

Items Sterilized by Saturated Steam Under Pressure

Steam sterilization is used for almost all metal items, most rubber goods, surgical trays, fabric packs, glassware, and some hard plastic items. Steam sterilization is also used for solutions. These items can all withstand the high temperature, pressure, and moisture associated with steam sterilization. Steam sterilization is more easily controlled, less expensive, and generally presents fewer safety hazards to personnel than other sterilization methods. Therefore, steam sterilization should be used preferentially for any item that will withstand the process.

Types of Steam Sterilization Cycles

A variety of steam sterilizer cycles are used in health care facilities. Each type has advantages and limitations. Any exposure times given in this chapter for steam sterilization are for normal situations. As explained in Chapter Five, there are some instrument sets for which manufacturers are recommending extended exposure times in certain sterilizer types.

GRAVITY-DISPLACEMENT CYCLES In a gravity-displacement cycle, steam enters at the top of the chamber and displaces the air within the chamber. (Air is heavier than steam and therefore sinks below the steam.) As the pressure in the chamber and packages increases, the steam pushes the air out the drain at the bottom front of the chamber. The pressure continues to rise until the steam at the chamber drain reaches a preset temperature. This is measured by a temperature-sensitive device in the drain line.

To speed up chamber heating, the jacket, an envelope around the chamber, has been filled with steam at the same pressure and temperature as the chamber is set to attain. The steam in the jacket heats the walls of the chamber, which helps to maintain a constant chamber temperature throughout the cycle and prevents condensation from forming on chamber walls. The jacket is filled with steam when the sterilizer is turned on, and stays there until the sterilizer is turned off. Therefore, when each sterilization cycle is started, the chamber walls are already heated. Caution must be taken to avoid getting burned by touching the chamber walls. A typical cycle would proceed as follows:

- *Phase 1 (Come-Up)* A valve opens and saturated steam is admitted into the chamber from a port in the top rear portion of the chamber. The steam pushes the air out the drain as it fills the chamber. The pressure and temperature inside the chamber and packages rise until the preset temperature, as measured by the temperature-sensitive device in the drain line, is reached; the drain valve then closes and the timer starts.
- *Phase 2 (Exposure)* The sterilizer maintains the temperature by periodically removing cooled steam in the form of condensate through the drain and replacing it with fresh steam at the top. This process continues until the sterilization time is completed.
- *Phase 3 (Come-Down)* When the timer reaches the end of the sterilization cycle time, the steam valve is shut off, the drain opens, and the steam is exhausted from the chamber.
- *Phase 4 (Drying)* When atmospheric pressure is reached within the chamber, the drying time begins. The chamber remains hot due to the steam contained within the jacket surrounding the chamber, and its dry heat slowly drives excess moisture out of the packs and dries them. After this drying phase, which helps prevent wet packs, a buzzer or other signal indicates that the cycle has been completed.

In a gravity-displacement cycle, air is gradually displaced by the incoming steam simply by gravity, without the aid of a pump. The relative difficulty of air removal also means that dense items may require extended drying times in a gravity-displacement cycle. The usual cycle parameters for gravity displacement cycles for wrapped devices are 23 to 30 minutes' exposure time, 250°F temperature, and 15 to 17 psig pressure.

STERILIZING LIQUIDS Only gravity-displacement liquid cycles may be used to sterilize *liquid loads.* Liquids should never be sterilized with other items, but rather in a dedicated load. Containers run in each liquid load should be the same size. The sterilization of liquids requires exhaust and cooling cycle parameters that differ from those of a conventional gravity-displacement cycle. Steam does not penetrate the liquid, but instead is used to heat the liquid to 250°F (121°C). Several minutes are required for the liquid to attain this temperature, which must then be maintained for an additional time to achieve sterilization. (The volume of liquid in each container dictates the total steam exposure time; for example, 75 to 250 ml, 20 minutes; 500 to 1,000 ml, 30 minutes; 1,500 to 2,000 ml, 40 minutes.) Because the sterilization temperature is above the boiling point of water at atmospheric pressure, the chamber pressure must be released slowly to allow the liquid to cool to below 200°F (93°C) before the sterilizer door is opened. If this is not done, the solution containers will explode when the door is opened, possibly causing serious injury to the sterilizer operator or others in the vicinity. It is also very important that the containers (Pyrex) and caps used for this process be *specifically designed* for sterilization of liquids and that they be used properly. A typical cycle for a liquid load is as follows:

- *Phase 1 (Come-Up)* Steam is admitted into the chamber, pushing air out as it fills the chamber. The pressure and temperature inside the chamber rise until the preset temperature is reached. The timer then starts.
- *Phase 2 (Exposure)* The sterilizer maintains the temperature until the exposure time is completed.
- *Phase 3 (Come-Down)* Steam is cut off and the drain opened slightly, allowing the steam to escape very slowly. Also, the jacket pressure is released slowly so that the temperature drops gradually. This process can take 30 or more minutes. When the steam is all out and the chamber temperature has fallen to below 200°F, the door can be opened. Special care in moving the hot bottles and liquids must be taken at this point, because some of the bottles may boil over or even explode. After cooling, flasks with nondisposable caps should be "burped" (listen for the "water hammer" click) by tapping on the cap. The purpose of this procedure is to check for proper seal. Disposable caps will appear concave if properly sealed.

Sterilization of liquids must be evaluated to determine the feasibility in the facility. Commercially prepared sterile solutions are readily available. A cost analysis for in-facility and commercially prepared sterile solutions should be conducted to determine the most cost-effective method. Another consideration that must be taken into account is personnel safety.

PREVACUUM CYCLES In prevacuum cycles, a vacuum system pulls most of the air from both the sterilizer chamber and the load contents out through the drain in the bottom front floor of the sterilizer. As in gravity-displacement cycles, a jacket surrounding the chamber is filled with steam at the same pressure and temperature as the chamber is set to attain, so that a uniform chamber temperature can be maintained. A typical sequence of events in a prevacuum cycle is as follows:

- *Phase 1 (Come-Up/First Prevacuum)* The vacuum system pumps approximately 90 percent of the air out of the chamber.
- *Phase 2 (Come-Up/Conditioning)* Steam is admitted into the chamber for several seconds, thereby beginning to heat the contents of the load and to help drive air out of hard-to-reach areas.

- *Phase 3 (Come-Up/Second Prevacuum)* The vacuum system comes back on and removes about 90 percent of the remaining air. Together, the two vacuum phases remove almost 99 percent of the original air.
- *Phase 4 (Exposure)* A valve opens and saturated steam flows into the chamber. The preset temperature setting is reached and held fairly constant for the exposure time. The temperature is held steady by automatic evacuation of cooler steam and condensate at the bottom of the chamber and replacement with fresh steam at the top.
- *Phase 5 (Come-Down)* After the sterilization period, the drain opens and the chamber empties of steam.
- *Phase 6 (Drying)* After most of the steam pressure is out of the chamber, the vacuum system comes on and again draws a 90 percent vacuum. Then, with the vacuum system still running, a timer starts timing a drying period. This hold time allows excess moisture to be removed from the packs by means of the dry heat in the chamber due to steam contained within the jacket. When the drying phase is over, the vacuum is released by allowing filtered air into the chamber and the cycle is complete.

The vacuum system of a prevacuum steam cycle provides very efficient air removal. Therefore, overall cycle time is shorter than for gravity-displacement cycles.

Another version of the prevacuum cycle is the prevacuum pulsing cycle. The main difference is that instead of the two prevacuums discussed above, up to five partial vacuums are drawn, with only the final one a 90 percent vacuum. Between each vacuum, steam is allowed into the chamber, just as in Phase 2 above. This process serves to efficiently drive out any entrapped air and to thoroughly precondition the load. In all other respects, the two types of prevacuum cycles are the same. The usual cycle parameters for prevacuum cycles for wrapped devices are 4 minutes' exposure, 272°F temperature, and 28 to 30 psig pressure.

Because achieving the proper vacuum is so critical to the use of the shorter prevacuum cycle times, the performance of the vacuum system is routinely evaluated by using a Bowie-Dick test. This test (named after the scientists who developed it) is performed daily, usually before sterilization loads are run. If the sterilizer is used continuously, the test can be performed any time, but at the same time each day. After major repairs, any interruption in the steam supply, new sterilizer installation, or relocation of the sterilizer, three consecutive Bowie-Dick tests should be performed with uniform color change before the sterilizer is put back into operation. The three BIs that must be done in these instances are done in separate cycles from the Bowie-Dick tests because there are different cycle parameters for each one.

Commercially prepared air-removal tests are available from several manufacturers. Department-produced packs used for this test consist of folded absorbent towels with a Bowie-Dick test sheet in the center of the pack. The test sheet may consist of several strips of heat-sensitive autoclave tape applied in a criss-cross pattern to an otherwise plain sheet of paper, or it may be one of several commercially available test sheets with heat-sensitive ink imprinted in a pattern. The test pack is made by folding laundered huck towels (a coarse absorbent cotton or linen fabric) to dimensions of about 9 by 11 inches. These towels are placed one on top of each other, alternating the folded edges, to form a stack approximately 10 to 11 inches high. The total number of towels needed may vary from test to test, depending on towel thickness and wear (24 to 30 towels). The test sheet is placed between the towels in the center of the pack. No other items are to be placed in the pack. The stack of towels is then wrapped loosely with only one wrapper (see Figure 7.3).

The size and density of the pack affect the results of the test, so it is important that CSD technicians follow these instructions carefully in preparing the test pack. Also, some manufacturers of prevacuum sterilizers make available special test devices that can be used to measure the efficiency of the vacuum system.

To test the sterilizer, the Bowie-Dick test pack is placed horizontally on the bottom of the sterilizer rack, near the door and over the drain, in an otherwise empty chamber. A special prevacuum cycle is run, with the following parameters:

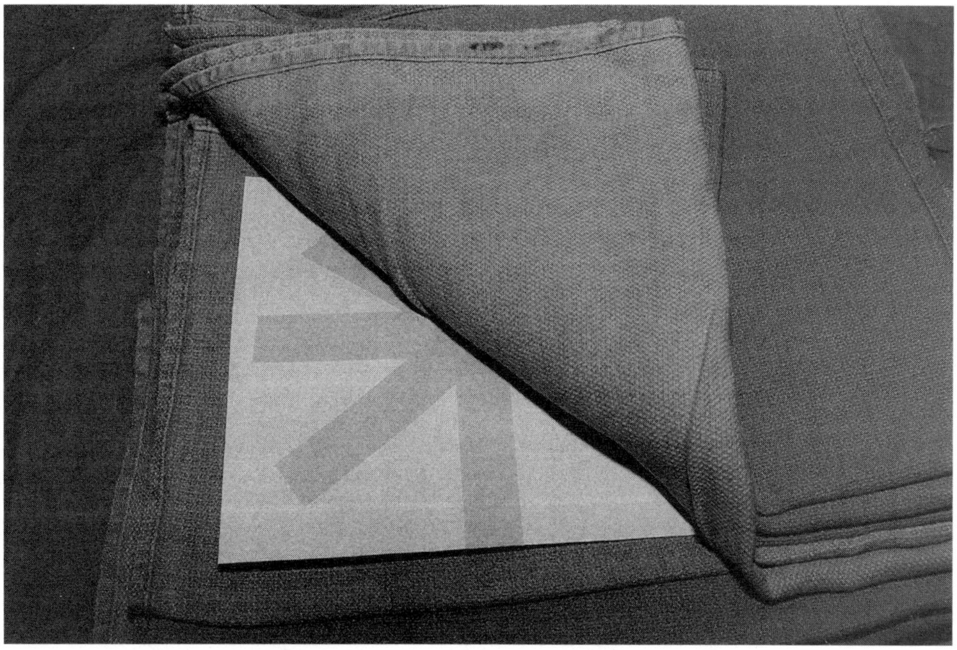

Figure 7.3. The Bowie-Dick Test Pack.

an exposure time of at least 3 minutes but no longer than 3.5 minutes, a temperature setting of no more than 273°F (134°C), and no drying time. Check the parameters recommended by the sterilizer and test pack manufacturer.

Immediately after the cycle has been completed, the test sheet must be examined. Sterilizer vacuum performance is acceptable if the test sheet shows a uniform color change. Entrapped air will cause a spot to appear on the test sheet, due to the inability of the steam to reach the chemical indicator. The time and temperature are critical to allow the chemical to change properly where steam contacts it and to prevent any entrapped air from getting hot enough to change the indicator even though steam is not present.

It must be remembered that the Bowie-Dick test is not a sterilization test, but rather a test of the effectiveness of the vacuum system of the sterilizer. It is never performed on gravity-displacement sterilizers (because these sterilizers do not have a vacuum system), and it is not a substitute for biological monitoring or for routine chemical monitoring of packaged items.

STEAM-FLUSH PRESSURE CYCLES In the steam-flush pressure cycle, there is a repeated sequence consisting of a steam flush and a pressure pulse that rapidly removes air from the sterilizer chamber and materials using steam at above atmospheric pressure. A vacuum is not required for this cycle. Advantages of this type of sterilizer include that conditioning is at pressures above atmospheric pressure, air cannot be drawn back into the chamber during the conditioning phase, and a Bowie-Dick test is not required. Cycle phases and parameters are based on the materials being processed.

ABBREVIATED STEAM-STERILIZATION CYCLES Flash sterilization is a sterilization method used for sterilization of medical devices needed in the event of an emergency. The devices are not wrapped or are put into special flash containers before being sterilized. Because of the difficulty of transferring unwrapped items to the sterile field after sterilization without contaminating them, this process is only to be used when wrapping devices and using other sterilization methods are not possible, such as when a one-of-a-kind instrument is dropped during surgery. Flash sterilization is not recommended for implants. Devices that have been contaminated with prions cannot be flash sterilized because the exposure time, and in some cases temperature, is not adequate to kill the prions. There are specific BIs designed to monitor flash cycles.

Items to be flash sterilized must be disassembled and *thoroughly* cleaned with detergent and water to remove any soil, blood, body fats, etc. After proper cleaning, items with lumens must be flushed with distilled water. During the sterilization process this water will become steam and will displace the air in the lumen. The composition of the item to be flash sterilized, not the size or shape, is what determines the exposure time used (unless otherwise indicated by the manufacturer).

Medical devices composed of all metal or glass, nonporous, and with no lumens that are placed in an unwrapped perforated tray are to be sterilized in a high-speed gravity-displacement or prevacuum flash sterilizer at 270°F (132°C) for an exposure time of 3 minutes with no dry time. Items with lumens, porous items, or towels placed in perforated trays with medical devices require 10 minutes of exposure at 270°F (132°C) in a gravity-displacement flash sterilizer for 4 minutes at 270°F (132°C) in a prevacuum flash sterilizer. The cleaned medical device to be flash sterilized is placed in a flash pan with an appropriate chemical sterilization indicator so that the portion of the indicator to be read is visible. Flash sterilization can be performed in either a gravity-displacement or prevacuum cycle.

Recently, containers have been manufactured for use in flash sterilizers. These containers make it possible to transfer the instruments from the flash sterilizer to the sterile fields without contaminating the items. Follow the manufacturer's directions carefully for the type of sterilizer (gravity displacement or prevacuum) that can be used and the required exposure time.

Loading Steam Sterilizers

Gravity-displacement and prevacuum cycles are loaded in the same manner. No items should touch the chamber walls. Linen packs should be placed on their sides on the carrier cart or sterilizer rack, leaving space for air and steam circulation (at least enough space so that a flat hand can be inserted between items). To permit air and steam circulation and to allow moisture to drain out freely, basins and solid-bottom trays are placed in such a position that if they contained a liquid, it would pour out (Figure 7.4). The total number of basin sets per load should be evaluated to ensure dry sets. Instrument container systems and perforated or mesh-bottom surgical trays are placed flat on the carrier shelf or sterilizer rack (Figure 7.5). Instrument trays must not be stacked. Container systems can be stacked only if this is documented by the manufacturer. Individual instrument packages should not be stacked.

Pouches should be placed loosely on edge with paper side to plastic side in a perforated or mesh bottom surgical tray or held in place by a peel pouch rack. If the load is a mixture of fabrics and metal items, the metal items should be placed below the fabrics, so that condensation from the metal will not wet other items in the load. The sterilizer must not be overloaded. There must be room for the sterilant to circulate between, above and below, and into all packages. If the load is to be biologically monitored, the test pack is placed in the lower portion of the chamber, over the drain, in an otherwise routinely loaded sterilizer (see Figure 7.6).

Operating Steam Sterilizers

Sterilizer models vary considerably in their performance characteristics and safety features. Therefore, any steam sterilizer should be operated strictly in accordance with the manufacturer's instructions and the CSD procedure manual instructions.

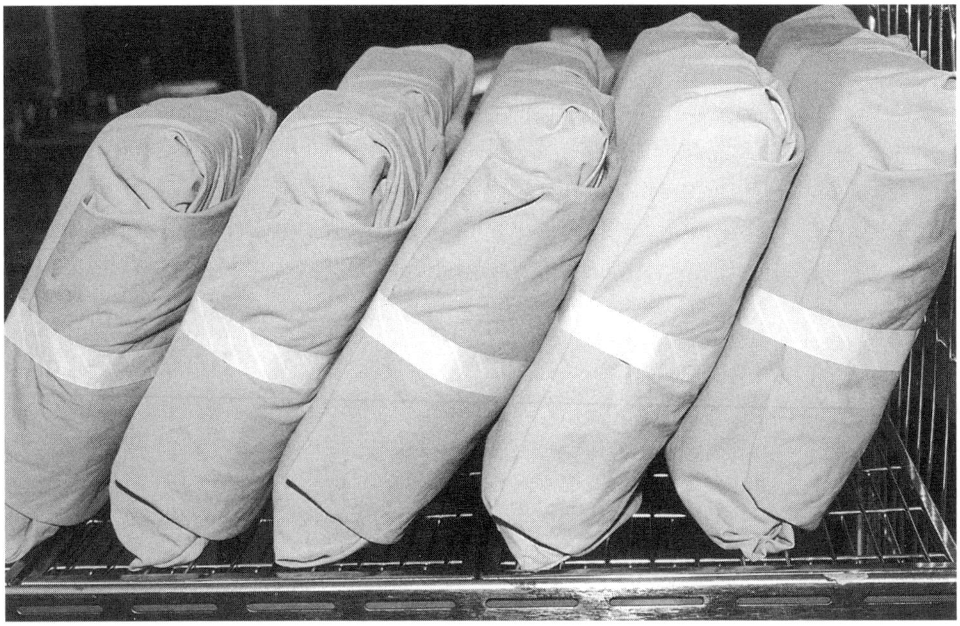

Figure 7.4. A Sterilizer Cart Correctly Loaded with Basin Sets.

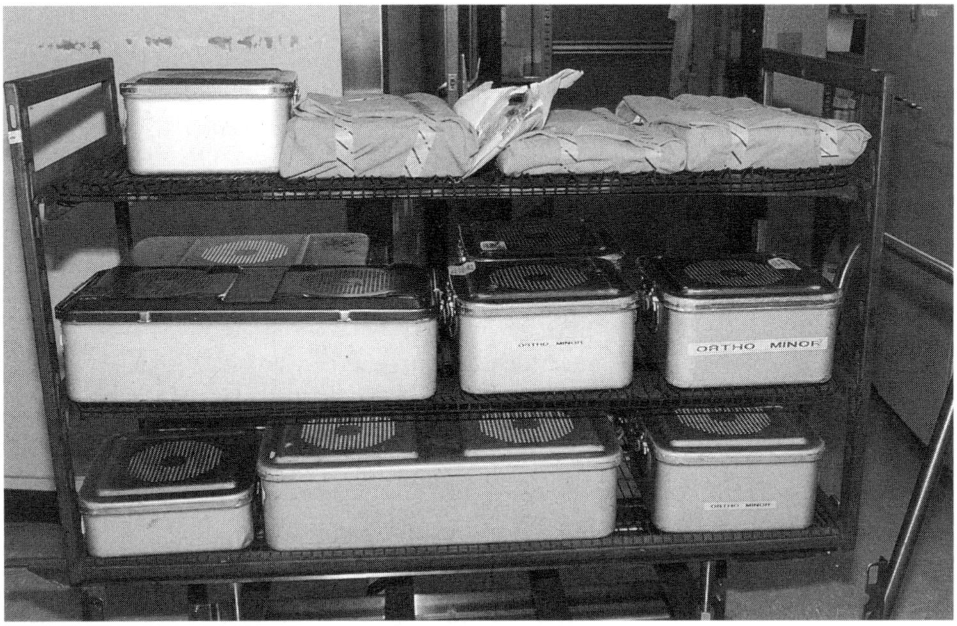

Figure 7.5. A Load of Instrument Trays with Mesh or Perforated Bottoms.

At the beginning of a cycle, the pen or printer must be checked to see if it is functioning properly. At the end of each cycle, the printout or graph must be examined to verify that the cycle parameters (temperature, time, pressure) were met for sterilization. This check step must be documented on the printout or graph by the person checking it.

Unloading Steam Sterilizers and Inspecting Sterile Supplies

The sterilizer cart or container is removed from the sterilizer and placed in a sterile holding area or other low-traffic area, where it should remain until the load is cool. This can take 30 minutes or more, depending on the type of devices and metal mass in the load. The cart should not be placed near air vents or fans, because air currents may cause condensate to form by cooling the packages too fast. Sterile items should not be touched while cooling. Hot packages will quickly absorb moisture and, as a

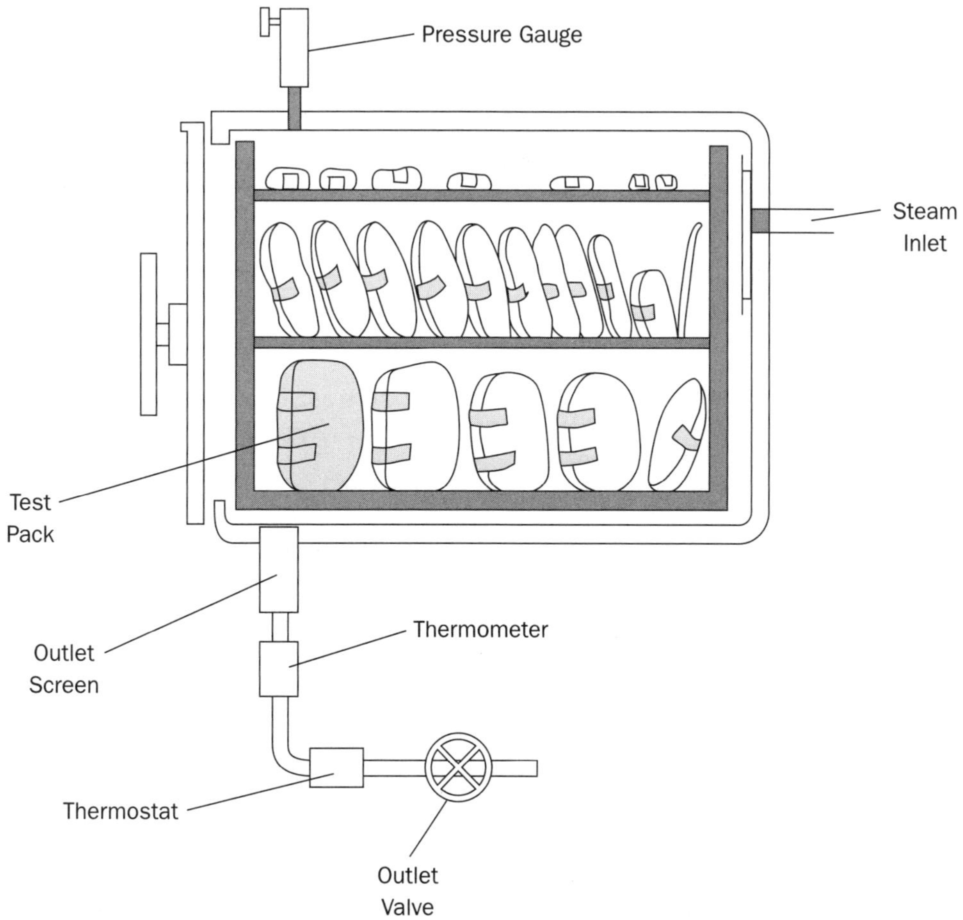

Figure 7.6. Placement of the Biological Indicator Test Pack in a Load to Be Steam-Sterilized.

Copyright © 1980 by the Association for the Advancement of Medical Instrumentation.

result, bacteria from the hands will be wicked into the package, contaminating the contents. Freshly sterilized items should never be placed on metal or cold surfaces before they have cooled completely. When hot and cold surfaces are brought together, moisture will condense both from within the package and from out of the air. Consequently, the package will become damp, and its contents will be contaminated.

As the cooled items are removed from the sterilizer cart, they must be visually inspected. Check the chemical indicator tape on each package for color change, which verifies the item has been exposed to sterilizing parameters. When color change has not happened on the chemical indicator tape, the load should not be used. The cause of an inadequate color change must be investigated (for example, is it a tape manufacture problem or were the sterilizer cycle parameters not met?). Any items with torn or stained packaging or with packaging that appears to be wet should not be used. These items should be returned to the assembly/preparation area for inspection and repackaging. Linen packs should be disassembled and relaundered. All linen items must be laundered between sterilizations in order to rehydrate them. If they are too dry, porous items such as linens will absorb large amounts of moisture from the steam during the sterilization cycle, which may interfere with sterilization. It must be remembered that steam sterilization requires contact with both heat and moisture.

Sterilized items must be cooled before being placed inside a plastic dust cover (sterility maintenance cover) or other protective barrier. Any moisture remaining in a package covered in plastic cannot evaporate and will condense on the inside of the dust cover, which is not sterile. This moisture, now unsterile, will wick into the packaging of the sterile item. Sterility maintenance covers must be labeled such that no one mistakes one as a sterile cover. These covers should be placed on the items right after they are cooled and kept on until the item is used. Not all items are dust covered, and individual facility policies should be followed.

Wet Packs

If packs are wet at completion of the steam sterilizer cycle, the cause must be identified and corrective actions initiated. Some of the causes for wet areas on the outside of the packages are condensate dripping from carriage shelves, condensate collected in and blowing through steam lines, and metal items on an upper shelf dripping condensate onto items below. If the inside of packs are wet, some causes are overloading of the sterilizer, items improperly placed on the load, too many instruments in the set (more condensate produced than can be revaporized), and fabrics wrapped too tight. Mechanical problems that can be the cause of wet packs include an obstructed chamber drain (screen should be cleaned daily), improper drying time, and improper steam pressure from steam generator to sterilizer. Any package that is wet when touched should be considered contaminated (moisture acts as a vehicle to carry microorganisms inside the pack).

Care and Maintenance of Steam Sterilizers

Steam sterilizers must be cleaned and maintained in accordance with the manufacturer's instructions. Failure to do so can result in processing problems. For example, if a sterilizer chamber is not properly cleaned, mineral deposits condensing from the steam will accumulate on the walls and may stain items in the load, especially surgical instruments. If the chamber drain is not cleaned, it will eventually interfere with air and steam evacuation, and may result in wet packs.

EtO Sterilization

Ethylene oxide (EtO) is a colorless gas that has an odor similar to ether in concentrations (greater than 700 ppm), but that is odorless at lower concentrations. This chemical has properties that make it an ideal sterilant for heat-sensitive medical devices. EtO gas will kill all known microorganisms by means of a process called alkylation, a chemical reaction that interferes with the metabolism of all types of microbial life, including bacterial spores. EtO is noncorrosive and nondamaging to plastics and rubber and is an effective sterilant at temperatures and pressures that are tolerated by these heat-sensitive items. The gas readily penetrates commonly used packaging materials and diffuses rapidly to contact all surfaces of items.

EtO sterilization does have some disadvantages. First, the process takes many hours due to the need for lengthy exposure and aeration periods. Second, it is more expensive than steam sterilization. This is due to the cost of purchasing and maintaining the equipment, the cost of ventilation systems and other monitoring devices for safety, and the cost of the gas. Third, EtO in its pure form is extremely flammable. To minimize fire and explosion hazards, special precautions must be taken in its storage and use. For this reason, 100 percent EtO is available to health care facilities only in small cartridges. Fourth, due to the toxicity of EtO, sterile items must be aerated for a specified time to allow the residues to escape. (EtO is absorbed into all medical devices except those made of glass or metal.) If EtO-sterilized items are not properly aerated, patients and staff can be exposed to toxic levels of the gas and suffer both short-term effects (such as chemical burns) and long-term effects (such as those listed in the next paragraph).

There are serious health hazards associated with inhaling EtO gas. OSHA has designated EtO as a known carcinogen (it may cause cancer), and there is concern that it may cause birth defects as well. In addition, acute overexposure to concentrations above 500 ppm may cause dizziness, respiratory distress, nausea, vomiting, and headache. EtO is a poisonous gas; it otherwise would not be useful as a sterilant. Rigorous ventilation and other engineering controls to remove the gas from the air must be maintained, and many safety precautions must be scrupulously observed to prevent excessive exposure of the health care worker to the gas.

Because of the toxicity and health hazards, EtO sterilization should only be used to process devices that will not withstand steam sterilization or when the device manufacturer specifies EtO sterilant. OSHA's current permissable exposure limit (PEL) for EtO is 1 ppm TWA (time-weighted average) (exposure in an 8-hour period). In addition, less health screening and monitoring is required if the level can be maintained at or below 0.5 ppm TWA (called the ation level). OSHA has also set a limit beyond which a person should not be exposed over a short time period. This level is called the excursion limit (EL), and it is set at 5 ppm in a 15-minute period. For further information, consult *Ethylene Oxide Use in Hospitals: A Manual for Health Care Personnel* (third edition), or the OSHA standard limiting occupational exposure to EtO. The OSHA document is required by law to be available for employee review in all CSDs where EtO is used as a sterilant.

Unless special equipment is attached, the gas from the sterilizer chamber and aerator is exhausted outside the facility where it rapidly disperses. Many states now regulate the amount of EtO that can be released into the environment outside the facility. To comply with these regulations, equipment (an abator) is attached to the EtO sterilizer and aerator to convert the EtO exhausted from the chamber to nontoxic chemicals.

Parameters of EtO Sterilization

The parameters (conditions) essential for EtO sterilization are EtO gas concentration, moisture (in the form of humidity), temperature, and time. A change in any of these parameters requires that the others be changed accordingly. For example, if the temperature is lowered, the exposure time must be lengthened.

The concentration of EtO in the sterilizing chamber is measured in terms of milligrams per liter (mg/l) of chamber space. A concentration of 450 mg/l of chamber space is usually recommended. Doubling this concentration will reduce the necessary exposure time by almost one half, because the lethal activity of EtO increases with concentration. However, there are limits on how much the chamber concentration can be increased without creating an explosion hazard. The specified concentration must be maintained throughout the exposure phase of the cycle. Therefore, most EtO sterilizers are equipped to automatically add more gas to compensate for absorption of EtO by the materials in the load.

Moisture is essential to the sterilizing process. Ethylene oxide cannot penetrate the cell walls of bacteria without sufficient moisture; water acts as a catalyst for the EtO reaction with cell components. Therefore, excessively dry items will be more difficult to sterilize than properly preconditioned items. However, too much moisture, in the form of water droplets, is also a problem. Free water will combine with EtO to form ethylene glycol, a byproduct that may be toxic and cannot be eliminated by normal aeration. In most EtO sterilizers, water vapor is injected into the chamber to obtain a relative humidity of 50 to 75 percent in the chamber. (The amount of water vapor necessary for this purpose is not sufficient to cause water droplets and thus cause ethylene glycol to form.)

The temperature of the cycle affects the sterilizing efficiency and penetration of the EtO gas. Temperatures of 130°F (54°C) to 140°F (60°C) are typically recommended for large-chamber sterilizers. Sterilizers using 100 percent EtO usually have a "warm cycle," which runs at 145°F (63°C), and a "cold cycle," which runs at 85°F (29°C) to 100°F (38°C). Its ability to sterilize at these relatively low temperatures (compared with steam sterilization) makes EtO suitable for processing heat-sensitive items that could be damaged at higher temperatures.

The exposure time must be long enough to allow thorough gas penetration of all items in the load. This time varies with the gas concentrations and temperatures used and with the type of product being processed. Because of variations in density, thickness, configuration, and permeability of materials, standard sterilizing cycles for hospital EtO processing have been established to accommodate the most difficult processing requirements. For a given sterilizer, the manufacturer's instruction manual should be consulted to determine the appropriate exposure time.

Items Sterilized by EtO

EtO sterilization is used for items that are sensitive to heat or moisture and thus will not withstand steam sterilization. Items commonly sterilized by EtO include delicate microsurgery instruments, electrical equipment, anesthesia and respiratory therapy supplies, cardiac catheters, and the endoscopes and other lensed equipment introduced into the body for diagnostic purposes.

EtO Sterilizers and Gas Sources

Two types of EtO sterilizers are most commonly used in U.S. health care facilities: devices that typically use "single-dose" cartridges of 100 percent EtO, and units that typically use tanks or cylinders of EtO diluted with a carrier gas, which reduces the flammability and eliminates the potential for explosion.

Ideally, EtO sterilizers should be located in a separate room with minimum traffic. It should be designed to be as far away from the flow of traffic and work centers as is practical. The purpose of isolating the sterilizers in this way is to minimize personnel exposure to the gas. Due to space or funding limitations, it may not always be possible to put EtO sterilization equipment in a separate room. A well-designed ventilation system can minimize EtO exposure and thus reduce the hazard. CSD technicians should adhere strictly to established procedures for loading and unloading sterilizers and aerators, traffic control, and authorized entry to the area housing EtO sterilizers.

The EtO or EtO mixture is supplied by the manufacturer in liquid form. The pressurized liquid vaporizes when it reaches room temperature. The pressure within the container injects the mixture into the sterilizer chamber, where adequate temperature is required to maintain a satisfactory vaporized state at the chamber pressure. Ethylene oxide gas will diffuse at atmospheric pressure, but most EtO sterilizers are designed to operate at a higher or lower pressure. Some EtO sterilizers have vacuum systems, and some operate at higher than atmospheric pressure.

There are a number of manufacturers of EtO sterilizers, and each manufacturer offers several individual models. The specific cycle characteristics of the sterilizer designs vary, but many EtO sterilization cycles consist of the following phases:

- *Phase 1 (Vacuum)* A partial vacuum is drawn for a brief period to remove most of the residual air from the chamber and from the packaged items in the load. When the vacuum has been attained, steam is injected into the chamber and diffuses throughout the load, beginning a 20- to 30-minute conditioning period during which the contents of the load reach a relative humidity of 50 to 75 percent and the desired temperature (for example, 130°F).
- *Phase 2 (Charge)* The EtO gas or gas mixture is admitted, and as the sterilant is injected, the chamber pressure rises to the proper pressure.
- *Phase 3 (Exposure)* The sterilizer remains in the exposure phase for the predetermined time. During this time, the chamber load is maintained at the correct pressure, humidity, and temperature. After the exposure phase is completed, a final vacuum (called the *purge cycle*) is drawn, removing the gas or gas mixture from the chamber and exhausting it to the outside atmosphere or to a device that converts the EtO to non-toxic chemicals.
- *Phase 4 (Air)* After the chamber exhaust and evacuation, some sterilizers draw fresh air into the chamber through a bacteria-retentive filter and then reevacuate the chamber, removing most of the EtO. Filtered air is again admitted, and this air wash continues for a period of 10 to 30 minutes. It is at this point that some machines begin aeration in the chamber. These machines allow for aeration to be accomplished without movement to a separate aeration chamber.
- *Phase 5 (Off)* At the end of the air-wash or in-chamber aeration period, the machine returns to atmospheric pressure. An audible or visible indicator signals that the cycle is completed. Some sterilizers continue the filtered air purge until the door is opened.

For each EtO sterilizer used in the CSD, the manufacturer's specific operating instructions must be followed carefully to ensure both effective sterilization and personnel safety.

Care and Maintenance of EtO Sterilizers and Aerators

Sterilizers and aerators should be cleaned and maintained in accordance with the manufacturer's instructions. It is recommended that the interior walls be wiped with a damp cloth after each use.

Loading EtO Sterilizers

The packaged items to be sterilized should be placed on metal sterilizer carts or in wire baskets. The use of metal carts or baskets minimizes handling of sterile items and, because metal does not absorb EtO, allows safe transfer of the items from the sterilizer to the aerator. In facilities with in-chamber aeration capabilities, there may be occasions where a load may have to be transferred to an aerator to make room for the volume of items needing to be sterilized in a day.

When the cart or basket is loaded, the items to be sterilized should be arranged loosely to ensure that the sterilant will circulate freely and reach all surfaces. The items must be arranged so that they will not touch the sterilizer chamber walls during the sterilization cycle or the operator's hands when the cart or basket is being removed from the sterilizer for transfer to the aerator. Heavy packages should not be stacked. Pouches should be on edge.

Instrument pans with perforated or mesh bottoms should be used to hold delicately constructed devices such as flexible fiberoptics.

The biological test pack should be placed in the approximate center of the load, because this is the area in EtO sterilizers where it is most difficult to achieve sterilization.

At the beginning of a cycle, the printer must be checked to see if it is functioning properly.

Unloading EtO Sterilizers

At the end of each cycle, the printout must be examined to verify that the cycle parameters (time, temperature, humidity) were met for sterilization. This check step must be documented on the printout by the person checking it.

Many of the newer EtO sterilizers have the capability of in-chamber aeration, which starts right after the completion of the sterilization cycle. When aeration of EtO-sterilized items must take place in a separate aerator, procedure steps must be carefully followed to avoid employee exposure to EtO.

If the sterilizer has a purge cycle, the sterilized items should be *immediately* removed from the sterilizer and transferred to an aerator when the cycle is completed; otherwise, EtO levels will build up in the chamber because of desorption (gas being released) from the load. If the sterilizer does not have a purge cycle, common practice is for the operator to crack the sterilizer door 2 to 8 inches and leave the area for a specified time (usually 15 minutes). This allows the dedicated exhaust and room ventilation systems to remove from the air most of the EtO being released from the sterilizer chamber. If an exhaust hood is used over the door, it is important not to open the door too far or the escaping gas will not be captured by the hood.

Sterilizer carts should be pulled, not pushed, to the aerator, so that the CSD technician can avoid inhaling EtO being released from the sterilized items. Gloves need not be worn, because the technician touches only the metal carts or metal baskets. If any of the packages have to be touched or handled in any way, neoprene gloves should be worn to avoid possible reaction from EtO residuals. If it is necessary to remove the biological test pack from the load and retrieve the BI prior to aeration, extra care must be taken. Neoprene gloves are to be worn to help prevent contact with EtO. The packaging material should also be aerated when the CSD technician is finished retrieving the BI. Opinion differs as to whether the BI should be retrieved before or after the test pack is aerated; different procedures are used in different health care facilities. If the BI is aerated, the culture results are not known as soon as they would be if the indicator were not aerated. This may be an important factor in scheduling the use of implantable items. The CSD technician should thoroughly wash his or her hands to remove any possible gas residue. For sterilizers that use 100 percent EtO gas cartridges, the used gas cartridge from each cycle must be removed from the sterilizer and aerated prior to disposal or left in the sterilizer if the load is being aerated in the chamber.

Aerating EtO-Sterilized Items

Most materials commonly sterilized by EtO will absorb varying amounts of the gas (except metal and glass), and it is essential that this residual gas be allowed to dissipate before the sterilized items are handled and used. *All packaged EtO-sterilized items must be aerated;* even if the item itself does not absorb EtO, the packaging will retain residuals. If the load must be resterilized due to failure of the process, the load must be aerated before repackaging and sterilization. This will prevent employee exposure to residual EtO.

Medical device manufacturers sometimes aerate sterilized products by ambient or room aeration; that is, the sterile items are placed in an isolated, well-ventilated area at room temperature, and the gas is allowed to dissipate slowly over a period usually of several days. Residual testing is performed to validate removal of EtO to safe levels. In health care facilities, mechanical aerators are used. These aerators provide controlled air flow and air exchanges at elevated temperature, which speeds up the dissipation of the gas from the sterilized items. Room aeration is not an acceptable practice in health care facilities because of the possible exposure of workers to unacceptable levels of EtO.

Some materials absorb and retain more EtO than others. Generally, aeration times are set for a given temperature, based on the most-difficult-to-aerate product and packaging materials. The higher the temperature, the faster the EtO gas will desorb from the product and the shorter the time needed for aeration. Typical aeration times and temperatures are 12 hours at 122°F (50°C), 10 hours at 130°F (55°C), and 8 hours at 140°F (60°C). The device and sterilizer/aerator manufacturer's instructions for aeration should always be consulted. The aeration time and temperature should be recorded on a printout or graph. This must be checked for adequate aeration time at temperature and documented by the person checking it.

It is important not to overload the aerator cabinet, because air must circulate freely. One inch of space should be left between items and between items and cabinet walls. To begin the aeration cycle, the power is turned on and the timer is set for the appropriate duration. The cycle will then proceed automatically, and the completion of the cycle will be signaled by a visible or audible indicator. The date and time of completion of the aeration cycle should be recorded by the operator. When the cycle is completed, the sterilizer cart or wire basket should be removed from the aerator and the sterile items allowed to cool.

As the cooled items are removed from the cart or wire basket, they must be inspected. Check the chemical indicator tape on each package for color change, which verifies the item was exposed to sterilizing conditions. Check each package for tears, holes, broken seals, stains, and wet areas. Reject and reprocess any items where packaging is compromised or color change did not occur on the chemical indicator.

Aerators should not be opened until the entire cycle time has elapsed. Even though some items will give up all of their residual EtO fairly quickly, opening the aerator and sorting through the load to retrieve these items will expose the CSD worker to unacceptable levels of EtO.

Dry-Heat Sterilization

Dry-heat or "hot-air" sterilizers are used only for specialized purposes in modern health care facilities. Dry-heat sterilization involves very high temperatures that will damage most items ordinarily sterilized in health care facilities. Also, the long exposure times that are often required make the process an impractical one for most purposes. Packaging materials are problematic as well. Papers and plastics cannot withstand the heat. Cotton muslin and glassine pouches or envelopes char. Aluminum foil is recommended, but it presents difficulties in sealing and is not tamperproof.

Another challenge of dry-heat sterilization is the biological monitoring. *Bacillus atrophaeus* is recommended, but conventional self-contained indicators will melt at the higher temperature. Dry spore strips in glassine envelopes may be recommended. Follow the directions of the sterilizer or biological indicator manufacturer.

Consequently, the only items for which dry-heat sterilization is appropriate are those that cannot be sterilized by steam or EtO because they cannot be penetrated, or will be damaged, by moisture or because the items must be pyrogen-free.

In moist-heat (steam) sterilization, bacteria die from the coagulation or denaturation of their protein constituents. Dry-heat sterilization actually burns up (oxidizes) microbial cells, whereas steam kills but leaves cellular debris behind. This debris can be pyrogenic (fever causing) in patients.

Dry-Heat Sterilization Cycle Parameters

The two basic parameters of dry-heat sterilization are time and temperature. The higher the temperature, the shorter the exposure time needed to achieve sterilization. Typical time and temperature settings are 30 minutes at 356°F (180°C), 1 hour at 340°F (170°C), 2 hours at 320°F (160°C), 2.5 hours at 300°F (150°C), 3 hours at 285°F (140°C), and 6 hours or overnight at 250°F (121°C). These times are *exposure times* only and do *not include* the time needed to heat an item to the desired temperature; this heating time varies with the type of item and its composition. As in all sterilization processes, the effectiveness of the cycle parameters relies heavily on proper preparation, packaging, and loading of the items to be sterilized.

Items Sterilized by Dry Heat

Among the items suitable for sterilization by dry heat are hypodermic needles (which must be pyrogen-free) and petroleum ointments, powders, petroleum gauze, and other oil-based items, which will not allow adequate penetration of moisture. Many such items are now commercially available in sterile, single-use form.

Types of Dry-Heat Sterilizers

The two basic types of dry-heat sterilizers (commonly called *hot air ovens*) are the gravity convection sterilizer and the mechanical convection sterilizer.

In a gravity convection sterilizer, air passively circulates according to the temperature differential in the chamber. Hot air rises from the heating elements in the bottom of the chamber, loses some of its heat to the load and the chamber walls, and then descends as it cools. The air that is exhausted through the vent at the top of the chamber is replaced by fresh air from the air intake at the bottom of the chamber. Because this method of air circulation is relatively slow and passive, it takes a much longer time (compared with mechanical convection sterilizers) for a gravity convection sterilizer to bring a load up to the desired temperature, and the temperature is not distributed very uniformly throughout the chamber. Consequently, gravity convection sterilizers are only used for items that do not require precise temperature control.

Mechanical convection sterilizers provide forced air circulation. This more precise control of air velocity, direction of circulation, and heat intensity results in more uniform temperature distribution throughout the load.

In some health care facilities, especially those where very few items are dry-heat sterilized, steam sterilizers have been modified for use as dry-heat sterilizers. Special precautions are needed, however, to ensure that the temperature can be monitored and documented adequately and to avoid spills of oil-based materials that will interfere with steam sterilization of subsequent loads. The sterilizer manufacturer should be consulted about proper written procedures in this situation.

Loading and Operating Dry-Heat Sterilizers

The operating procedures for dry-heat sterilizers vary with design, manufacturer, and model. In all dry-heat sterilizers, the temperature must be regulated and monitored to ensure that the load is neither overheated (and possibly damaged) nor underheated (and possibly nonsterile). External chemical indicators are sometimes used to verify that items have been exposed to dry heat.

Perkins (1983) described the following general procedure for loading and operating a dry-heat sterilizer: "Never load the chamber to the limit. Allow some space between each packaged article and between each basket or container of supplies. Keep all articles well away from chamber sidewalls, so that the free circulation of air is not cut off. After placing load in sterilizer, check the thermometer to see that it is properly inserted in top of chamber. Adjust the air flow damper to MEDIUM position and partially open the air inlet and exhaust vents. The heat should then be turned on and the thermostat set to maintain the desired temperature range. Time the exposure only when the thermometer shows the correct temperature. Avoid opening the door during the exposure period because the chamber will cool rapidly" [p. 301].

Unloading Dry-Heat Sterilizers and Inspecting Sterile Supplies

The procedures for unloading dry-heat sterilizers and inspecting sterile supplies are the same as those used in steam sterilization.

Care and Maintenance of Dry-Heat Sterilizers

Dry-heat sterilizers must be cared for and maintained in accordance with the manufacturer's instructions.

Liquid Chemical Sterilization

Liquid chemical sterilization is accomplished by the complete immersion of items in a sterilizing solution in the concentration and for the time recommended by the manufacturer. Sterilant disinfectants are capable of killing even highly resistant bacterial spores if contact time is prolonged.

Because of the difficulty of maintaining the sterility of an item when rinsing off the sterilant solution and transferring the item to its point of use, liquid chemical sterilization is not suitable for processing items such as implantables, for which absolute sterility is critical.

Parameters of Liquid Chemical Sterilization

The primary parameters of liquid chemical sterilization are the concentration of the active chemical and the length of time that items are immersed in the solution. Temperature may also be a factor, in that some chemicals may be heated to shorten exposure time. However, heating the liquid creates fumes, which can be toxic. The larger the number of microorganisms contaminating the item to be processed, the longer it will take to destroy them all. Therefore, items must be thoroughly cleaned before the sterilization procedure.

Types of Items Processed by Liquid Chemical Sterilization

Immersible surgical and diagnostic instruments, such as endoscopes and their components, anesthesia airways, and anesthesia masks are among the items that may be processed by means of chemical sterilization.

Types of Chemicals Used for Liquid Chemical Sterilization

GLUTARALDEHYDE Glutaraldehyde is a chemical compound that in its activated state takes 10 hours of contact on all surfaces of an item to sterilize at room temperature. It is typically used in an alkaline concentration of 2 percent in distilled water, although acid solutions are also available. The alkaline solution is generally noncorrosive, "instrument-safe," and compatible with metal, rubber, and plastic. Acid solutions are corrosive to metal and will damage some other items. Disadvantages of using glutaraldehyde to sterilize items include difficulty in maintaining an adequate concentration, toxic fumes, prolonged time needed to sterilize items, potential for contamination of sterile items during rinsing and transfer to user area, and no reliable method of monitoring the sterilization process.

Glutaraldehyde is highly toxic and must be used with care to avoid personnel and patient exposure to residues. After immersion, sterilized items must be thoroughly rinsed several times with fresh sterile water for each rinse, because contact with the solution can cause chemical burns of skin and mucous membranes.

The hazards, exposure limits, and proper use of glutaraldehyde were detailed in Chapter Four under types of disinfectants and antiseptics. All statements regarding glutaraldehyde that applied to disinfection also apply to sterilization of items. The differences when using glutaraldehyde to sterilize items are the extended contact time, rinsing with sterile water, and aseptically transferring the device to the user area. Review the information regarding glutaraldehyde in Chapter Four.

To sterilize items using glutaraldehyde, pour the solution into a sterile container and add the activator. The items to be processed must be thoroughly cleaned, dried, and then submerged in the solution for the period specified by the manufacturer (usually 10 hours). The items should be dry when placed in the solution to avoid diluting the sterilant solution. All surfaces of the device must have contact with the solution. After the specified exposure period, the items are removed from the solution and rinsed thoroughly several times with sterile water. Aseptic technique must be used.

When using sterilizing solutions, personnel should wear sterile butyl or nitrile gloves to prevent contamination of the items and to protect their hands. An organic vapor mask should be worn to avoid irritation to nasal passages and to prevent contamination of the processed items. Eye protection should be worn to protect the eyes from vapor irritation and from direct contact with the highly toxic solution, which may be splashed during the procedure. To minimize personnel exposure to the toxic fumes, the procedure must be carried out in a well-ventilated room, in a covered container, and preferably under an exhaust hood. This equipment is designed to contain the toxic vapors in the glutaraldehyde. Filters in exhaust hoods must be changed according to manufacturers' recommendations. OSHA has not established permissible exposure levels for glutaraldehyde. The American Conference of Government Industrial Hygienists (ACGIH) has a recommended threshold limit value (TLV) not to exceed 0.2 ppm from vapors of either activated or unactivated solutions.

Solution containers should be clearly labeled with the name and concentration of the solution, the date on which it was prepared, and the expiration date. Detailed records of all items processed and the soak time must be documented. A large and small spill pan, including chemical neutralization, should be in place.

Glutaraldehyde becomes inactive over time, so it is very important that the solution not be used after the expiration time specified by the manufacturer. The expiration date placed on a newly activated container of glutaraldehyde only indicates when that solution is no longer active. However, once the solution is poured into a container and activated, it will gradually become diluted with water and accumulate contaminants as items are processed, thereby losing its effectiveness.

Commercially available products should be used to check the concentration of the active ingredient in glutaraldehyde solutions daily. This process is called minimum recommended concentration (MRC) testing. Although these products do not monitor the actual sterilization process, they are useful in assessing the effective life of the solution. When the test strips are used, the results should be recorded.

PERACETIC ACID Peracetic acid (peroxyacetic acid) is a neutral-pH liquid chemical solution that destroys microorganisms and is used as a low-temperature sterilization process. The peracetic acid solution has anticorrosive agents in it, so there is no harm to instruments. After the sterilization process the end product is acetic acid, water, and oxygen, which can be disposed of in the sanitary sewage system. This method of sterilization provides just-in-time (items sterilized just before use) availability of sterile devices. The types of devices this process can be used on are immersible surgical instruments and miniature video cameras.

Peracetic acid sterilization is dependent on thorough cleaning and preparation of devices prior to sterilization. All exterior and interior surfaces of devices must come into contact with the sterilant solution for sterilization to occur. The cleaned devices are positioned within specifically designed processing trays and containers to hold them in the correct position. Internal channels of endoscopes are connected to fluid flow connector sets to ensure sterilant contact to all surfaces. The manufacturer's recommendations must be followed for preparations of devices prior to sterilization and for use of correct adapters for each type of scope.

Prior to use, a diagnostic cycle must be run in the processor. If the system passes the diagnostic cycle, the processor can be used. If it fails the diagnostic test, repeat the test. If the test fails again, the processor must be shut down and be checked by a service representative.

To sterilize items using peracetic acid, place the cleaned item in the proper container or tray, close the lid, and place the container in the processor along with the container of sterilant. Press the start button. The processor will automatically advance through the stages of the sterilization cycle. The devices are exposed to the liquid sterilant at 122 to 131°F (50 to 60°C) for 12 minutes. This is followed by 4 sterile water rinses. The total cycle is approximately 30 minutes. Sterilization occurs throughout the entire processor (devices, processing chamber, and tray or container). The containers have tortuous pathways to protect sterile instruments from contamination during transport to user area. Verify the cycle parameters on the printed document after each cycle. Specific biological and chemical monitoring devices should be used for this process.

Cleaning and maintenance of the peracetic acid processor must be done in accordance with the manufacturer's recommendations.

Gas Plasma Sterilization

Gas plasma is used for low-temperature sterilization of heat- and moisture-sensitive items. This sterilization system does not require aeration or have the hazards, expense, and required safety devices that are needed for low-temperature sterilization using EtO.

Gas plasma sterilization is a relatively new technology and potential users must examine carefully what devices can be sterilized using this method. Items that are typically looked at to see if they can be processed by gas plasma include sterotactic equipment, endoscopic instruments, laser hand pieces, fibers and accessories, ophthalmic lenses, external and internal defibrillators, fiberoptic and pacemaker cords, esophageal dilators, transducer cables, surgical power equipment, and electrocautery and metal instruments. An advantage to using gas plasma is the shorter turnaround time.

Gas plasma is composed of ions, electrons, atoms, and free radicals. The electrons and free radicals are responsible for the destruction of microorganisms. Introducing vaporized hydrogen peroxide into the sterilizer under very low vacuum generates gas plasma. The gas is then exposed to an electromagnetic field (radiofrequency [RF] energy), which generates electrons and free radicals that have biocidal properties. After the plasma exposure time is complete, the electromagnetic field and chemical precursor (hydrogen pyroxide) stops, the vacuum removes the residual precursor, filtered air is introduced, and the articles can then be removed from the sterilizer. Process time varies with the nature of the items being sterilized and runs from 54 minutes to 74 minutes. The temperature ranges from 104°F (40°C) to 131°F (55°C).

Toxic residuals on articles are very low. The precursor vapor breaks down to nontoxic chemicals such as water and oxygen.

Cellulose-based materials (paper, linens, towels, cotton, paper, cardboard, huck towels, gauze sponges, or any items containing wood) cannot be used due to their propensity for absorbing the sterilant precursor. In addition, items that contain copper or copper alloys should not be used. Items that absorb liquids should also not be used. (An item must be dry in order to be run through this sterilization cycle.) What may be used is plastic polypropylene sterilization wrappers, instrument trays designed specifically for this process, or Tyvek pouches. Specifically designed chemical and biological indicators for this system must also be used.

Cycle parameters are recorded and should be examined at the end of each cycle. Depending on the type of sterilizer purchased, the system goes through five basic phases: vacuum, injection, diffusion, plasma, and venting. The size and length of lumens are important, and each item to be sterilized should be approved by the manufacturer of the product and the sterilizer manufacturer.

Ozone Sterilization

Ozone, another low-temperature sterilization method, is the most recent entry in the hospital sterilization arena. Ozone is an oxidizing agent and is used commercially as a bleach for waxes, oils, and textiles. As a powerful germicide, it is used to sterilize air, foods, and drinking water. Due to ozone's oxidative action on organic matter such as bacterial spores, viruses, and fungi, it is a powerful sterilizing agent.

Like gas plasma, this sterilization method does not require aeration or have the hazards, expense, and required safety devices that are needed for low-temperature sterilization using EtO. An advantage to using ozone is the lack of toxic residuals from the sterilization process. At the end of the cycle, the ozone goes through a catalytic converter in the sterilizer. This results in the residual products of oxygen and purified water vapor that are returned to the atmosphere. The chamber is under a vacuum during the cycle; therefore, if there is a leak air would enter the chamber.

Items must be clean before packaging and ozone sterilized. Ozone must contact all surfaces of items.

Ozone sterilization is compatible with most medical items. Exceptions include sealed ampoules (which may burst), natural rubber or latex (ozone degrades them), textiles, implants (not validated), flexible endoscopes (not validated), liquids, copper and its alloys, zinc, nickel, container systems with cellulosis filters, and polyurethane (ozone processing can cause physical changes). Lumen inside diameter and length restrictions are

> 2mm dia < 250mm length

> 3mm dia < 470mm length

> 4mm dia < 600mm length

Further validation studies may change the exceptions and lumen restrictions over time. CSD staff considering this method of sterilization must keep current on what is and is not compatible for ozone sterilization. *Each* item to be sterilized should be approved by the manufacturer of the product and the sterilizer manufacturer.

Packaging materials that can be used for ozone sterilization include uncoated, nonwoven material, polyethylene pouches, and commercially available anodized aluminum containers using noncellulose disposable filters.

Ozone is a metastable product: it decomposes in minutes at ambient temperatures and in seconds at higher temperatures. The sterilizer generates the ozone (O_3) on-site, during each cycle, using U.S.P.-grade oxygen (O_2) and electricity. Sterilizer hookup to a water supply is also needed for humidification of the load. The cycle is approximately 4 hours long at 85°F to 94°F (30°C to 35°C) and includes the following two half cycles:

FIRST HALF CYCLE

- Vacuum
- Humidification phase

- Ozone injected into chamber (ozone created by oxygen being released into the ozone-generating unit and subjected to an electrical field)
- Beginning of sterilization process

SECOND HALF CYCLE

- The previous four steps are repeated
- Ventilation phase (removes ozone from the chamber and packaging)

Process parameters are printed and should be examined at the end of each cycle. The critical parameter for ozone sterilization is the ozone concentration (dose) admitted into the chamber, unlike with steam and EtO, where the critical parameter is time. A dose is expressed as a concentration of ozone in milligrams per net-chamber volume (mg/L).

A specifically designed ozone chemical indicator should be put inside each package. The sterilizer manufacturer recommends that a biological test be run with each load. There is a specifically designed self-contained OZO-TEST biological indicator (BI). This should be put in a test pack per the manufacturer's instructions. The self-contained BI contains spores of *Geobacillus stearothermophilis.* The capsule will fit in most of the tabletop incubation units currently used for steam sterilization BI capsules. Incubate capsules and readout according to the manufacturer's written instructions.

The sterilization agent is safe for employees, patients, and the environment. OSHA exposure limits are a permissible exposure limit (PEL) of 0.1 ppm over 8-hour time-weighted average (TWA) and a short-term exposure limit (STEL) of 0.3 ppm for a period of 15 minutes. Ozone has a pungent smell at levels of 0.003 to 0.01 ppm.

Summary

Chapter Seven has presented the complexities of the sterilization process and the techniques used to ensure the sterility of processed items. Sterilization methods used in health care facilities were reviewed, including the applications and limitations of each. New sterilization methods were reviewed. Others are being developed and the CSD technician must take responsibility for becoming familiar with these processes as they become commercially available.

Chapter Eight will focus on how sterility is maintained between the time items are sterilized and when they are used.

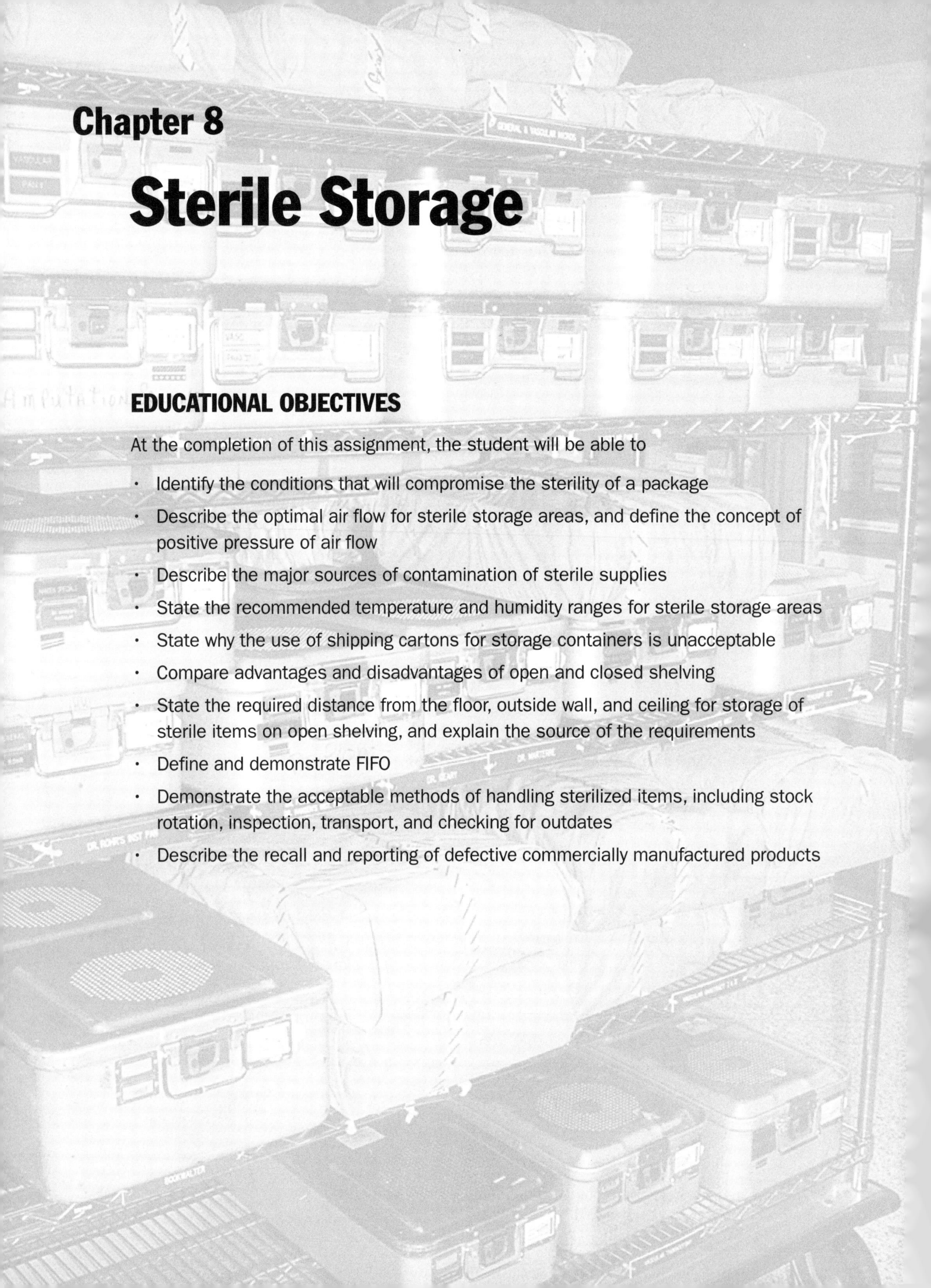

Chapter 8

Sterile Storage

EDUCATIONAL OBJECTIVES

At the completion of this assignment, the student will be able to

- Identify the conditions that will compromise the sterility of a package
- Describe the optimal air flow for sterile storage areas, and define the concept of positive pressure of air flow
- Describe the major sources of contamination of sterile supplies
- State the recommended temperature and humidity ranges for sterile storage areas
- State why the use of shipping cartons for storage containers is unacceptable
- Compare advantages and disadvantages of open and closed shelving
- State the required distance from the floor, outside wall, and ceiling for storage of sterile items on open shelving, and explain the source of the requirements
- Define and demonstrate FIFO
- Demonstrate the acceptable methods of handling sterilized items, including stock rotation, inspection, transport, and checking for outdates
- Describe the recall and reporting of defective commercially manufactured products

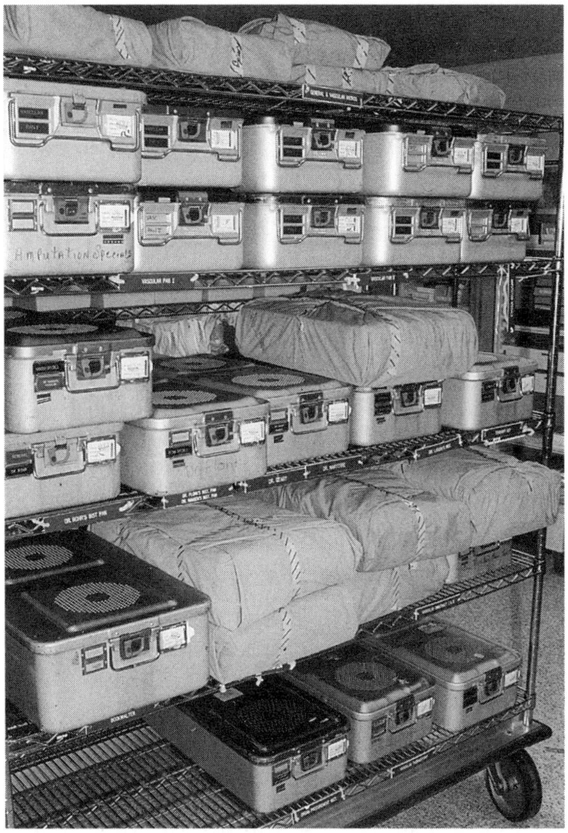

STERILE MEDICAL DEVICES and supplies must be stored temporarily until they are needed for use in patient care. Sterile items are constantly being moved in and out of the sterile storage area of the CSD, and care must be taken to ensure that they are protected from damage or contamination. Most materials used to package medical/surgical items for sterilization and storage do not necessarily provide a complete barrier against contamination. Consequently, the environment of the sterile storage area must be carefully controlled, and CSD technicians must strictly adhere to established procedures for the handling of sterile items.

Sterilized items must not only remain sterile and functional, they must also be available promptly when needed. Therefore, it is important that good inventory and storage techniques be practiced and that the shelf life and sterility maintenance of sterilized items be closely monitored. This chapter describes the principles of and procedures for the storage and handling of sterilized items.

Maintaining Product Sterility

Three conditions can compromise the ability of a package to maintain the sterility of its contents: moisture, soil, and physical damage to the package such as cuts or tears. These conditions can be virtually eliminated with the following safeguards:

- Careful attention to environmental control
- Correct placement of supplies and use of storage systems
- Proper inventory control systems
- Proper handling of sterile items

Environmental Control

In most CSDs, the sterile storage area is usually an enclosed area that limits personnel traffic and minimizes the entry of airborne contaminants from elsewhere in the department.

It is important that the air in the sterile storage area be as clean and dust-free as possible; consequently, air entering the area via the ventilation system is usually filtered. The air is under positive pressure in relation to adjacent areas and is exchanged a certain number of times per hour. (Ten air exchanges per hour are generally recommended for the sterile storage area. *Positive pressure* means that air flows out into other less clean areas, which are under *negative pressure* relative to the sterile storage area.)

Moisture is a major cause of contamination of sterile items. As explained in Chapter Six, some packaging materials can be penetrated by moisture, which will carry microorganisms into the package contents and cause them to be unsterile. Too much (or too little) environmental humidity can adversely affect package seals and the adherence of sterilization indicator tape and other labels, causing packages to become unsealed or making it impossible to verify that packages have been in the sterilizer. (If the environment is moist enough to affect label and seal integrity, it will also accelerate the growth of microorganisms and thus will be unsuitable for sterile storage purposes.) For these reasons, sterile storage areas should have controlled temperature and humidity. Common practice is to maintain the room temperature in the range of 68° to 73°F and the relative humidity in the range of 30 to 60 percent, not to exceed 70 percent.

Another potential source of contamination is people. All people carry microorganisms on their bodies and clothing; for this reason, sterile storage areas should be located away from general traffic. This is also the reason for enforced handwashing, restricted entry to the sterile storage area, and strict departmental policies on personnel access to the area. Proper attire, healthy staff members, and good personal hygiene are also important. Only authorized personnel should enter the sterile storage area (or any part of the CSD).

All CSD technicians should practice good personal hygiene. It is especially important that those assigned to the sterile storage area maintain clean hair, body, nails, and clothing at all times. In particular, it is vital that they wash their hands frequently and thoroughly. Departmental policy on personnel attire and health should always be observed.

The third major source of contamination of the sterile storage environment is shipping containers and transportation vehicles. Sterile items arrive at the sterile storage area from several locations. Reusable items and other hospital-sterilized items come from the sterile processing area and are typically transported in sterilization containers or carts. Transportation vehicles gather contaminants from the air and the floor, so it is important that all parts be cleaned and disinfected frequently, especially the wheels.

Clean or sterile disposable items also come from the receiving area. These items must be removed from their outer shipping cartons and placed in clean transportation containers or vehicles for transfer into the sterile storage area. Shipping cartons must not be allowed in either a clean storage area or a sterile storage area, and they should never be used as storage containers in these areas. Shipping cartons are often very dirty from the shipping process, and they may contain insects. In particular, corrugated cardboard boxes harbor dust and bacteria in the grooves and are frequent sources of fungal contamination and bacterial spores.

Storage Systems

The two basic systems for storing sterile items are open shelving and closed shelving.

OPEN SHELVING Open shelving, the most common method for storing sterile items (see Figure 8.1), is economical and easy to keep clean, allows ready access to supplies, and conserves floor space. However, open shelving provides little protection for the supplies. Strict environmental control and frequent cleaning of the shelves with a disinfecting agent are necessary.

Open shelving must be designed so that the sterile items can be placed at least 8 inches from the floor, at least 2 inches from outside walls, and at least 18 inches from ceiling fixtures (for example, sprinklers). It is particularly important that sterile items be stored away from outside walls, because the difference in temperature between the outside and the inside of the building can cause moisture to condense on the inside surfaces of the walls. In addition, sterile items should not be stored against interior walls, because the walls may be damaged by the storage containers and the sterile items can pick up contaminants from the wall surfaces.

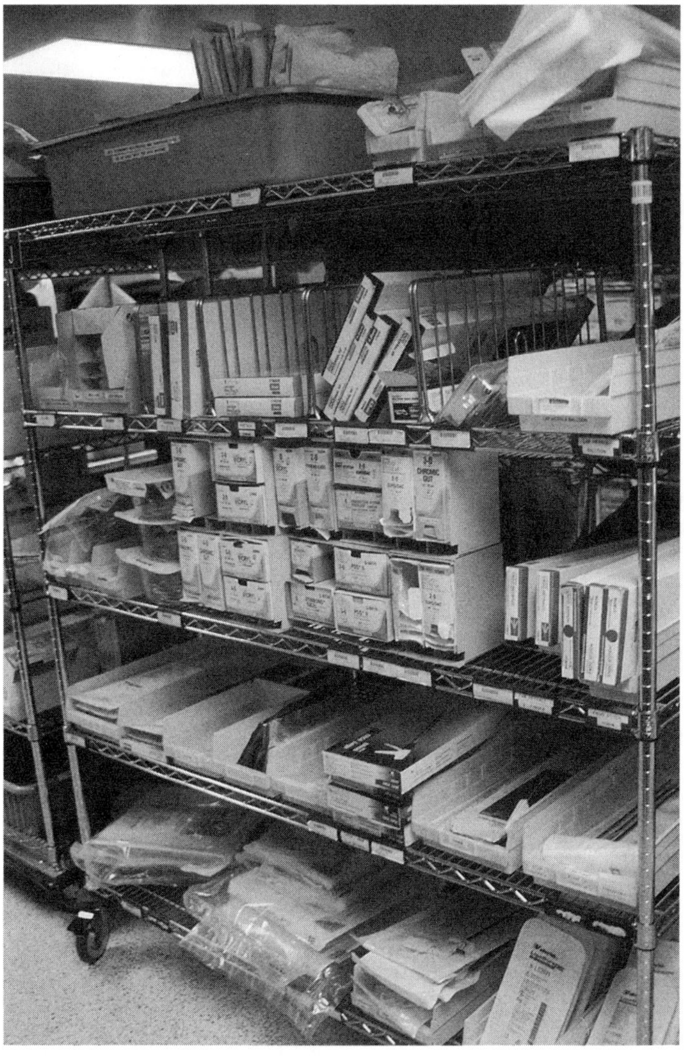

Figure 8.1. Open Shelving.

Sterile items on open shelving or in open containers should always be stored away from sinks, windows, doors, exposed pipes, and vents. A barrier between the items on the bottom shelf and the floor is necessary. This barrier may be a solid bottom shelf, covered tote boxes, a sheet of heavy-gauge plastic, or other means. Items on top shelves of open shelving units must be protected from contaminants falling from the ceiling,

ceiling fixtures, or the ventilation system. This may be accomplished in much the same way as discussed above for the bottom shelf.

CLOSED SHELVING Closed shelving or cabinet storage (see Figure 8.2) provides better protection of sterile items against damage and, if used correctly, against contamination. Care must be taken to open cabinet doors slowly, because rapid air movement can draw in contaminants and defeat the purpose of using an enclosed storage system. Because closed shelving is more expensive than open shelving, many CSDs tend to use closed cabinets mainly for storage of seldom used supplies.

Whichever storage system is used, freshly sterilized items must be thoroughly cooled before storage. As explained in Chapter Seven, contact between hot and cold surfaces will cause condensation of moisture on packaging and hence contamination of the package contents.

To provide maximum protection of sterile items from contamination, a sterility maintenance cover (dust-cover) is often used to overwrap hospital-sterilized packages. This cover should be designed for this purpose, be 2 to 3 millimeters thick, be labeled as a sterility maintenance cover, and be able to completely enclose the item and be properly sealed. Such a cover can compensate for improper environmental conditions, storage techniques, or handling procedures, but CSD technicians should still observe proper handling and storage practices.

It is important that enough space is available to easily accommodate the normal inventory level. Crowding, stacking, and compression of sterile items on the shelves can result in damage to packaging or contents as staff move through the aisles. Also, there should be enough space between storage units so that personnel can avoid accidental contact with storage shelving, storage containers, or sterile items.

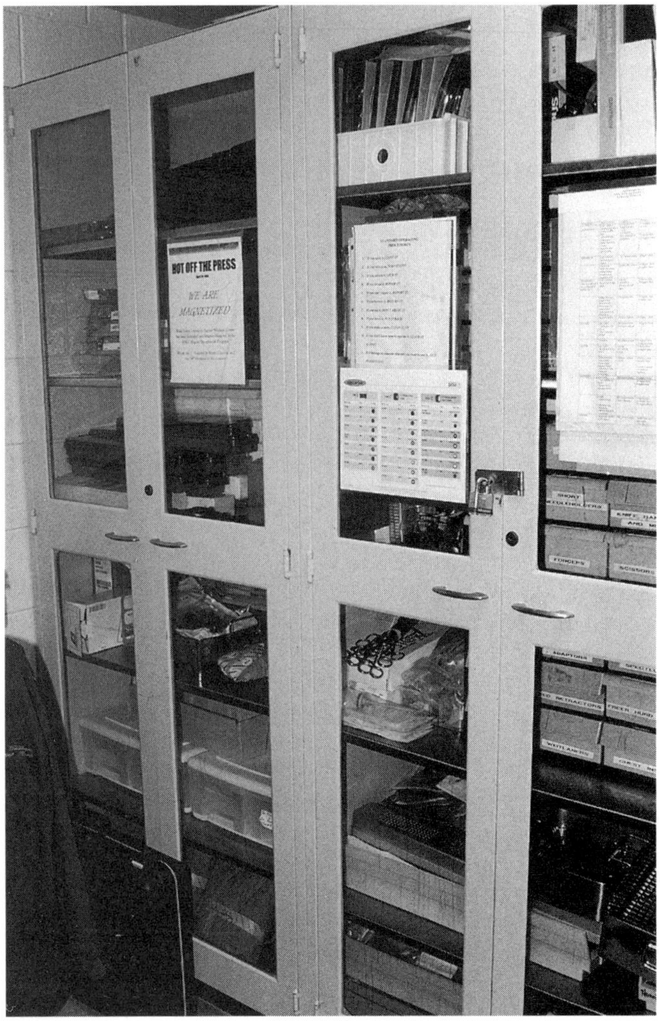

Figure 8.2. Cabinet Storage.

OTHER SHELVING CONFIGURATIONS There are many variations in shelving configurations made by several manufacturers. For example, among the open and closed shelving available, there is a variety of materials they can be made of, including sheet metal, plastic, and plastic and chrome impermeable finishes. There are also many ways to adjust the size, position, and number of shelves in a unit.

Shelving can be all solid material or wire. There are a variety of sizes and configurations of bins to fit on shelving to accommodate the containment of items. Some shelving units have drawers that can be mounted on the shelves to accommodate small items (see Figure 8.3). Some shelving can be mounted on tracks that allow the shelving to be moved so supplies can be obtained (see Figure 8.4). This system of shelving provides fewer aisles; therefore, more items are stored in less space.

The storage system used in a particular facility or area within the facility depends on space, the types of items being stored, ease of retrieval, and customers' needs. When needs change, the type of storage system may change.

Handling and Inspection of Sterile Supplies

Packages should be handled only when absolutely necessary. Inventory counting should be accomplished with as little handling of the supplies as possible. Sterile items should be distributed to patient care areas in baskets or covered carts. Personnel

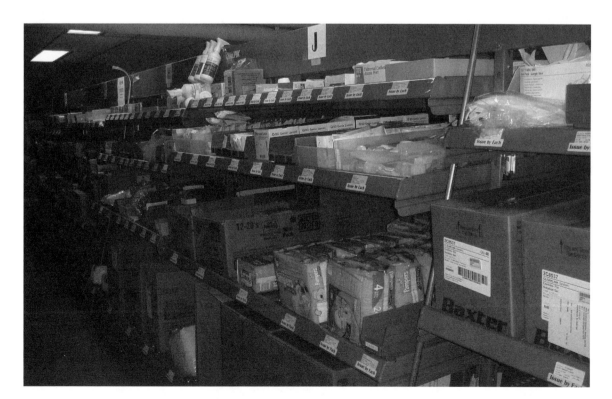

Figure 8.3. Open Shelving, Vertical High Density.

may carry sterile items in their hands, but never under their arms or cradled in their arms. Whenever a sterile item is moved or is selected from inventory for distribution, the packaging should be inspected to verify that it is intact and dry. This check ensures that compromised packages will not be issued. Any package that appears soiled, compressed, torn, or wet should be removed from stock and either reprocessed or discarded. Any package that has fallen or been dropped on the floor must be inspected for damage to the packaging or contents. The package should be considered contaminated, even if there is no apparent damage, because the fall and landing can force unseen air and dust into the package.

If the packaging has been damaged, the item must be considered contaminated. If reusable, the item must be reprocessed before it can be used. If disposable, it may have to be discarded. Wet packs must be dismantled and the contents completely reprocessed.

Housekeeping

Environmental cleaning should start in the sterile holding area and move to the dirtiest part of the area. The sterile storage area must be maintained in the cleanest possible condition, because dust, insects, and vermin all serve as carriers for microorganisms. Any spill should be cleaned up immediately. The floor should be damp-mopped or wet-vacuumed daily (never dry-mop in any area of the CSD), and all work surfaces should be cleaned with an EPA-approved germicidal solution. Storage shelving and containers should be damp-dusted routinely and as needed. When cleaning storage shelving and containers, care should be taken to avoid excessive handling of supplies, and surfaces should be thoroughly dried before the supplies are placed back on shelves.

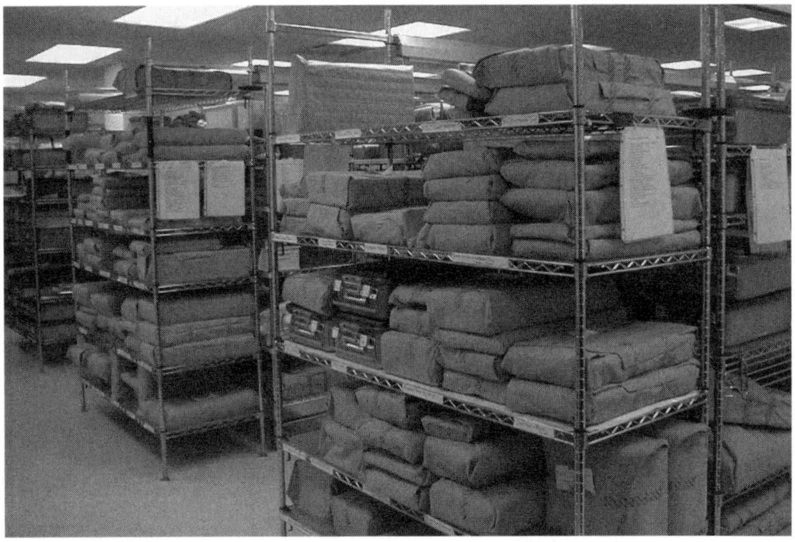

Figure 8.4. Open Shelving, Track-Mounted High Density.

Walls, ceilings, vents, and ceiling fixtures (such as lights, sprinklers, and exhaust fans) should be inspected regularly for accumulated dust, lint, and debris. These areas should be damp-dusted monthly or as often as needed. Transportation carts and containers should also be cleaned on a regular basis, either by hand or in a cart washer, using a detergent followed by a disinfecting agent. Records of the dates of all cleaning activities should be maintained.

Stock Arrangement, Rotation, and Shelf Life

Efficient arrangement of stock, correct stock rotation, and careful monitoring of product shelf life are important factors in ensuring prompt availability of sterile items for use in patient care areas and in minimizing reprocessing costs. Central service department employees should notify the appropriate person if the quantity of an item becomes too depleted.

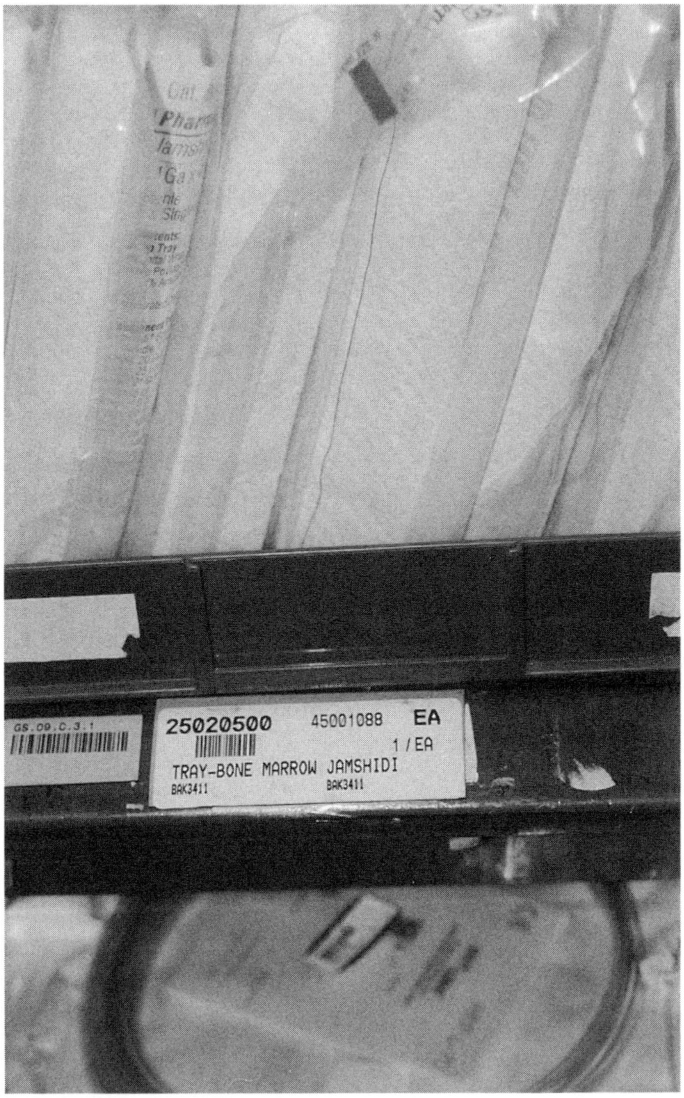

Figure 8.5. An Example of Stock Location Labeling.

Stock Arrangement

Sterile devices, equipment, and supplies must be stored where they can be readily located for distribution. Stock may be arranged functionally (that is, with related items grouped together), alphabetically by item name, or numerically by stock number. Whatever the system, each storage container or shelf location should be labeled with a description of the items stored there, including item name, issue unit stock number (if applicable), patient chargeability, and reorder information (see Figure 8.5). To promote safety and ergonomics, heavy items such as large instrument trays should be stored on middle and lower shelves and lighter, less bulky items on top shelves.

Stock Rotation

It is important to issue the "oldest" supplies first, because many have dates indicating when they can no longer be considered safe for use. Correct stock rotation minimizes waste by reducing the number of sterile items that will have to be reprocessed or discarded. More important, it helps ensure that devices that may have had their sterility compromised will not be used.

"First in, first out" (FIFO) is the principle to follow in the removal and replacement of sterile items in sterile storage; that is, when a particular type of item is requisitioned, the "oldest" item of that category is issued first. The key to ensuring FIFO rotation is consistency in stock placement and issue. Stock should always be rotated from left to right or from back to front; that is, items are placed on the left side of the shelf or cabinet when initially stored and removed from the right side when needed for distribution (or placed in the back of the shelf or cabinet and removed from the front). Freshly sterilized items are placed on the left or at the back, and the older stock is moved on the shelf to the right or front. Items to be issued are then taken from the right or front of the shelf.

Shelf Life

The shelf life of all sterilized items must be indicated on the packaging. There are several methods for identifying the shelf life of sterilized items. The most common is to use a manufactured date, which is shown on the quality-control or lot-number label affixed to the package prior to sterilization. Some facilities still use an expiration date that depends on the type of packaging used, storage, and the amount of handling. All sterile items must be stored in such a way that this label is clearly visible.

Manufacturers of sterile disposable items generally claim an indefinite shelf life that depends only on the integrity of the package. Some commercially sterilized items, however, do have a fixed shelf life, mainly those that contain pharmaceuticals or materials such as latex, which deteriorates over time.

In-house sterilized items are generally assigned a shelf life. With the development of better packaging materials and improvement in sterility assurance controls, event-related, open-ended expiration dating has become more feasible in health care facilities. The maintenance of sterility depends on many variables, and inventory control needs and techniques vary considerably. Therefore, policies and procedures for determining shelf life must be developed at each health care facility, according to its own particular set of circumstances. (See Chapter Six for further discussion of shelf life.)

OUTDATES Outdates are sterile items that have surpassed their expiration date. Sterility is event-related, not time-related. However, if a time-related outdate is used, expired product should not be issued from the CSD. Therefore, all sterile items should be checked for an expiration date before being distributed. Through the rotation methods discussed above and careful control of inventory levels, the number of outdates can be kept to a minimum. Outdated items should be reprocessed the same way as used items. This means that outdated disposable items must be discarded unless the manufacturer supplies written cleaning and resterilization instructions. Reusable items must be unwrapped and reprocessed. Textiles must be relaundered before being sterilized again. Outdates are costly to the health care facility because these items must be completely reprocessed, which could increase the amount of lost revenue charges in many CSDs.

Reprocessing outdated items can become very expensive. Before outdated items are reprocessed, it should be verified that they are needed. If proper stock rotation procedures are being followed, numerous outdates may indicate that certain items are being overstocked, that they are obsolete, or that they need not be supplied sterile. Medical/surgical procedures are often changed, and the CSD is not always notified that use of a particular item has been discontinued. Usually, items identified for use in emergency procedures should be reprocessed without question when they become outdated. However, if certain items repeatedly become outdated, consideration should be given to eliminating them from inventory.

RECALLS Occasionally the manufacturers of commercially sterilized items will notify the facility of a quality assurance problem with their product. Directions from the manufacturer for return, disposal, and replacement must be followed and documentation of actions kept on file.

When the facility discovers a quality assurance issue in a commercially prepared product or equipment, which potentially could cause serious harm or death, this must be reported to the FDA. If serious harm or death was caused by use of a defective product, it must be reported and documented according to the Safe Medical Device Act. Each facility should have policies and procedures with steps to follow and a person assigned to report incidents and deal with the disposition of defective products.

Summary

After an item has been packaged and sterilized, it must be protected from contamination until it is needed. Chapter Eight has shown how environmental control, correct placement and rotation of stock, proper materials handling and, above all, cleanliness are important in maintaining the sterility of sterilized items.

Chapter Nine will discuss the procedures and systems for delivering items to the areas of the health care facility where they will be used in patient care.

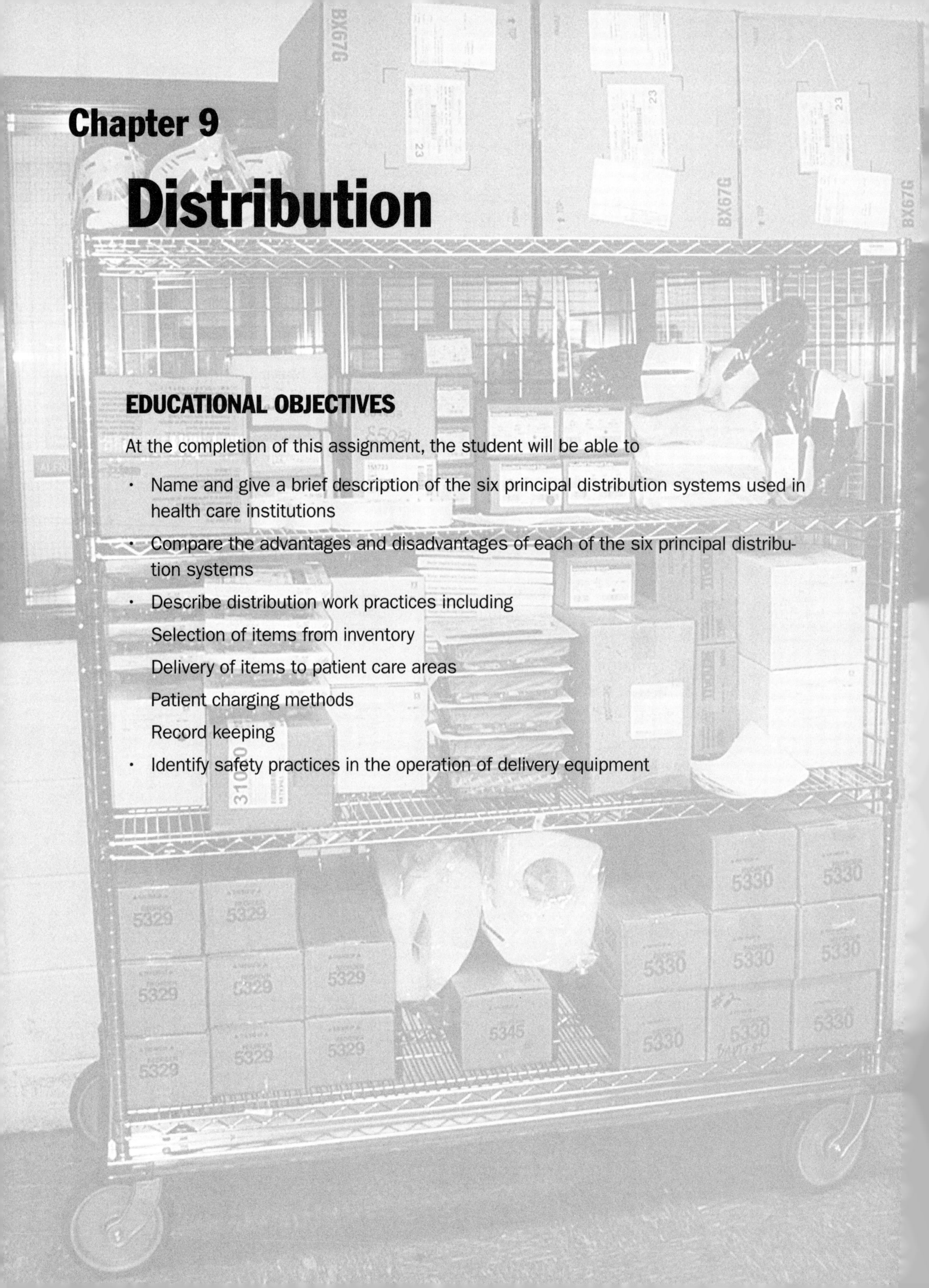

Chapter 9

Distribution

EDUCATIONAL OBJECTIVES

At the completion of this assignment, the student will be able to

- Name and give a brief description of the six principal distribution systems used in health care institutions
- Compare the advantages and disadvantages of each of the six principal distribution systems
- Describe distribution work practices including
  - Selection of items from inventory
  - Delivery of items to patient care areas
  - Patient charging methods
  - Record keeping
- Identify safety practices in the operation of delivery equipment

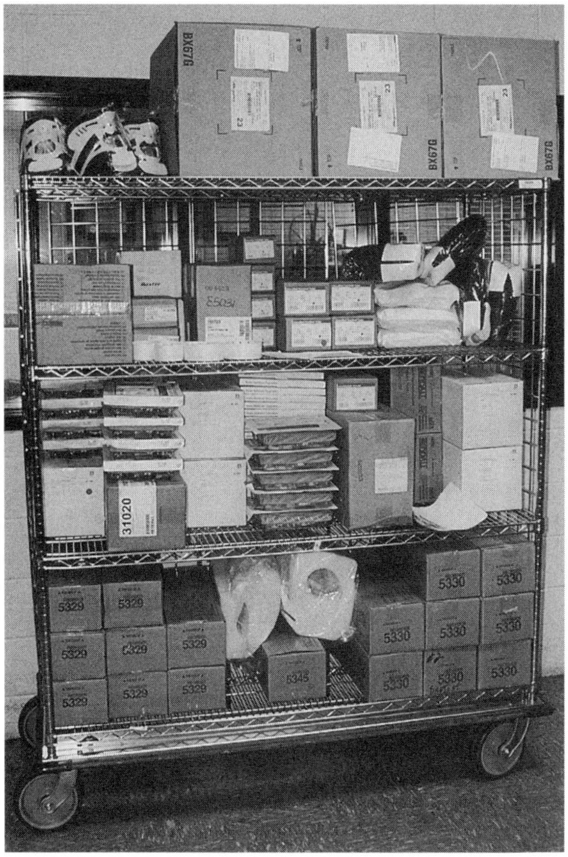

WHEN CLEAN OR STERILE ITEMS are needed in patient care, they must be transferred from the CSD to the user department. The distribution of items throughout the health care facility must be timely and accurate, and care must be taken to ensure that the function, cleanliness, and sterility of the items are not compromised during transport. A variety of distribution systems have been developed within health care institutions to meet these needs. This chapter presents the major types of distribution systems, as well as delivery methods, distribution work practices, patient charging, and record keeping.

Types of Distribution Systems

The seven main types of distribution systems are demand, par-level restocking, automated dispensing systems, exchange-cart, case-cart, specialty-cart, and stockless or "just-in-time," also referred to as JIT. Which system or combination of systems is used at a given health care facility depends on the needs of the customers, the services the facility provides, and its size, physical design, age, and financial resources and goals. Because these factors can change over time, hospital management must reevaluate and modify their distribution system(s) periodically to ensure optimum efficiency and cost-effectiveness. Considerations in evaluating a distribution system are provision for supply forecasting, the timeliness and accuracy of supply availability, and the effectiveness of capturing charges of patient-chargeable, revenue-producing items.

It is important that CSD technicians be familiar with the basic characteristics and the generally accepted advantages and disadvantages of each of the major types of distribution systems. In this way, they can better understand why a particular system is used at their own health care facility and how they can help make distribution as efficient, reliable, and cost-effective as possible.

Demand Distribution Systems

Every health care facility has at one time or another used a demand distribution system (also termed a requisition and delivery distribution system), and at some institutions this system remains the predominant method of distributing medical or surgical items and supplies. In this system, the nursing staff or the various customers within the health care facility are responsible for maintaining an adequate level of supplies for use in that department. When these supplies must be replenished or when an individual item is needed, customers request the necessary items from the CSD. The CSD staff fills the order (Figure 9.1) and delivers it to the requesting department, where the customer is responsible for storing the items or transferring them to the point of use. This process may be carried out on a regularly scheduled basis or as necessary (hence the term *demand* distribution system).

The demand distribution system is simple and has fulfilled the needs of many health care facilities for a long time, although it does have some disadvantages. This distribution method is very labor-intensive and thus is generally unsuitable for high-volume distribution in a large institution. Also, customers have many other responsibilities and priorities; they may not be able to commit sufficient time to inventory management and probably will not have had special training for this function. Consequently, there is sometimes a tendency to maintain very high levels of inventory by customers, so that every possible contingency will be covered and so that the staff will not have to take time from other responsibilities for frequent requisitioning and documentation. Even in the best case, the demand distribution system requires some duplication of inventory. Maintaining excessively high inventories can be very costly, which will be shown in Chapter Ten.

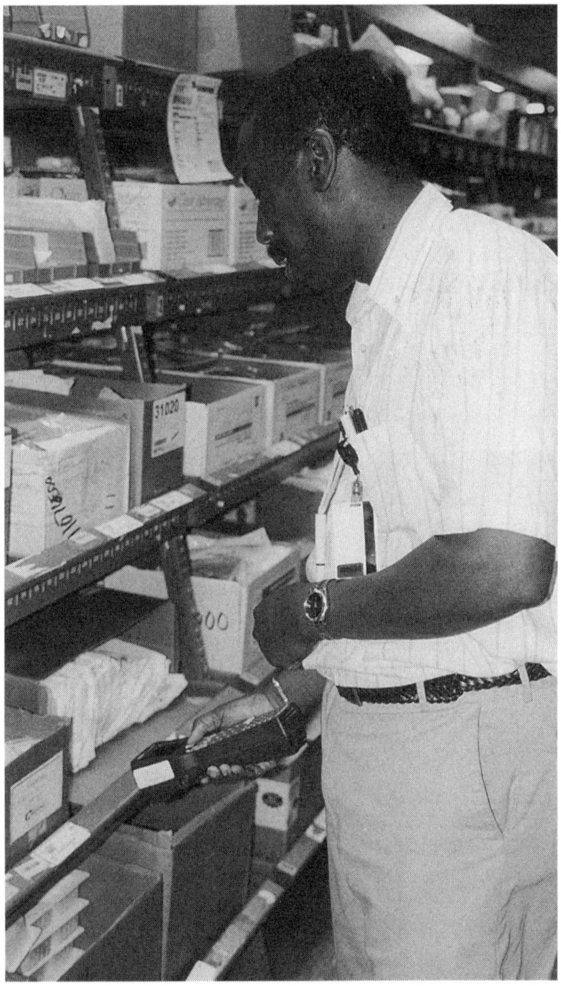

Figure 9.1. Filling an Order in a Demand Distribution System.

Par-Level Restocking Distribution Systems

In this type of system, an optimum level of stock for each item used on a regular basis is determined for each customer. These levels are reviewed frequently and changed as necessary to reflect actual usage. The supplies are stored in the storage space available in each unit. Carts, cupboards, closets, or shelving may be used for storage; usually, storage containers are kept in one area for effective replenishment. These stocks of supplies are then maintained by the CSD or other supply department.

A typical procedure for maintaining stock is when a CSD technician with a large cart of items moves throughout the health care facility, from department to department, and replenishes each area back to the desired, preset *par levels.* This procedure is carried out on a frequent, regularly scheduled basis. In some health care facilities, the procedure is to make an entire round of the customer supply areas, document the required items (either on a list or by use of bar code technology), and gather them all at once or notify the CSD for replenishment stock, which is then delivered. Bar code technology allows CSD technicians to use a device to swipe the bar code on a shelf label for a needed item and punch in the needed quantity. The bar code equipment is then plugged into the computer system, which produces the list for replenishment. With this system, the user department no longer has the time-consuming task of maintaining its inventory, and levels can be maintained more efficiently than in the demand system. This system provides a good means of tracking the use of patient-chargeable items and facilitates revenue collection.

However, this system also has some drawbacks. Distribution can be quite slow, especially if the institution is large or spread out or the volume of supplies needed is high. In such cases, the technician often has to return several times to the CSD to gather more supplies.

Automated Dispensing Systems

A variation of the par-level system is a locked supply cabinet. The supplies for each area are locked in cabinets. These locked cabinets are connected to a computer network in order to send usage information to a replenishment system. The user enters information (ID or password) into the computer. The cabinet door where the supply is kept unlocks, the user removes item(s), and the door locks when it is closed. The patient's name and other information can be accessed from the database. The item needed and the quantity are controlled by button or keypad pushing. The information is sent automatically to the computer in the replenishment area and to the billing area. The CSD can get a report for restock of supplies from the computer in CSD and deliver these supplies to bring the area back to par level. This system is less labor-intensive, supply loss is controlled, patient billing is automated, and less paperwork is involved for users, CSD, and the billing area.

Exchange-Cart Distribution Systems

In this system, similar to the par-level restocking system, the customer works with the CSD to determine the types and amounts of items that will be needed for regular operation of the unit. The required inventory levels must be reviewed frequently to remain effective. Once the cart inventory has been established, two identical carts are created, which are exchanged on a daily basis by a CSD technician (see Figure 9.2).

The exchange-cart system has a number of advantages. It is practical, flexible, dependable, and easily managed. It can be used in small or large institutions and in general or specialty hospitals. The system allows thorough documentation, good control of supplies, and ready identification of lost stock. Some of the disadvantages of the system are the duplication of stock and the need for large amounts of space for the storage and handling of carts in the CSD. These costs, as well as the large capital expenditure needed for the establishment of the system, can be formidable.

Case-Cart Distribution Systems

In a case-cart system, the operating room, labor-delivery room, and other such service departments are provided with carts that carry selected supplies, often including instruments, that will be needed for particular procedures. There are various methods of specifying what should be stocked on each cart. Physician procedure cards, computer printouts, and requisition forms are all means of identifying the items that individual physicians desire for specific procedures. After a cart is prepared, it is stored until needed for a procedure and then delivered to the customer.

A major incentive for using the case-cart system is the efficiency and economy that can be gained by concentrating processing and inventory management expertise and equipment in the CSD. This centralization frees the physicians, nurses, and other medical staff to focus on patient care and avoids costly duplication of processing, effort, and inventory.

In some health care facilities, the physical age and design of the institution are such that it would be prohibitive to establish a case-cart system. Similar to exchange-cart systems, a considerable amount of storage space is needed for the carts. A study must be conducted to determine if space and resources are available before this type of system is implemented. The case-cart system also requires a higher level of communication between the staff in areas using the system and CSD personnel to achieve uniform functioning than do the other systems.

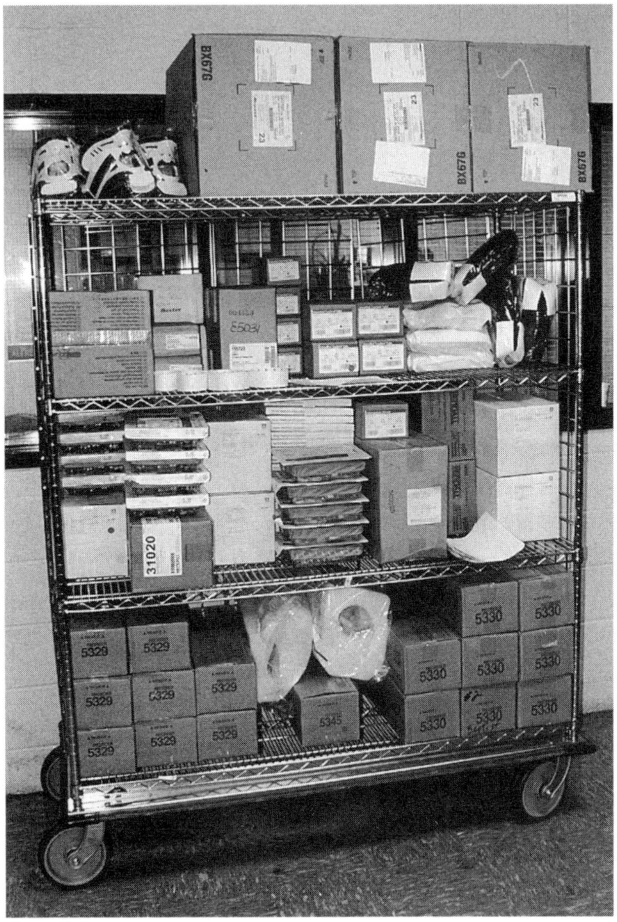

Figure 9.2. An Exchange Cart.

Specialty-Cart Distribution Systems

Supplies needed only in specific emergency situations are often placed on carts so that they can be taken to the point of use and any necessary items will be readily available (Figure 9.3). The two most frequently used types of specialty carts are code (also called crash) carts and disaster carts.

Code or crash carts (Figure 9.4) contain the supplies necessary to revive victims of cardiac and respiratory arrest. The carts are restocked after each use by following an inventory list of medical/surgical supplies and refilling set quotas. Billed carts are stored where they can be retrieved quickly and rushed when needed to the site of the cardiac arrest.

Disaster carts are used when a health care facility receives a rapid influx or large number of patients due to a natural or manmade disaster. It is considered a disaster situation because of the extraordinary efforts required to care for the patients properly. Large amounts of supplies (especially bandages, intravenous supplies, and splints) are needed in these instances. These supplies are stored on disaster carts so that they can be taken quickly to the arenas where the victims are being treated. The carts are filled according to an inventory list.

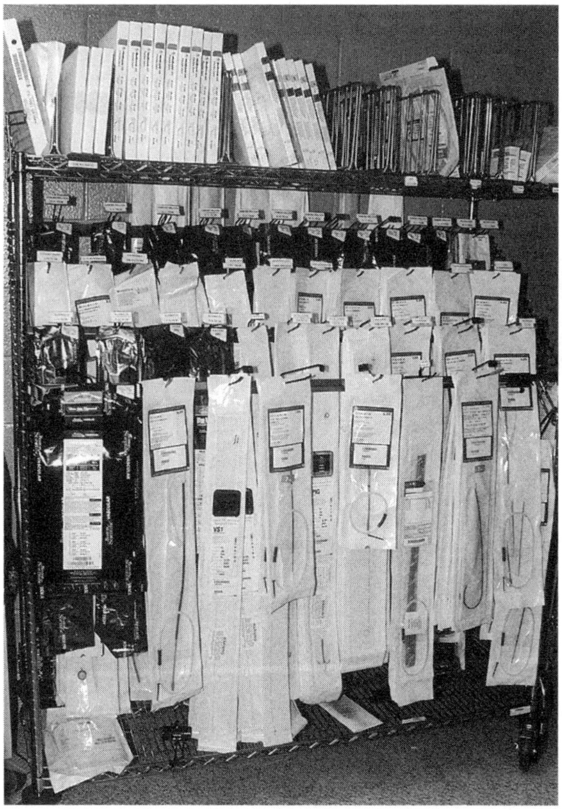

Figure 9.3. A Specialty Cart.

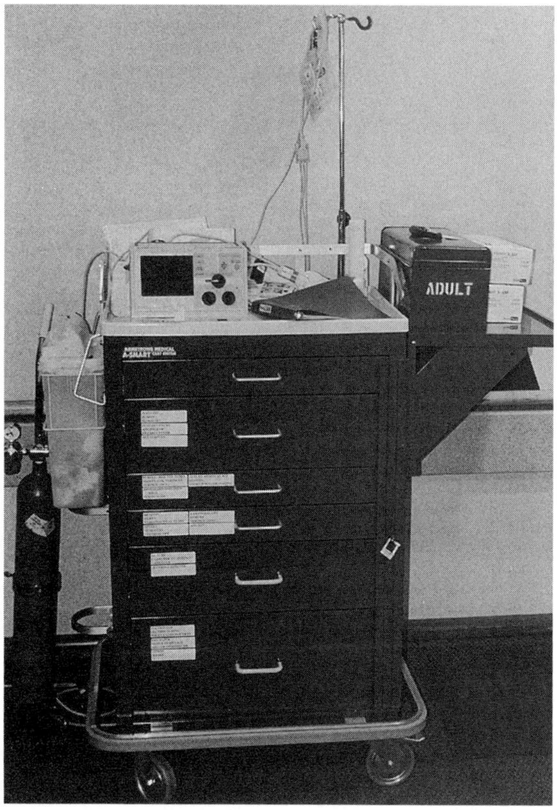

Figure 9.4. A Crash Cart.

It is important that all hospital employees know their roles during a code arrest or disaster. Detailed instructions should be identified in the facility policy and procedures.

Stockless or Just-in-Time Distribution Systems

A stockless or "just-in-time" distribution system is a modification of the par-level restocking system. Similar to that system, the types and amounts of supplies that will be needed for regular operation of the department are determined by the customer and the CSD. An entire round of all areas is made to document the required items needed to replenish the stock. This information is sent to the health care facility's supplier, who picks and delivers the supplies to the institution. The items are then taken to the customer areas and put away. In some instances the supplies are taken to the customer areas by the supplier.

The advantage of this system is the reduction of in-house inventory and freeing of space for other uses. The disadvantages of this system are that it may require additional personnel for smooth and efficient operation, and the ability to provide additional supplies quickly may be adversely affected.

Delivery Methods and Equipment

A variety of methods and types of equipment are used for the transport, delivery, and storage of items. Distribution carts are the most common means of transport and storage. *Nurse servers* are personal cupboards in patient rooms that are stocked, usually by general supply personnel, with basic items such as basins and linens and all patient care items. Dumbwaiters and pneumatic tubes are mechanical devices used to transport, upon request, small quantities of items to customers. Dumbwaiters and pneumatic tubes are often used for *stat* (immediately needed) items. It should be noted that mechanical devices may be harmful to fragile items. Mechanical devices carrying totes and containers must be cleaned routinely with a germicidal solution to avoid contamination. Window distribution is a method by which customers obtain items directly from the CSD.

Some health care facilities use tracked automated systems to supplement or replace manual delivery methods. Large institutions may use large mechanical or robotic devices to assist (with or without human guidance) in the transportation of supply carts or bulk quantities of materials. These systems can be quite advantageous in large institutions, but they are very expensive. An automated system can usually only be considered during the building of a new hospital; the acquisition and installation cost otherwise may be prohibitive. The cost of ongoing maintenance and the backup systems needed when the automated equipment is not functioning must also be considered, as well as the labor costs for supply replenishment.

Routine cleaning of the physical storage areas, equipment, and the transport vehicles with an EPA-approved germicidal solution is essential and should be documented.

Distribution Work Practices

Common to all distribution systems is the need for accurate selection, careful handling, and timely delivery of the items needed. If distribution is unreliable, customers may lose confidence in the system and begin hoarding supplies, resulting in wasteful and costly duplication of inventories and in poor accounting of items. Patient safety can be jeopardized if items are not available promptly, in sufficient quantity, and in good condition.

Selection of Items from Inventory

The distribution process begins with the receipt of a requisition for one or more items. The items are then removed from their storage location. Every picking, packing, and transportation step requires that the items should be handled carefully to avoid damage or contamination. The type and quantity of items selected should be verified against the requisition. Sterile items should be inspected to ensure that they are complete and appropriately packaged and that the packaging is not damaged, stained, wet, or soiled. If a chemical indicator is present, the package should be checked to verify that the item was subjected to the sterilization process. The expiration date or other shelf-life indication should be inspected. Distribution personnel should also make sure that the item is properly labeled in accordance with department standards.

Delivery of Items

Clean or sterile medical/surgical items should be covered, enclosed, or otherwise protected from contamination, physical damage, and loss during transport. Distribution carts should have a solid-bottom shelf or other barrier between the items being transported and the wheels of the cart and the floor. If an item falls on the floor, it should not be used; it should be returned to the CSD for inspection and, if appropriate, reprocessing. Transportation vehicles and containers must be cleaned between uses and must never be used to transport anything other than clean or sterile items. Contaminated or used supplies must be transported by a separate vehicle.

Distribution carts can be heavy and unwieldy; when manipulating them, CSD technicians should take care to observe the principles of good body mechanics and to avoid other traffic control problems.

Central service departments should have written policies and procedures defining the transportation routes to be used in distributing supplies. These routes are designed to be as direct as possible, while avoiding areas of the health care facility where there is heavy traffic or other potential sources of contamination. Distribution personnel should adhere strictly to these established routes. Distribution vehicles or containers should never be left unattended during transit because contamination of items or theft of supplies can occur.

Patient Charging

Each health care facility has an established policy regarding patient charges. Most facilities utilize some method of patient charges. Some facilities, such as health maintenance organizations (HMOs), may not charge for individual items. Health care facilities' dependence on reimbursement for individual supply expenses is decreasing over time. The responsible manager must determine, in consultation with the finance department, which items to designate as patient-charge items, and must develop an effective system for identifying these items on the patient's bill. Some of the methods used to accomplish this are requisitions attached to the item, adhesive labels identifying charges that are attached to the item, and a computerized request system in which charges are automatically made to the appropriate patient. In any method, the most critical factor is the physician, nurse, or other person who uses the item in patient care. They must place the requisition or label in the proper place or enter information into the computer as required by written procedure. It is very important that CSD technicians understand and follow strictly the procedures for identifying and charging items to patients, because patient charges for equipment, devices, and supplies are a vital source of revenue to the institution.

An equipment-tracking system should provide information on where each piece of patient care equipment is being used or stored. The system should also identify the patient, the length of use, revenue, and costs. It should be routinely verified that equipment is being used properly and that patient charges are correct. All of this information can be documented manually or computerized.

Record Keeping

The high cost of products used in health care facilities makes it essential that accurate and current records be kept of all supplies distributed throughout the institution. Many sources of revenue and costs can be identified if good documentation is provided by the CSD to the financial department of the hospital.

The hospital's accountability to third-party payers such as insurance companies and auditors is another reason every department in the supply chain must keep accurate records. Record keeping can be expedited by the use of computers. However, even in a computerized system, certain data-entry procedures must still be done manually. Continued improvements, in equipment such as bar codes, light pens, PDAs (personal digital assistants, such as a PalmPilot), and audio-input terminals, and in programming software are making these tasks faster and more accurate.

Bar coding is also making patient-charge revenue easier to assess. Bar codes are symbols consisting of rectangular bars and numbers that are used to designate the type and cost of an item. Bar codes can be read by a computer, enabling charge information to be processed quickly and accurately without the need for personnel to enter the data by hand. Bar codes are making data capture faster and more accurate.

Summary

Chapter Nine has explained the systems used to maintain supply levels to immediate area(s) of users, how items are transported to their ultimate destination, and the importance of accurate record keeping. Chapter Ten will present the final subject of managing inventory.

Chapter 10

Inventory Control

EDUCATIONAL OBJECTIVES

At the completion of this assignment the student will be able to

- State the rationale for good inventory control practices
- Name and give a brief description of the four principal types of inventory control systems
- Compare advantages and disadvantages of each of the four principal types of inventory control systems
- Describe work practices in inventory control activities

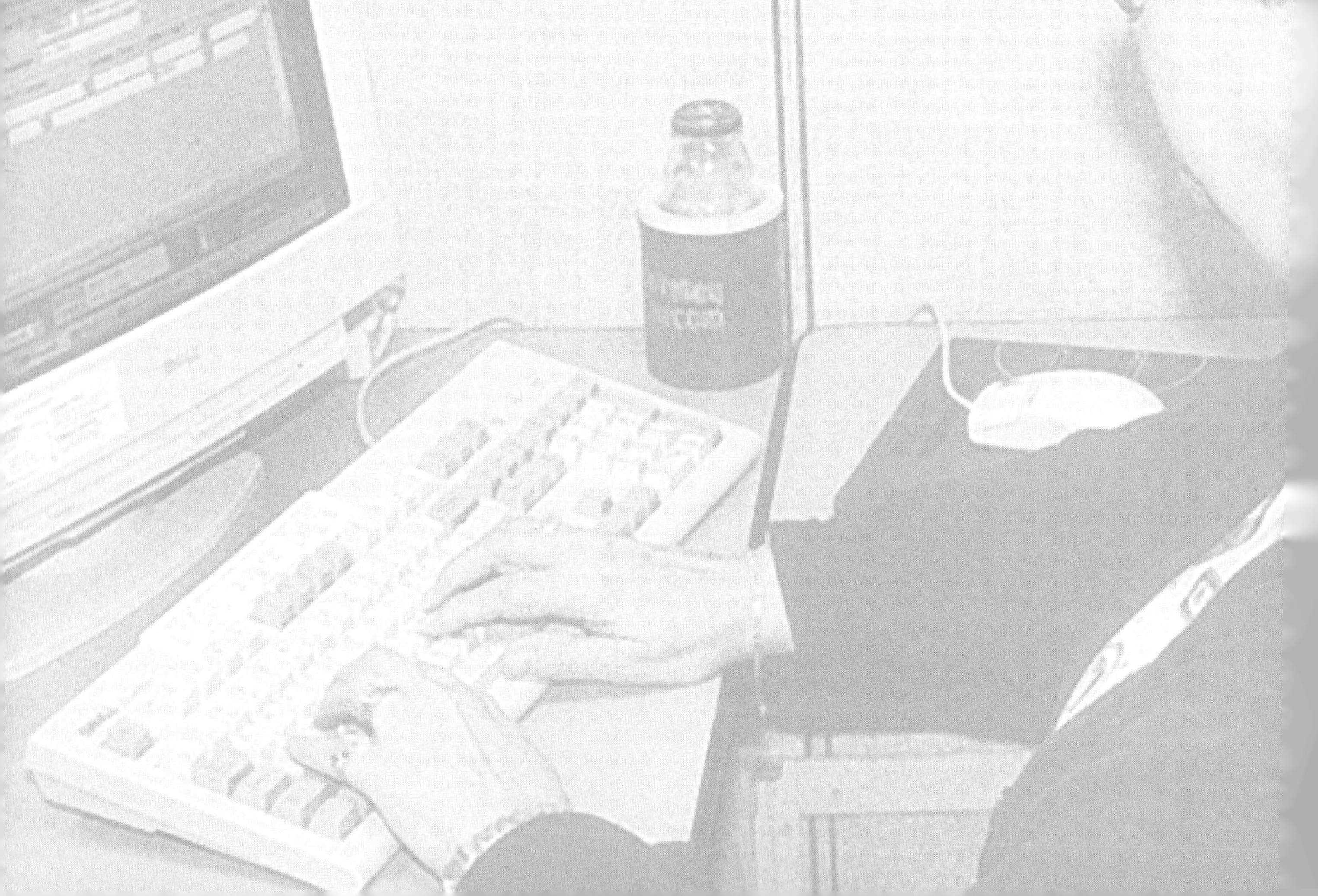

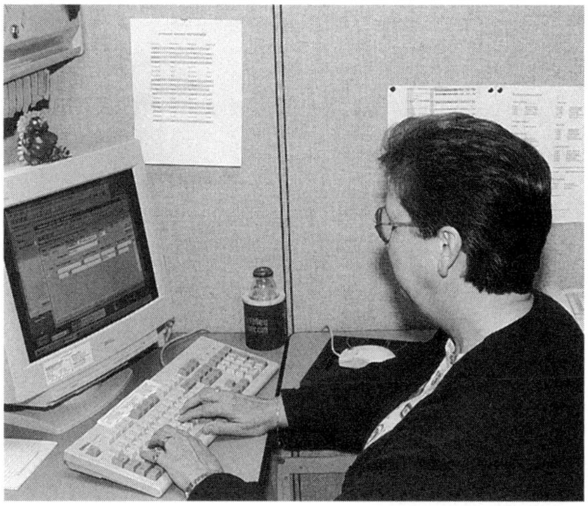

MODERN HEALTH CARE requires an ever-expanding variety of equipment, devices, and supplies. While health care facility investment in materials has grown and cost-containment pressures have intensified, more and more attention has focused on improving inventory management.

Inventory management is the effort to meet the health care facility's need for supplies while minimizing the overall cost of acquiring, handling, and maintaining supplies in storage. Minimizing the overall cost requires a careful balance among the various cost components. For example, the cost of acquiring a product (including both the purchase price and the cost of processing the purchase order) can often be reduced by ordering a large quantity of the product. However, buying a large quantity of a product can result in high storage costs. This includes the cost of the space to store the product, the cost of the money tied up in the product (money that could be used for some other purpose), and the cost for shrinkage (losses from damage, pilferage, or obsolescence). Thus, the initial cost savings that could be achieved by purchasing a large quantity needs to be analyzed to see if it offsets the additional costs associated with the storage of the large quantity.

Also, while central service strives to manage its inventories, one key question always needs to be asked: How will its decisions affect the inventories in other departments? Often, the combined inventories in patient care areas, such as surgery, radiology, respiratory therapy, and inpatient care units, are many times higher than the total inventory in the central storage areas. Central service can help each department reduce its inventories and run more efficiently by delivering materials in frequencies and quantities that match the usage patterns in each department. In this way central service can prove itself a reliable source of supply for each department.

Measuring Inventory Performance

Two measures of the performance of an inventory system are inventory turnover and line-item fill rate.

Inventory turnover is defined as the annual dollar value of the items issued from a storeroom, divided by the dollar value of the supplies stored in the storeroom.

Line-item fill rate is defined as the percentage of ordered supplies that are filled from stock on hand.

Taken together, these two measures give a good indication of the performance of a health care facility's inventory management system. Inventory turnover indicates if stock is being ordered in appropriate quantities and how much of the inventory is "dead" or nonmoving stock. The line-item fill rate indicates how well the CSD meets the needs of its customers.

Managing Inventory

Inventory is managed primarily by means of the following two functions:

- Reordering when supplies are depleted
- Disposing of obsolete (or nonmoving) stock

These functions must be performed well in order to achieve a high level of performance, that is, high inventory turnover and high line-item fill rate.

Most of this chapter discusses the various issues and systems concerning the reordering of supplies. Before discussing these aspects of inventory management, it is pertinent to look at the appropriate methods for identifying and removing obsolete stock from inventory. The result of neglecting obsolete stock is that it rapidly becomes worthless and a total loss for the health care facility. However, there are three ways to obtain value from an obsolete product:

- Use up the remaining (obsolete) product before totally converting to the new product or procedure.
- Return the product to a vendor for full, or at least partial, credit.
- Sell the product to another health care facility that is still using it.

Good inventory management requires constant vigilance regarding the usage patterns for all items in all departments. Departments can make decisions to change their procedures without giving thought to the impact their decisions will have on supply usage, but product standardization committees have been created in part to make this less likely. Good communication with customers should allow this situation to be addressed before a supply or procedure change occurs. An item that has been used at the rate of several cases per month might suddenly be used at the rate of only a few cases per month. As soon as such a change becomes apparent, the appropriate employee should question customers to determine why the usage pattern has changed.

Sometimes the reason will be a temporary phenomenon; for example, a unit is closed while under renovation. But, usually a dramatic drop in usage indicates that there has been a fundamental change, and usage of that item will not return to former levels. In this case, an effort should be made either to use up the excess inventory before abandoning the previous system, return the excess to the vendor, or sell the excess to another health care facility.

Reordering Stock

The reordering function involves the following two decisions:

- At what inventory level will each item be reordered (the reorder point)?
- How much of the item will be ordered when the inventory of the item reaches its reorder point (the order quantity)?

The reorder point must be high enough that it is unlikely that the stock will be depleted before the next order arrives. But the reorder point should not be so high that there is still a large stock of the item when the next order is received. The reorder quantity should be set low enough to result in an appropriate inventory turnover for the item, but high enough so that too much labor is not spent on repeatedly ordering it.

Order-Processing Systems

After reorder points and reorder quantities are established, it is necessary for the storeroom to have a system to determine when items reach their respective reorder points, and to place an order for the needed supplies. Many systems accomplish this, from simple manual systems to sophisticated computer systems. Some of the most popular systems are described below.

TWO-BIN SYSTEM With the two-bin system, a quantity of each item equal to that item's reorder quantity is segregated (held in reserve) from the stock picked routinely. When the stock picked routinely becomes depleted, then the item has reached its reorder point and must be reordered. The reserve stock will be sufficient to last until the next order arrives. For example, if the reorder point for Huber needles is three boxes, then three boxes of Huber needles would be segregated. The stock of Huber needles might be stored in a bin with a divider. Three boxes (the reserve) would be placed behind the divider. Additional boxes would be stocked in front of the divider. When the last box is picked from the quantity in front of the divider, then the order should be placed for the item. The three boxes behind the divider can then be used while the order is placed and delivered.

The two-bin system is an elegantly simple system that works very well, particularly for small, slow-moving items. It can be clumsy, however, when applied to large items, because it can require considerable extra space to effectively segregate the reserve stock.

PERIODIC-REVIEW SYSTEM With a periodic-review system, an inventory of stock on hand is taken at regular intervals. Items at or below their reorder points are ordered. Often, an experienced employee can conduct such an inventory very rapidly by walking through the storeroom "looking for open shelves" (items that are nearly out). The main problem with this arrangement is that chaos often results whenever the experienced employee is on vacation or sick.

TRAVELING-REQUISITION SYSTEM With both the two-bin system and the periodic-review system a method for processing orders for items that fall below the reorder points is required. An effective method is the traveling-requisition system. With the traveling-requisition system, there is a card (the traveling requisition) for each item in inventory. Figure 10.1 is a sample traveling requisition. Note that the top half of the requisition displays all of the information required to process an order for the item. The bottom half has lines that are filled out for each item order. The storeroom or central service personnel fill out the date submitted and the quantity to be ordered. The traveling requisition is then submitted to the purchasing department, which places the order and fills in the order date, expected delivery date, and any changes in unit price or vendor information. The traveling requisition is then returned to the storeroom or CSD.

A significant benefit of this system is that a complete ordering history is developed for the item on the traveling requisition. This may be the source of information for producing critical reports, such as the listing of inventory items sorted by decreasing annual usage.

PERPETUAL-INVENTORY SYSTEM With a perpetual-inventory system, a record is kept of each receipt into and issue from the supply area. After either transaction (receipt or issue), if the quantity on hand falls below the reorder point, an order can be placed.

Perpetual-inventory systems can be maintained manually, usually with a Kardex file. With a Kardex file system, there is a stock card for each line item in inventory. The top portion of the stock card, like the traveling requisition, contains the information necessary to place an order for the item. The bottom portion of the stock card has lines for entering the transactions that change the level of stock for the item, both receipts and issues. After each transaction, the quantity on hand is manually updated on the stock card. When the on-hand quantity falls below the reorder point, the card serves similarly to a traveling requisition. It is submitted to purchasing for ordering and subsequently returned to the supply area.

COMPUTERIZED PERPETUAL-INVENTORY SYSTEMS Many health care facilities now use computer systems to maintain perpetual inventory for their supply storerooms. Computer systems can simplify some of the mundane tasks involved in maintaining a perpetual inventory, and can provide reports that help the health care facility do a much better job managing its inventory. The computer can automatically generate reports such as the following:

- Suggested reorder points and reorder quantities for each item
- Inventory turnover and line-item fill rate trend information
- Purchase orders for items below their respective reorder points
- Expense accounting information for the finance department that shows the dollar value of supplies issued to each cost center in the health care facility

TRAVELING PURCHASE REQUISITION

Product Description

______________________________ ☐ Chargeable ☐ Taxable

______________________________ ☐ Non-Chargeable ☐ Non-Taxable

Manufacturer Information			**Purchase Order Information for Purchasing Use Only**			
Name	Product No.	Packaging	Vendor No.	Name	Product No.	Purchase Unit
			(1)			
			(2)			
			(3)			

Department Information — Name ______ Cost Center ______ Charge Code ______

Authorizations — Supervisor ______ Director ______ Administrator ______

Department Request					Purchase Order Information for Purchasing Use Only								Dept. Receipt Information		
Date	Requested By	Date Needed	Qty.	Unit	Date	Qty.	Unit	Unit Cost	Del. Date	Vendor No.	Purchase Order No.	Buyer	Date	Qty.	Unit

Requesting Department to Complete All Except the Shaded Areas

Figure 10.1. A Sample of a Traveling Requisition.

The information available from a computerized inventory system can be used to significantly reduce the inventory and improve service to the customers. This information can help save money by making it easier to negotiate better supply contracts, by identifying departments that may be using excessive quantities of supplies, and by specifying which items should be investigated to see if there are more cost-effective alternatives. Being able to obtain these benefits from the computer system depends on the accurate and timely entry of information into the system.

The need for accurate and timely entry of information into a computer system cannot be overemphasized. A computer system with accurate data that are wisely used will result in significant savings. However, a system that is not kept current with good data not only can consume considerable effort but also can lead to poor decisions that result in increased costs and decreased service to customers. For example, if issues are not promptly entered into the computer system, then the data will indicate that stock levels are higher than they actually are, so that items may not be ordered when they fall below their reorder points. This can lead to a higher level of stockouts and inadequate service to customers.

To ensure that the computerized perpetual-inventory system is effective, all receipts into and issues from the supply areas must be accurately entered into the computer prior to placing orders for additional stock. For example, if purchasing places orders for stock starting at 8:00 A.M. each day, then the previous day's receipts and issues must all be entered into the computer before 8:00 A.M.

For continued accuracy of the inventory levels, many health care facilities conduct cycle counts. Cycle counts are checks of the inventory on hand against the inventory level shown on the perpetual-inventory system for some fraction of the line items. Different items are checked on each successive cycle count until all items have been reviewed. Then the process begins again with the first group of items. For example, for a supply area containing 1,000 line items, 100 items could be checked each week. All items would be reviewed once every 10 weeks.

For cycle counts to be accurate, they must be done after all past receipts and issues have been recorded, and when there is no picking activity occurring. An employee might be scheduled to arrive at work one hour early to perform the cycle counts on a day when all receipts and issues for the previous day have been recorded. If there have been any transactions that have not yet been logged when the cycle occurs, then the inventory level would have to be adjusted to account for that activity.

If the cycle count finds a discrepancy between the on-hand level and the level shown, then the cause of the discrepancy needs to be investigated. Often the discrepancy can be traced to a single error; for example, a box of 22-gauge needles was issued, but a box of 20-gauge needles was entered for that issue. Once the error is discovered, it can be corrected to bring the inventory into balance with the cycle count. In cases where no explanation can be found for an error, the on-hand inventory as shown should be corrected.

Summary

Inventory management is the effort to meet the health care facility's needs for materials, while minimizing the costs of acquiring, storing, and handling. Two aspects of inventory management are identifying and disposing of obsolete stock, and reordering stock at the right time and in the right amount. Changes in the usage patterns for items must be monitored.

Simple but effective manual reordering systems include the two-bin system and the periodic-review system. With these manual reordering systems, a traveling-requisition system can be effective for processing the actual orders.

Another effective reordering system is based on a perpetual inventory, in which the inventory of each item is tracked continually. This can be done manually with a Kardex file. Many health care facilities use computer systems to support a perpetual-inventory system. Computer systems can be an excellent source of information to develop strategies to save money. However, computer systems can only be as good as the accuracy and timeliness of the information entered. Cycle counts can be used to verify the accuracy of the information in a perpetual system.

Appendix A
Central Service Terminology

A

AAMI Association for the Advancement of Medical Instrumentation.

abdomen The part of the body between the chest and the pelvis.

abdominal bag An adherent plastic pouch used to collect fluid and waste material from an abdominal stoma.

abdominal pad (ABD pad) Used over large abdominal suture sites and heavy drainage areas.

abduction Position away from midline of the body.

abortion Termination of pregnancy before the fetus is capable of survival out of the uterus.

abrasive A substance that tends to scrape or wear down by friction.

abscess A localized collection of pus in any area of the body.

absorbent A material that draws up and incorporates another substance.

acid A substance that liberates hydrogen ions in solution; turns litmus paper red; has a pH less than 7.

adaptor A device used for connecting two parts of an apparatus; for example, catheter or syringe.

adduction Position toward the midline of the body.

adenoid Glandular tissue located in the nasopharynx.

adenoma A tumor of glandular tissue.

adhesive Adhering, sticky, or gummed substance adjoinment of surfaces.

adhesive tape A tape coated on one side with an adhesive.

adhesive ties Adhesive tapes with ties attached used to secure abdominal dressings; for example, Montgomery straps or ties.

administration set Tubing used to deliver or dispense fluids; for example, blood or intravenous set.

adrenal Glands that produce hormones essential to life; located above each kidney.

aerate To expose items to warm, circulating air for de-gassing.

aerator A mechanical device designed to remove gaseous residuals from items by subjecting them to warm, circulating air.

aerobe A microorganism that needs the presence of free oxygen to live and grow.

aerosol A suspension of fine solid or liquid particles in the air.

agar Common name for agar-agar; a gelatinous seaweed extract that is added to bacterial media to make it semisolid or solid.

AIDS Acquired immunodeficiency syndrome; disease caused by HIV (human immunodeficiency virus).

air The gaseous mixture that surrounds the earth, which includes invisible, odorless, tasteless gases such as oxygen and nitrogen.

air count The number of bacteria or microbes in a select quantity of air; also called air sampling.

airflow regulator A meter or gauge used to control the amount of air or other gas administered.

air freshener A mechanical device or scented wick or substance used to eliminate odors.

airway A rubber or plastic device that is inserted into the mouth or nose, which reaches to the back of the throat to keep the air passageway open; may be a hollow tube or grooved device.

alcohol prep Sponge saturated with isopropyl alcohol, which is used to clean and disinfect the skin.

alimentation The process or act of giving or receiving nourishment.

alkaline A substance that accepts hydrogen ions; turns litmus paper blue; has a pH greater than 7 (base).

allergen Substance causing an allergy or introducing hypersensitivity.

ambu bag A ventilation bag used to restore breathing in a patient whose respirations have ceased.

amniocentesis Removal of a sample of amniotic fluid from a pregnant uterus via abdominal perforation.

amniotic fluid Fluid that surrounds the fetus.

amputation Removal of a limb or other body appendage, especially by surgery.

anaerobe A microorganism that lives and grows in the absence of free oxygen (open air).

anal Relating to the anus, the rectal opening on the body surface.

anatomy The study of the structure of the human body; the science of the shape and structure of organisms and their parts.

anemia Decreased red cell count or blood hemoglobin level.

anesthesia Partial or complete loss of feeling as a result of disease, injury, or the administration of a gas or drug.

anesthesiologist A physician specializing in the medical study and application of anesthetics.

anesthetic An agent that produces anesthesia. Anesthetics can be general (producing a sound sleep) or local (rendering a specific area insensitive to pain).

anesthetist Person trained to administer anesthetics. The term *nurse anesthetist* refers to a registered nurse with additional training in anesthesia.

aneurysm A sac formed by disease or weakness of the walls of the blood vessels, usually an artery, which fills with blood; associated with life-threatening risk of rupture.

angiocatheter An intravenous catheter used for the administration of intravenous fluids.

angiogram Introduction of a contrast material (radiopaque dye) into the blood vessels for an x-ray photograph.

anhydrous Containing no water.

anionic Carrying a negative charge.

ankle support An elasticized cloth support used to stabilize a sprained or injured ankle.

anoscope An endoscope or speculum used to examine the anal canal.

antibacterial Destroying or stopping the growth of bacteria.

antibody Immunoglobulin, a serum protein developed in response to, and interacting specifically with, an antigen. The antigen-antibody reaction forms the basis of immunity.

anticoagulant Agent that prevents blood coagulation.

anti-embolism Elastic support hose sized to a patient, used to prevent clotting of blood by stockings maintaining continuous pressure on the legs.

antigen A substance introduced into the body, or produced by the body, that induces the formation of antibodies. The antigen-antibody reaction forms the basis of immunity.

antiseptic Chemical that inhibits growth of microorganisms on living tissue.

AORN Association of Operating Room Nurses.

aorta The trunk of the arterial system of the body; the great artery that rises from the left ventricle and carries blood to all arteries of the organs and limbs.

aortogram tray A set of instruments and supplies necessary for introduction of a contrast material (radiopaque dye) into the aorta for an x-ray photograph.

appendectomy Removal of the appendix.

applicator A wooden, plastic, or metal stick with an absorbent tip used for applying a substance.

aquathermia Application of warm or cold water for therapy.

aquathermia control unit A unit containing distilled water powered by an electrical motor, with a temperature gauge on one side and two coupling outlets at the base. These outlets attach to a pad that has recirculating coils. The unit continuously heats the distilled water and pumps distilled water through the pad.

aqueous Water; prepared with water.

arm board A flat piece of wood, plastic, or metal used to stabilize an arm at the wrist or elbow to promote the administration of blood or intravenous feedings.

arteriogram tray A set of instruments and supplies necessary to inject a contrast medium (radiopaque dye) into the bloodstream for an x-ray photograph of an artery or the arterial system.

artery A blood vessel that carries oxygenated blood from the heart to the tissues.

arthrogram The injection of a contrast medium (radiopaque dye) into a joint for an x-ray photograph.

asepsis Freedom from germs, infection, or infectious material; sterile.

aseptic technique Procedure used to maintain sterility or prevent contamination.

asepto syringe A glass or plastic syringe with an attached bulb used for aspiration, irrigation, and feeding.

aspirating tubes Tubes used to obtain and collect fluids for a specimen.

aspiration Act of drawing in by suction.

aspirator A device or instrument that removes fluids or gases from a space by suction; a suction pump, especially used medically to evacuate a body cavity.

athletic supporter Also called "jockstrap"; elastic support for the male genitals.

atomizer A device used to produce a fine spray; nebulizer.

autoclave A device for sterilization by means of saturated steam under pressure.

autoclave film A continuous roll of paper or transparent plastic tubing used for packaging items for steam sterilization.

autoclave tape Tape printed with ink sensitized for heat and moisture used for packaging items for steam sterilization. The ink changes to a dark color during the sterilization process (external indicator).

automatic A self-acting or self-regulating mechanism.

autopsy Examination of a dead body to determine the cause of death; postmortem examination.

axilla The armpit.

axillary Pertaining to, or located near, the armpit.

B

bacillus, bacilli A rod-shaped bacterium.

Bacillus Atrophaeus (formerly called *Bacillus subtilis*) A spore-forming microorganism used in spore form on commercially prepared strips for checking sterilization effectiveness in ethylene oxide, gas plasma, and hot-air sterilizers.

bacteria Plural of bacterium.

bacterial count A method of estimating the number of bacteria in a sample.

bactericide An agent that kills bacteria.

bacteriology The study of bacteria, particularly in relation to medicine and agriculture.

bacteriostasis The stopping or inhibition of bacterial growth and reproduction.

bacterium A single-celled microscopic plant; sometimes pathogenic.

bandage Fabric or gauze used as a protective covering for a wound or other injury.

Band-Aid Trade name for an adhesive bandage with a gauze pad in the center; used as a protection for minor wounds.

bar code A printed array of contrasting bars and spaces that encodes information in a machine-readable form, used to identify materials.

barium sulfate A fine white powder, bulky when mixed with water, used as an opaque medium for x-ray examination of the digestive tract.

barrier Anything that prevents or obstructs passage.

base A substance that accepts hydrogen ions; turns litmus paper blue; has a pH greater than 7.

basin An open, rounded vessel used especially for holding water and other fluids.

bed board A wooden or plastic device, the length and width of a mattress, placed atop bed springs under the mattress to provide very firm support; used especially to treat back problems.

bedpan A metal or plastic receptacle used for receiving urine and feces from the patient confined to bed.

bedsore Decubitus ulcer; an ulcer-like pressure sore over a body prominence due to prolonged confinement in bed or continuous pressure that limits the nutrition of the affected area.

Bennett respirator A mechanical pressure device used to substitute for or assist with breathing in a patient.

benzoin A balsamic resin used as a local antiseptic, a stimulant to promote healing, a protective coating for decubitus ulcers, an expectorant, and an inhalant used in steamers for treating respiratory disorders.

Betadine Trade name for povidone-iodine preparations; used for antiseptic purposes such as handwashes and surgical scrubs and preps.

bevel The angle at which the point of a needle is ground.

bile A yellowish or greenish alkaline fluid secreted by the liver and stored in the gallbladder; used to aid digestion and promote absorption of fats.

bile bag Plastic pouch used to collect bile following gallbladder surgery.

binary fission A form of asexual reproduction of microorganisms; splitting of a nucleus into two nuclei, followed by similar division of the whole cell body.

binder A large band of cloth or elastic worn around the abdomen or chest for support; types of binders include abdominal-elastic, scultetus, breast, chest, and t-binders.

bio Word element meaning life or living.

bioburden The amount of microbial contamination; associated with specific items prior to sterilization.

biological indicator Measured amount of microorganisms on a strip used to show that sterilization conditions were met.

biology The scientific study of plants and animals.

biomedical engineer A person professionally trained in biotechnology and the repair and maintenance of biomedical equipment.

biomedical technician (BEMT) A person trained in the technical aspects of repair and maintenance of biomedical equipment.

biopsy Excision of tissue and the microscopic examination of that tissue.

biopsy needle Needle used for the extraction of tissue for microscopic examination.

biotechnology The engineering and biological study of human beings as related to machines.

Bird respirator A mechanical device used to substitute for or assist in breathing for a patient.

bladder A membranous sac that serves as the receptacle for a liquid; especially the urinary bladder.

bladder irrigation The washing of the urinary bladder with cleansing or therapeutic solutions.

Blakemore esophageal tube A tube with an inflatable balloon used to control esophageal hemorrhaging.

blocking The process of obstructing or deadening.

blood The fluid that circulates throughout a vertebrate animal via the heart, arteries, capillaries, and veins carrying nourishment and oxygen to and removing waste product from all parts of the body.

blood administration set A special tubing used to dispense blood products to a patient.

blood bank Place where blood is typed, tested, and stored until it is needed for transfusion.

bloodborne pathogens Microorganisms that are present in human blood and can produce disease in humans.

blood collection set A special tubing used to extract and collect blood.

blood gas tray A collection of supplies and equipment necessary to determine the oxygen and carbon dioxide levels in the blood.

blood pressure Pressure exerted on the blood vessels by the blood.

blood pressure cuff A secured band positioned on an arm above the elbow, with tubing attached to a sphygmomanometer, used to apply pressure against an artery to measure the blood pressure of the artery wall.

blood pump Cuff with hand pump; used for rapid infusion of blood.

blow bottles Containers used for intermittent positive pressure exercises for the lungs.

body restraint A device such as a belt, vest, or net used to safely immobilize a patient.

boil To heat a fluid to the point of bubbling and turning the fluid into a gaseous state; furuncle, a pus-filled, painful swelling of the skin and subcutaneous tissue caused by bacterial infection.

bone marrow The soft, sponge-like material in the cavities of bones made up of blood vessels, connective tissue, fat, and blood-producing cells.

bone marrow needle Needle used to extract marrow from a bone for examination.

boric acid A white or colorless crystalline powder used in solution as a mild antiseptic, especially for the skin and eyes. Boric acid ointment is used for mild skin irritations such as blisters; for external use only; highly toxic if taken internally.

borosilicate Silicate glass used especially in heat-resistant glassware (Pyrex).

bowel Intestine; the digestive tract below the stomach.

Bowie-Dick Test A test, originated by J. H. Bowie and J. Dick, designed to challenge the vacuum pump in a prevacuum steam sterilizer.

box lock The point where two parts of the instrument jaws or blades connect or pivot.

breast binder A supportive band of cloth or elastic device that holds the breasts firmly in proper position; used postpartum and postoperatively.

breast prosthesis An internal or external replacement of, or addition to, a breast by an artificial substitute.

breast pump A device used to extract and collect milk from the breast.

bulb syringe Rubber or plastic syringe used for suctioning and irrigating ears, or the nasal and oral cavities of infants; an asepto syringe.

butterfly anal dressing Butterfly-shaped, moist, medicated gauze dressing dispensed from a jar; used for anal cleansing and analgesic and anal surgery.

butterfly infusion set A scalp vein set; short intravenous catheter with tubing used for intravenous fluid administration.

C

CABG See *coronary artery bypass graft.*

cadaver A dead body usually intended for dissection.

Caesarean section See *cesarean section.*

calcium gluconate A compound used in solution to replenish calcium in the body.

cannula, canula A tube used for insertion into a body cavity to drain fluid or inject medication.

capillary A minute blood vessel that connects the smallest arteries to the smallest veins.

carbon dioxide (CO_2) A heavy, colorless gas used with oxygen to stimulate respiration.

carcinogenic Having the ability to produce or cause cancer.

cardiac arrest Sudden and often unexpected stoppage of the heartbeat.

cardiologist A physician who specializes in cardiology.

cardiology The study of the heart and its functions and diseases.

cardiovascular Pertaining to the heart and blood vessels.

carotid angiogram The injection of radiopaque dye into the bloodstream to observe the blood circulation to the brain by means of x-rays.

carotid artery Either of two principal arteries of the neck that carry blood to the head.

carpal Refers to the bones in the wrist.

carrier A person or an animal harboring pathogenic microorganisms that is at least temporarily immune to the organisms but transmits them directly or indirectly to others.

cataract Cloudiness of the lens of the eye.

catheter A slender, flexible tube made up of such materials as rubber, plastic, or metal, used for draining a body cavity or injecting fluids through a body passage; intravenous, nasal, and urinary catheters.

catheter care kit A set of instruments and supplies used to clean the genitalia surrounding an indwelling urinary catheter.

catheter guide An instrument used to direct catheters into position in the body cavity.

catheter irrigation tray A set of instruments and supplies used for the cleansing of a canal such as the urinary bladder.

catheterization The introduction of a catheter into a body passageway.

cationic Carrying a positive charge.

caudal anesthesia A regional anesthesia used in childbirth. An anesthetic agent is injected into the caudal area of the spine via the lower end of the sacrum, deadening nerves affecting the cervix, vagina, and perineum.

cautery A method of destroying tissue by electricity, heat, or caustic chemicals; used to treat decubitus ulcers and to seal blood vessels (bleeders) during a surgical procedure.

cavitation The rapid formation and collapse of low-pressure bubbles in liquids by means of mechanical forces; the process used by an ultrasonic cleaner in which the bubbles implode (burst inward) and dislodge the soil off the instruments.

CBC Complete blood count; commonly performed group of hematological tests.

CDC Centers for Disease Control.

ceiling limit (CL) An airborne concentration of a hazardous substance that should never be exceeded.

cell The smallest structural unit of living organisms capable of performing all the basic functions of life.

Celsius A temperature scale having the freezing point of water at 0 degrees and boiling point at 100 degrees, developed by Anders Celsius; also called Centigrade.

central service department (CSD) The department that processes, stores, and distributes medical and surgical supplies and equipment; also referred to as supply processing distribution (SPD).

central venous pressure set (CVP) A device used to measure pressure within the veins.

centrifuge A machine using the centrifugal force of rotation to separate substances of different densities.

cervical Referring to the neck; a neck-like part of an organ.

cervical collar An extra firm, contoured band of molded foam rubber or a similar synthetic material covered with stockinette; used to support neck injuries such as a whiplash.

cervical halter A traction device prescribed for certain neck injuries or surgical procedures.

cesarean section Incision into the uterus through the abdominal wall to deliver a fetus.

chafing A reddened irritation of the skin caused by friction.

chamber An enclosed space or cavity of a sterilizer.

charge system A method of accounting for each item issued and charged to a patient or department.

chelating agent Chemical reaction which prevents soaps or detergents from reacting with the minerals in water.

chemical indicator A device used to monitor certain parameters of a sterilization process by means of a characteristic color change; for example, chemical-treated paper strips, pellet sealed in a glass tube.

chest stripper Instrument used to remove tissue from rib bones.

chest trocar Thoracic trocar; a large-handled instrument with a sharp triangular tip used with a cannula to remove fluid from the chest cavity.

chiropractor A specialist in treating disease by manipulation of the spinal column.

chloride A compound of chlorine and another element.

cholangiogram The injection of a radiopaque dye to observe the common bile duct by means of x-rays.

chronic A constant, continuous, long-term illness.

cidal Word element meaning having the power to kill, such as bacteriacidal (will kill bacteria).

circular electric bed An electrically powered, circular framed bed that promotes circulation in a bedridden patient by slow, continuous rotation of the body.

circulation Continuous movement of blood through the vessels of the body resulting from the pumping action of the heart.

circumcision Excision of the foreskin of the glans of the penis.

CL Abbreviation for "ceiling limit"; an airborne concentration of a hazardous substance in the work environment, which by law should never be exceeded.

clamp A surgical device such as a hemostat used to compress blood vessels or tubing.

clean catch urine A urine sample collected after the urethral opening and surrounding tissues have been cleansed.

cleft lip A congenital separation or division of the lip.

clinical case Pertaining to actual observation and treatment of a patient as a clinical or bedside case as opposed to a theoretical or experimental case.

clip remover An instrument used for the extraction or removal of metal clips from surgical wounds.

coagulation Formation of a fibrin clot to help stop bleeding.

coagulation factors Proteins present in plasma that interact to form a fibrin clot.

coccus, cocci Spherical or oval-shaped bacterium.

collar, cervical See *cervical collar.*

collodion A gluey substance used as a protective coating for some skin conditions and to hold surgical dressings in place.

colon The large intestine.

colony A visible, circumscribed mass of bacteria growing in or on a solid or semisolid medium; assumed to have grown from a single organism. A collection of microorganisms in a culture.

colony count A method of estimating the number of bacteria in a sample.

colostomy The surgical creation of an opening made at the surface of the abdomen for the purpose of evacuating the bowels and to act as a substitute for the rectum and anus.

colostomy appliance set A ringed plastic bag, surgical adhesive, and an elastic waist belt used to cover the colostomy for fecal collection.

colostomy belts An elastic waist band that fits around a patient to hold the colostomy bag for fecal collection.

colostomy irrigation A kit containing a plastic irrigation bag and tubing, catheter, connector, and appliance collection bag for fecal material; used for irrigation to regulate the colostomy.

colostomy pouch A ringed, adhesive backed, plastic bag that fits over the stoma of the colostomy to collect fecal material.

combustible Ability to undergo a chemical process accompanied by the emission of heat, typically by combination with oxygen.

commode Portable toilet.

commode pan A pail-like removable receptacle for a portable toilet.

communicable disease An illness that can be transmitted from one person to another, directly or indirectly.

complication An added difficulty, such as a secondary condition developing in addition to the primary disease.

compress Material such as gauze or cloth folded and firmly pressed to a body part to prevent hemorrhage or moistened with water or medication to reduce inflammation or pain.

compressed air Air under greater than atmospheric pressure.

compression The act of squeezing together.

compressor A machine that compresses gases such as air.

concentration The amount of a specified substance in a unit amount of another substance.

condom A rubber sheath designed to cover the penis during sexual intercourse to prevent infection or conception.

condom drainage unit A device used as an external catheter for males.

conduction heating Heat is transmitted in solids from molecule to molecule.

connecting tubing Rubber or plastic tubing used to connect catheters and tubing to pump or drainage units.

contagious Transmitted or communicable by contact.

contaminated linen Any linen that has been soiled with blood or other potentially infectious materials.

contaminated sharps Any contaminated object that can penetrate the skin, including, but not limited to, needles, scalpels, broken glass, broken capillary tubes, and exposed ends of dental wires.

contaminated waste Potentially infectious materials disposed of by health facilities, such as soiled dressings, sharps, and fluids.

contamination The presence of pathogenic microorganisms on or in an object.

continuous quality improvement (CQI) An organized system to continually improve process outcomes and service.

contrast agent Medium used by a radiologist in reading x-ray film; administered to the patient before the x-ray procedure.

convalescence A period of recovery from an illness, operation, or injury.

convection heating The transfer of heat in fluid from one place to another by motion of the fluid.

copious A large amount; overflowing.

coronary artery bypass graft (CABG) A surgical procedure to restore the blood flow to the heart by bypassing clogged coronary arteries, usually with a saphenous vein graft taken from the leg.

corrosion Process of wearing away the surface of a solid.

cot, finger See *finger cot.*

cotton balls Circular spun-cotton pledget used to cleanse, apply medications, or absorb discharge from a wound.

cotton elastic bandage A pressure dressing made of stretchable cotton fabric with interwoven strands of rubber.

cotton-tipped applicators Firmly wound tufts of cotton bonded to a stick used to cleanse or apply medications.

Coude catheter Olive-tip catheter with a single drainage eye; used for male patients with urinary strictures.

cranial Pertaining to the cranium.

craniotomy Opening of the skull to allow surgery of the brain.

cranium Skull; bony covering of the brain.

Creutzfeldt-Jakob disease (CJD) A chronic, fatal disease of the central nervous system; it is very difficult to destroy the prion that causes this disease.

cross-contamination The transfer of contaminants from one person or object to another.

cross-infection Infection transmitted among hospital patients or staff infected with different pathogenic organisms.

crutch An artificial support made of wood or metal to aid a patient unable to walk due to injury, disease, or other defects.

crutch pad A rubber pad used over the arm piece of a crutch to cushion the underarm.

crutch tip Rubber tip used on the bottom of a crutch to reduce slipping.

cryotherapy The use of low temperatures for medical therapy to a part of the body.

CT scan Computed tomographic scan that provides images of the inside of the body.

culture To cultivate bacteria in a nutrient medium; a mass of growing bacteria.

culture tube A glass or plastic tubular container used to house microorganisms for growth.

curette, curet A scooped or spoon-shaped surgical instrument used for scraping dead tissue or growths from a body cavity.

cutdown A procedure creating an incision in order to reach a vein; used for passage of an intravenous catheter to administer intravenous (IV) fluids or transfusions.

CV Cardiovascular.

CVP Central venous pressure.

cycle time A time interval during which a succession or recurring series of events is completed.

cysto Word element meaning bladder or cyst.

cystodrape Drape used to cover the area surrounding the genitalia for genitourinary surgery.

cystogram Injection of a radiopaque dye into the bladder for an x-ray photograph.

cystoscope An endoscope fitted with a light; designed to pass through the urethra to visually examine the bladder and ureters.

cystoscopy Visual inspection of interior of the bladder and examination of adjacent structures by means of an instrument introduced through the urethra.

D

debridement The surgical removal of dead or nonliving tissue.

decontamination Process that removes or reduces the number of infectious agents on items and renders reusable medical products safe for handling.

Decontamination Area The designated place in central service in which instruments, supplies, and equipment are made safe for handling.

decubitus ulcer See *bedsore.*

defibrillator A device used to apply a brief electroshock to restore the rhythm of a defibrillating heart.

degree C A reading of a Celsius or Centigrade scale.

degree F A reading of a Fahrenheit scale.

density Quality of being massed close together.

depigmentation Loss of skin color.

detergent A water-soluble cleaning agent that has wetting and emulsifying properties.

detergent/germicide An agent that combines cleaning and disinfecting actions.

dextrose Glucose; a sugar considered one of the most important carbohydrates, making up 80 percent of all simple sugar absorbed into the bloodstream.

dextrose 5 percent lactated Ringer's solution An intravenous solution used for fluid and electrolyte replacement.

dextrose 5 percent saline solution An intravenous solution used for fluid and body salt replacement.

dextrose 5 percent 0.25 saline An intravenous solution used for fluid replacement in dehydrated patients.

dextrose 5 percent 0.33 sodium chloride An intravenous solution used to open a vein before administering whole blood.

dextrose 5 percent water An intravenous solution used as a source of calories and water.

dextrose 10 percent saline An intravenous solution used as a calorie and salt supplement.

dextrose 20 percent water An intravenous solution, diuretic in action, that may be used to reduce edema.

dilation and curettage (D&C) Surgical procedure to scrape the inner walls of the uterus.

dilator An instrument or drug that expands an organ or body part.

disease A condition of a living animal or plant body or of one of its parts that impairs the performance of a vital function.

disinfectant A chemical agent that destroys, neutralizes, or inhibits the growth of pathogenic microorganisms on inanimate objects.

disinfection The process of freeing from infection by destroying microorganisms.

disposable An item or product designed to be used only once and discarded.

distillation The process by which a liquid such as water is heated to a vapor form, cooled, and then collected as a condensate with impurities removed.

distilled water The condensate collection of water boiled (distilled) to remove impurities.

distribution The act or condition of allotting, dispensing, and delivering medical and surgical supplies and equipment.

douche A stream of water or a vapor directed against a body part or cavity for cleansing and medical applications.

drain A tube inserted into the opening of a wound or cavity to promote discharge of fluids.

drainage bag A plastic bag with connecting tubing used to collect fluid from patients with indwelling drains.

drape Woven or nonwoven protective cloth used to maintain sterility.

dressing A bandage or covering for an external wound.

dry-heat sterilizer Hot-air sterilizer; an oven-like apparatus powered by electricity to sterilize items by subjecting them to high temperatures for long exposure periods.

dust cover A plastic cover placed over packaged sterilized products to help maintain sterility by protecting the package from the environment.

dysentery Inflamed condition of intestines accompanied by pain and diarrhea.

dysfunction Impaired or abnormal function.

E

ear syringe A ringed syringe used for irrigation of the ear.

ectopic pregnancy Pregnancy in which the fertilized ovum is implanted outside the uterus.

EL See *excursion limit.*

elastic bandage A flexible, stretchable fabric made with interwoven strands of rubber; used as a pressure dressing.

electrocardiogram (EKG) The tracing or recording of the electric impulses of the heart.

electroencephalogram (EEG) The tracing or recording of the electric impulses of the brain.

electrolytes Ionized salts in blood, tissue fluids, and cells, including salts of sodium, potassium, and chlorine.

electronic thermometer An electric device with disposable probe used to take oral and rectal temperatures.

electron irradiation Procedure used by some manufacturers for commercial sterilization.

emergency room, emergency department (ER or ED) Area in which patients are received, evaluated, and treated; usually involves treatment for disease or injury that cannot wait for a visit to a doctor's office.

Emerson suction pump A three-bottle suction unit with a variety of pressures used for thoracic suction.

emulsion A mixture of two liquids not mutually soluble; the process of breaking up oils and fats into small particles, which are held in suspension, making it easier to clean items.

encephalogram The injection of air into the cerebrospinal canal to allow for an x-ray photograph of the brain.

endocardial Pertaining to or within the heart.

endoscope A device consisting of a tube with a lens used to examine a body organ or cavity.

endotracheal Pertaining to or within the trachea.

enema Injection of fluid into the rectum for cleansing.

engineering controls Items that isolate or remove such hazards as bloodborne pathogens from the workplace (e.g., sharps disposal containers, self-sheathing needles, etc.).

environment The circumstances, objects, or conditions by which one is surrounded.

enzyme Protein substance produced by living matter, which produces a reaction in another substance without changing itself.

epidemic disease An outbreak of sudden rapid spread and growth of an infectious disease.

epidemiologist A specialist in epidemic diseases.

epistaxis To bleed from the nose.

ergonomics The study of physical capacities in relation to the demands of various kinds of work.

esophageoscope An endoscope used to visually examine the esophagus.

ethylene oxide (EtO) A gaseous sterilant used for instruments and supplies that cannot withstand high heat or humidity.

ethylene oxide sterilizer A sterilizer with a locked chamber and humidity control used to sterilize instruments, supplies, and other items that cannot withstand high heat or humidity.

evacuation The act of vacating or emptying a body cavity, or an area (such as evacuating staff and patients from a hospital in a fire).

eye mask Covering used to keep dressings in position following eye or cataract surgery.

eye pad An oval gauze dressing used on the eye to absorb drainage.

eye shield A device used to cover and protect the eye.

exam gloves Disposable gloves made from a latex-free material or vinyl worn for protection during patient contact.

excrete To eliminate or separate waste matter from an organism.

excursion limit (EL) A certain amount of a hazardous substance beyond which a person should not be exposed to in a specified period—e.g., EtO EL is 5 ppm in 15 minutes.

expiration date A date assigned to sterile products to determine shelf life.

exposure The total time that materials are subjected to a sterilization process; the act of being subjected to potentially infectious or hazardous materials.

exposure incident A specific eye, mouth, other mucous membrane, or non-intact skin contact with blood, or other potentially infectious materials that results from the performance of an employee's duties.

F

Fahrenheit A temperature scale having the freezing point of water at 32 degrees and the boiling point at 212 degrees, developed by Gabriel Fahrenheit.

fallopian tube Tube extending from near the ovary to the uterus, which conveys the ovum from the ovary to the uterus.

FDA Food and Drug Administration; agency of the U.S. Department of Health and Human Services with the responsibility for protecting the public against poisoning, contamination, or any other health hazard in foods. This agency also ensures the safety and effectiveness of drugs, commercially manufactured medical devices, high-level disinfectants, and sterilants.

feces Bodily waste discharged from the intestine.

feeding tube A nasogastric tube used as a pathway to the stomach for the feeding of liquids and semisolid foods.

felt A fabric of matted, compressed fibers used as padding for orthopedic procedures.

femoral Pertaining to the femur or thigh bone.

fenestrated Having one or more openings.

fetal Pertaining to a fetus.

fetus The unborn child in the uterus from the third month of development to birth.

fever A rise of body temperature above normal.

fiberoptic A bundle of thread-like flexible, transparent fibers used in an instrument to transmit light and images (such as for viewing body cavities).

filiform Thread-shaped; used to dilate narrow ureteral strictures.

finger cot A small rubber shield placed over a finger for protection against soiling or infectious materials.

flatus Gas generated in the stomach or bowels.

flora Plant life; more specifically, plants adapted for living in a specific environment or period.

fluffs A postoperative dressing; loosely woven and folded gauze.

Foley catheter A double lumen rubber or plastic indwelling urethral catheter with a balloon, which when inflated holds the catheter within the bladder.

Foley catheter plug A stopper used to plug the lumen of a Foley catheter.

fomite An object, such as a book, an item made of wood, or an article of clothing that is not in itself harmful but is able to harbor pathogenic microorganisms and therefore may serve as an agent of transmission of infection.

footboard A device placed at the foot of a bed to support the proper alignment of the foot; used to prevent foot drop.

forceps Surgical instrument designed for extracting, grasping, or manipulating.

formaldehyde A chemical used chiefly as a preservative and disinfectant.

Fox postnasal balloon A device with an inflatable cuff used to stop nosebleeds.

fracture bedpan Receptacle designed for collection of urine and feces for patients with fractures or in body casts.

fungicidal A chemical that destroys fungi.

fungus A vegetative organism that lives off organic matter.

G

gag A device placed in the mouth to keep it open.

gamma radiation Used in radiotherapy and by some manufacturers for commercial sterilization.

gangrene Local death of soft tissues due to loss of blood supply.

gasket A seal such as is used around the inside of a sterilizer door to prevent the escape of steam or gas.

gastric connecting tube Tubing used to connect a nasogastric tube to a suction collection container.

gastric lavage tray A collection of instruments and supplies used to irrigate or wash out the stomach to remove ingested poisons.

gastric suction unit A device that aspirates gastric and intestinal contents.

gastric tube A tube made of rubber or plastic that is inserted into the stomach.

gastroscope An endoscope designed for passage into the stomach to examine its interior.

gauge A standard of measurement.

gauze A surgical dressing made of loosely woven cotton threads.

gauze roller A long strip of gauze in various sizes used to wrap around a dressing.

gavage Introduction of material into the stomach by means of a tube.

Geobacillus stearothermophilus (formerly called *Bacillus stearothermophilus*) A highly heat-resistant spore-forming microorganism used in spore form on commercially prepared strips for checking sterilization effectiveness in steam, ozone, and peracetic sterilizers.

geriatrics A branch of medicine that deals with the problems and diseases of old age and aging patients.

germ A microorganism that causes disease.

germicide An agent (such as liquid or gas) used specifically to destroy microorganisms on inanimate objects.

gland An organ that produces a certain substance and secretes this substance into the body.

gloves Covering for the hands; used to protect the patient or wearer.

glucometer Instrument to measure the glucose level in blood.

glucose A sweet, colorless, soluble sugar that occurs widely in nature.

glutaraldehyde A chemical compound used in aqueous solution as a disinfectant and sterilant.

glycerin Liquid used as a solvent, lubricant, and sweetener.

glycerin/lemon swab Small wad of material used for oral hygiene.

graduate A container marked with graduations; used for liquid measurement.

gram The basic metric unit of weight or mass.

Gram-negative Refers to bacteria that are decolorized in the Gram stain, and pink-red in color after counterstaining.

Gram-positive Refers to bacteria that retain the crystal violet dye in the Gram stain; purple-blue in color.

Gram stain A stain that differentiates bacteria according to the chemical composition of the cell walls.

gynecologist A doctor specializing in gynecology.

gynecology That branch of medicine dealing with diseases and disorders of the female reproductive system.

H

hazardous waste Waste material harmful to human health or the environment if not treated properly.

head halter An orthopedic device used to position the head for cervical traction.

health care The prevention, treatment, and management of illness and the preservation of mental and physical well-being through the services offered by the medical and allied health professions.

heart-lung machine A pump-oxygenator that temporarily takes over the functions of the heart and lungs during open heart surgery.

heat resistant An inanimate or animate object that is generally unaffected by the application of heat.

heat sensitive An organism that is readily affected or damaged by the application of heat.

heel/elbow cushion A padded covering designed to fit over the heel or elbow for prevention of pressure sores.

hematology The science concerned with the study of blood, blood cells, and blood-forming tissues.

hematoma The swelling of tissue around a vessel due to leakage of blood from the vessel into the tissue.

hematuria Presence of red blood cells in the urine.

hemiplegia Paralysis of one side of the body, usually caused by a stroke.

hemo Prefix meaning blood.

hemoglobin A red blood cell constituent, which is composed of heme and globin, and which carries oxygen.

hemorrhage Excessive or uncontrolled bleeding.

hemostasis Process of stopping blood flow.

hemostat A forceps used to clamp off a blood vessel.

Hepa A filter or respirator that does not allow very fine particles to pass through it; Hepa respirators are used when caring for patients with active TB.

heparin An anticoagulant.

hepatitis B (HBV) A bloodborne pathogenic virus that can cause inflammation of the liver. An infected person can be symptomatic or asymptomatic. Symptoms include jaundice, flu-like manifestations, and liver failure. The viral incubation period can vary from 4 to 25 weeks. An effective HBV vaccine is available.

hernia An abnormal protrusion of a body part through the containing structure.

hexachlorophene A phenol-based skin antiseptic used for handwashing; effective only against Gram-positive bacteria and relatively slow-acting compared to other skin antiseptics.

high-vacuum steam sterilizer Sterilizer that uses a vacuum pump to remove air from the chamber, making it faster than a gravity-displacement sterilizer to complete a sterilization cycle.

HIV Human immunodeficiency virus.

hospital An institution that provides medical, surgical, or psychiatric care and treatment for the sick or the injured.

hot pack Moist, heated dressings for therapeutic treatment.

humerus Bone of the upper arm from the shoulder to the elbow.

hydrogen peroxide An oxidizing and bleaching agent.

hygiene A science of the establishment and maintenance of health.

hypertension High blood pressure.

hyperthermia High fever; producing heat by physical means.

hyperthermia unit A device designed to pump heated or cooled water through a coiled pad to therapeutically raise or lower body temperature.

hypodermic needle A hollow needle used for injections or for obtaining fluid specimens.

hypotension Low blood pressure.

hypothermia Subnormal temperature of the body.

I

ice pack A rubber or plastic bag filled with ice to produce cold.

ileostomy appliance Device used to fit over a stoma for fecal collection.

immune Having a high degree of resistance to a disease.

immunity Resistance to disease or infection.

immunization Process by which an antibody is produced in response to an antigen, which protects against a specific disease.

impervious Material that resists fluids, especially body fluids, such as gowns, aprons, and surgical drapes.

implode Bursting inward.

inanimate Not alive.

incision A cut made by a knife, especially for surgical purposes.

incompatible Unsuitable for use together because of undesirable chemical or physiological effects.

incontinent pad Material placed under a patient to collect any drainage or excrement.

incubate To maintain bacterial culture under conditions favorable for growth.

incubator Temperature-controlled chamber into which inoculated media are placed so that bacterial growth will occur.

indicators See *specific indicator; i.e., biological, chemical, mechanical.*

indwelling (catheter) Held in place within a part of the body, especially in the bladder.

infection Invasion of pathogenic microorganisms on or into the body or body parts, which causes injury in susceptible persons.

infectious Spreading or capable of spreading germs rapidly to others.

infectious waste Waste that potentially contains sufficient numbers of pathogens with sufficient virulence so that exposure into a susceptible host could result in an infectious disease.

inflammation A tissue reaction to injury in which swelling is present.

infusion The continuous slow introduction of a solution into a vein.

injection To introduce a substance into the body.

inoculation The intentional introduction of certain organisms into the body to protect against subsequent infection.

inorganic Material composed of other than plant or animal substances.

insecticide An agent that destroys insects.

inspect To view closely in critical appraisal.

instrument A device used in medical procedures, especially surgery, normally handheld and made of stainless steel.

insulin Hormone produced by the pancreas responsible for the control of carbohydrate metabolism.

intermittent suction A suction device that starts and stops suctioning at periodic intervals.

internal On the inside.

intracatheter A plastic tube inserted within a vein for infusion, injection, or monitoring.

intravenous Within a vein; an injection or infusion introduced into a vein.

intubate The introduction of a tube into a hollow organ.

invalid ring An inflatable plastic or rubber ring used to relieve sacral pressure.

inventory The quantity of goods or materials on hand; stock; catalog or list of materials on hand.

iodoform A yellow crystalline, volatile compound with a penetrating, persistent odor used in an antiseptic dressing.

iodophor A complex of iodine and a surface-active agent that releases iodine gradually and serves as a disinfectant.

ion An atom or molecule with an electric charge; the atoms or molecules into which electrolyte molecules are divided in solution.

irrigation The flushing or cleaning of a body part or wound by means of a stream of solution.

isolate To set apart from others.

isolation To set apart or quarantine a patient with a communicable disease from others.

J

jaundice Yellowness of the skin and eyes; a symptom of hepatitis.

JCAHO Joint Commission on Accreditation of Healthcare Organizations. A regulatory organization whose purpose is to encourage the attainment of uniformly high standards of institutional medical care, establish guidelines for the operation of hospitals and other health care facilities, and conduct survey and accreditation programs.

jelly lubricant A water-soluble lubricant used to facilitate the introduction of catheters and tubes.

Julian calendar A calendar introduced in Rome in 46 B.C. establishing the 12-month year of 365 days, with each fourth year (called a "leap" year) having 366 days, and the months each having 31 or 30 days, except for February with only 28 days or in leap years 29 days.

just-in-time A distribution method that involves receiving materials just as they are needed. This type of system permits lower levels of inventory and overstock.

K

Kelly hemostatic forceps An instrument used for grasping.

kidney, ureter, and bladder (KUB) X-ray of the kidney, ureter, and bladder.

knee supporter An elastic binder used to support a weak or injured knee.

L

laceration A torn and ragged wound.

lactated Ringer's solution Mixture used for fluid and electrolyte replacement.

lancet A sterile, sharp, pointed blade, which can be used to perform a capillary puncture.

laparoscope A long, slender optical instrument for insertion through the abdominal wall, which is used to visualize the interior of the peritoneal cavity.

laryngoscope A device used for direct visual examination of the larynx.

laser Light amplification by stimulated emission of radiation; high-energy beam of light.

lateral Toward the side of midline of the body.

leg bag A plastic urinary drainage bag connected to a urinary catheter.

lens A transparent material curved on one or both sides, which spreads or focuses light.

lens paper A special nonabrasive material used to clean optical lenses.

lesion An abnormal change in structure of an organ or part due to injury or disease.

leukocyte White blood cell (WBC).

Levin tube Hollow tube used for gastric and intestinal aspiration or tube feeding.

limb holder A canvas device used to support an arm or leg.

linen pack Linens packaged together to be used for draping or donning by staff, usually for surgical procedures.

lipid Organic compound that contains fats.

liter A basic metric unit of volume; equal to 1,000 milliliters; slightly greater than 1 quart.

lithotripsy Crushing of calculi or stones in the bladder or urethra.

load control A number affixed to a sterilized item showing the date of sterilization, sterilizer number, and load number; used for stock rotation and recall.

lumen The open space within a tubular organ, catheter, or instrument.

lymphangiogram An injection of a contrast medium into the lymphatic channels to take an x-ray photograph.

M

magnetic resonance imaging (MRI) Imaging device that creates images by detecting the magnitude and behavior imaging of the hydrogen nuclei in the human body.

maintenance A program for controlling and keeping equipment in good working condition.

Malecot catheter Device with a particular retaining mechanism used for drainage of the body cavities, especially for suprapubic urinary drainage.

malpractice A dereliction from professional duty or a failure to exercise an accepted degree of professional skill.

mammogram X-ray photograph of the breast, sometimes with contrast medium injected into the breast.

mammoplasty Plastic repair of the breast to enlarge or reduce or to reconstruct after surgical removal of a tumor.

mask A protective covering worn on the face over the nose and mouth.

materials management The department that oversees and coordinates negotiations, purchasing, control, and distribution of medical supplies and equipment.

mechanical indicators Devices built into a machine used in identifying and preventing malfunctions and operational errors.

medical analyses The health profession concerned with the performance of laboratory technology used in the diagnosis and treatment of disease, as well as in health maintenance.

memory A general term referring to the recollection of what was once experienced or learned; space in a computer where data are stored; in CSD, wrapping material that tries to go back to its original position when unfolded has memory.

menopause The period during which the menstrual cycle slows down and eventually stops.

menstruation Discharge of blood and tissue from the uterus normally occurring every 28 days.

meter A basic metric unit of distance or length; one meter equals about 39.37 inches.

microbiology The science or study of microorganisms such as bacteria, fungi, and viruses.

microdrip An intravenous adaptor with a drop control that emits a drop 1/10 the size of a regular drop.

micron A unit of measurement equal to 1 millionth of a meter; also called a micrometer; 1/25,000 of an inch.

microorganism An organism of microscopic or ultramicroscopic size.

microscope Optical instrument consisting of a lens or combination of lenses for making enlarged images of minute objects.

micturition Passing of urine; urination.

midstream urine A urine sample collected in the middle of voiding.

moisture sensitive Unable to withstand dampness.

Montgomery straps Adhesive strips used to hold dressings in place; dressing can be changed without removing the strips.

morgue An area where bodies of deceased persons are kept until identified and claimed by relatives or released for burial.

MRI See *magnetic resonance imaging.*

MRSA Methacillin-resistant *Staphylococcus aureus;* a microorganism that is resistant to all but one (vancomycin) antibiotic.

MSDS Material safety data sheet; record containing specific required information (such as manufacturer's emergency telephone number, exposure limit, hazards, first aid, personnel protective equipment, spill procedure), which must be available to workers for each chemical—liquid or gas—that they are potentially exposed to.

mucous membrane The lining of passages and cavities of the body that open to the air.

mucus A viscid, slippery fluid secreted by the mucous membrane.

mutate A change in the nucleus of a cell that differs from the original cell and constitutes a new variety of cell.

myelogram An injection of a contrast medium (radiopaque dye) into the spinal cord to take an x-ray picture.

N

nasal Pertaining to the nose.

nasal cannula Device used for oxygen administration via the nose.

nasal catheter Catheter with side openings and an open end tip used for administration of oxygen via the nose.

nasal packing Material used for packing the nose to stop nasal hemorrhaging.

nasogastric tube Hollow tube used for feeding or aspiration of gastric contents.

natal Pertaining to birth.

needle A slender, hollow instrument for introducing material into or removing material from the body.

neonatal Concerning the newborn.

neurologist A doctor specializing in the treatment and diagnosis of disease of, or injury to, the nervous system.

neurology The branch of medicine that deals with the diagnosis and treatment of disorders or diseases of the nervous system.

nipple shield Cover worn over a nursing breast to protect the natural nipple.

nonionic Not carrying any electric charge.

nonwoven A fabric made by bonding fibers together as opposed to weaving of threads.

nosocomial infection Infection acquired in the hospital.

nuclear medicine Specialty dealing with moderate amounts of radioactive materials used in diagnostic procedures in radiology.

nucleus The vital part of a cell that controls metabolism, growth, reproduction, and transmission of characteristics of a cell.

nurse Professional skilled or trained in the caring for the sick.

O

OB pads Extra-long sanitary pads used to absorb vaginal flow following the birth of a child.

obstetrician A doctor who practices obstetrics.

obstetrics The branch of medicine that deals with pregnancy and childbirth.

occlude To close or bring together.

ocular Of the eye; eyepiece of an optical instrument.

opened but unused Single-use disposable device whose sterility has been breached or compromised or whose sterile package was opened even though the device had not been used on a patient or been in contact with blood or body fluids.

operating suite A room in surgery designed for performing a surgical procedure.

operation A procedure performed on a living body.

ophthalmoscope An instrument used to examine the inside of the eye.

oral hygiene swab Treated applicator used to clean the mouth.

oral suction catheter Hollow tube used to aspirate oral and nasal cavities.

oral suction machine A device used to suction liquids and mucus from the oral and nasal cavities.

organic Having the characteristics of living organisms.

orthopedic felt Material used for a cushioning effect under casts and splints.

orthopedics Specialty concerned with the correction or prevention of skeletal deformities.

OSHA Occupational Safety and Health Administration; a federal agency created to provide regulations and standard working conditions for all employees and to investigate possible hazards in the work environment, protecting the safety of workers.

osmosis Passage of a substance through a membrane that is separating different concentrations of solutions, from lower to higher concentration.

otoscope An instrument used to examine the inner ear.

ovum Female reproductive cell.

oxygen mask Covering used to facilitate the administration of oxygen.

oxygen saturation The ratio of oxygen volume carried by the blood to the potential oxygen-carrying capacity of the blood.

P

pancreas A large fleshy gland located behind the stomach that secretes a digestive fluid and insulin.

paracentesis Puncture of a cavity to remove fluid, often from the abdomen.

paramedic Person who works in a health care field in an ancillary capacity with a professional.

paraplegia Paralysis of the legs and sometimes the lower part of the body, usually caused by an injury to the spinal cord.

parenteral Denoting any route for introducing substances other than the alimentary canal.

passivation A process used during the latter part of the manufacture of stainless steel instruments, which provides a layer resistant to corrosion.

pasteurization Process of immersing cleaned items in a water bath heated to 160 to 180°F (65 to 77°C) for at least 30 minutes to achieve intermediate-level disinfection.

pathogen An organism or agent that causes disease.

pathogenic Causing or capable of causing a disease.

pathologist A physician especially trained in the cause and nature of disease.

pathology The study of the essential nature of diseases.

PCA Patient-controlled analgesia; a machine that dispenses a controlled amount of an analgesic.

pediatrics A branch of medicine dealing with the development, care, and diseases of children.

PEL Permissible exposure limits; an exposure limit to some form of hazard that is published and enforced by OSHA as a legal-limit standard.

pelvic sling A device that supports the pelvis.

pelvis A basin-shaped structure in the skeleton of many vertebrates that is formed by the pelvic girdle and adjoins bones of the spine.

pelvis traction Traction applied to the back by use of a belt that encircles a patient's waist with weights attached.

penicillin An antibiotic used to treat and prevent bacterial infections.

penile implant Surgical insertion of a prosthesis to enable the patient to obtain an erection.

Peracetic acid (peroxyacetic acid) A neutral-pH liquid chemical solution that destroys microorganisms and is used as a low-temperature sterilization process.

pericardial Area between heart and sac enveloping the heart.

Peri pad Mass of material used to absorb vaginal flow.

peristalsis The slow, synchronized contraction of the involuntary muscles that make up the walls of the alimentary canal.

personal protective equipment (PPE) Clothing and equipment worn as a barrier for personal protection by staff members who handle potentially infectious debris or chemical substances. Protective attire includes fluid-resistant gowns, rubber or plastic gloves, high-filtration-efficient surgical facemasks, protective eyeware, etc.

Petri dish A shallow, covered plate made of plastic or glass.

Pezzer catheter A device with a particular retaining mechanism used for urinary suprapubic drainage and drainage of body cavities.

pH A measure of the hydrogen ion concentration of a substance; a measure of acidity or alkalinity; a scale of 1 to 14 with 7 being neutral, below 7 being acidic, and above 7 being alkaline.

pharmacy The art or practice of preparing, preserving, compounding, and dispensing drugs.

phenol A chemical substance derived from carbolic acid used in disinfectants, resins, plastics, and drugs.

phlebotomist A health professional trained to draw blood.

phlebotomy Entry into a vein with a needle for the purpose of letting blood out of the body.

physical therapy Treatment of injury and disease by mechanical or physical means, such as exercise, heat, light, and massage.

physiology The study of the body's functions; science of the functions of cells, tissues, and organs of the living organism.

pipette A glass or transparent plastic tube used to measure and transfer small quantities of liquid.

piston syringe Instrument used for irrigation.

plasma The liquid part of the blood in which the cellular elements are suspended.

policy A selected course of action; what will be done.

porous Full of pores; permeable.

postnasal balloon Device used to stop nasal hemorrhaging.

postnatal Occurring after birth.

PPE See *personal protective equipment.*

ppm Parts per million.

prefix Modifying word or syllable(s) placed at the beginning of a word.

prenatal Occurring before birth.

preparation area Designated place for the assembling, wrapping, and packaging of articles, trays, and basins prior to sterilization.

pressure gauge A device for indicating pressure, such as of the sterilizer jacket or chamber.

prions Virus-like agents that can cause serious diseases, thought to differ from viruses by not having any DNA or RNA.

probe A slender instrument used for surgical exploration.

procedure A series of actions to accomplish a task; a certain step-by-step way of doing something.

proctology A branch of medicine dealing with the structure and diseases of the anus.

proctoscope An endoscope used for dilating and examining the rectum.

prosthesis An artificial device to replace a missing part of the body.

protozoa Single-celled animals with no cell wall or with one composed of chitin, some of which live as parasites in the blood or tissue fluids of humans and animals.

psychiatrist A physician who specializes in psychiatry.

psychiatry The branch of medicine that deals with the study, treatment, and prevention of mental illness.

psychologist Professional who studies the mind.

pulmonary Pertaining to the lungs.

pus Yellowish-white fluid matter formed by suppuration and composed of exudate containing tissue debris and microorganisms.

Pyrex A hard glass made of borosilicate.

pyrogen An agent that produces or causes fever.

Q

quadriplegia Paralysis that affects all four limbs.

quality assurance (QA) A program to monitor, document, control, and improve the quality of services provided.

quality control (QC) A system of checks designed to provide high-quality processes.

quats Quaternary; relating to organic compounds in which the central atom is attached to four functional groups; i.e., quaternary ammonium compounds.

R

radiologist A physician specializing in the use of radiant energy for diagnostic and therapeutic purposes.

radiology The science of radioactive substances and high-energy radiations.

radiopaque Being impenetrable to various forms of radiation.

radiotherapy The treatment of disease by means of x-rays or radioactive substances.

ratchets The part of a hinged instrument that locks it in a closed position.

reagent Substance used in laboratory analysis.

recording graph An apparatus designed for ongoing graphical recording of the time, temperature, and duration of a sterilization cycle.

rectal Relating to the rectum; for example, a rectal thermometer is an instrument that reads body temperature on insertion in the rectum.

relative humidity A ratio between the amount of moisture in the air and that which would be needed to saturate it, expressed as a percentage.

renal Pertaining to the kidneys.

repetitive motion Repeating the same movement(s) over and over again, which can potentially cause injury.

reprocessing To cause to undergo special or additional processing before reuse. All the steps that are performed (which may include cleaning, functional testing, repackaging, relabeling, disinfection, or sterilization) to make a contaminated reusable or single-use device patient-ready.

residual Pertaining to a residue. The quantity left over at the end of a process; for example, after EtO sterilization most products retain residual gas.

respirator A device used to replace or assist breathing in a patient with respiratory problems.

resterilization The application of a terminal process designed to remove or destroy all viable forms of microbial life, including bacterial spores, to an acceptable sterility assurance level, to a device that has previously undergone a sterilization process.

restraint A device used to immobilize or hold back a patient.

reuse The repeated or multiple use of any medical device, including those intended for single use, with reprocessing (cleaning, disinfection, or sterilization) between uses.

rib belt Belt providing compression of the thoracic area that may be used following surgery or rib fractures to resist expansion.

rickettsiae Gram-negative bacteria, which, like viruses, can only multiply when they are inside living cells.

Ringer's solution Solution of sodium chloride, potassium chloride, and calcium chloride in water used for topical cleansing and irrigation.

Robinson catheter Hollow tube used for urinary or wound drainage or aspiration.

S

salicylates Aspirin and aspirin-related compounds.

saline An isotonic solution of sodium chloride and distilled water.

salpingogram An injection of a radiopaque dye into a fallopian tube in order to take an x-ray picture.

salpingo-oophorectomy Excision of a fallopian tube and ovary.

salpingopexy Surgical fixation of a fallopian tube.

sanitary Characterized by or readily kept in a state of cleanliness.

sanitary napkin Material used during menstruation to absorb the uterine flow.

sanitation The promotion of hygiene and prevention of disease by maintenance of sanitary conditions.

saturated Chemical or liquid added to a point where a substance can absorb no more.

scalpel A small, straight, thin-bladed knife used in surgery.

scalpel blade A razor-thin blade that adapts onto the knife handle.

scalp vein needle A device used to administer fluids via a vein.

SCIDS Severe combined immunodeficiency syndrome.

scrotum The skin-covered sac that contains the testes and their accessory organs.

secretions Substances produced by a gland.

sedimentation The process of solid particles settling at the bottom of a liquid.

sepsis A toxic condition resulting from the spread of bacteria in the bloodstream.

septic Partial decomposition or decay of organic matter by the action of microorganisms.

serology Laboratory study of serum and the reaction between antigens.

serrations Grooves in the jaws of instruments.

serum The watery portion of the blood after coagulation.

sheet wadding Mass of material used for orthopedic padding.

shelf life The time during which sterility of a product is assumed to be maintained; event-related.

shroud Sheet or robe used to cover or protect a corpse.

sigmoidoscope A device used to examine the sigmoid colon.

single-use device (SUD) A disposable item that is intended for use on one patient during a single procedure. It is not intended to be reprocessed (cleaned, disinfected, or sterilized) and used on another patient. The labeling may or may not identify the item as single use or disposable and does not include instructions for reprocessing.

skin graft Excision of a flap of skin from one area of the body (donor site) to be transferred to another area.

sling A brace designed to give support to the arm and hand for bone and ligamentous injuries.

smear Material obtained from infected matter spread over solid culture media.

sodium Major portion of extracellular fluids; plays a central role in the maintenance of the normal distribution of water in the body.

sodium chloride injection A sterile, normal saline solution used to mix drug compounds for injection.

sodium chloride 0.45 percent An intravenous solution used for fluid and body electrolyte replacement.

sodium chloride 5 percent An intravenous solution used for fluid and body salt replacement.

sodium lactate An intravenous solution used for fluid and electrolyte replacement.

soluble Capable of being dissolved.

solute A liquid, gas, or solid that is dissolved in a substance to make a solution.

solvent The substance into which a solute is dissolved.

specific gravity A measure of density ratio of weight of a given volume of a solution to the weight of the same volume of water.

specimen A sample used for analysis and diagnosis.

specimen kit Container used for collecting specimens.

spectrophotometer An instrument that can be used to determine the concentration of a solution by measuring the light transmitted or absorbed by the solution.

sphygmomanometer An instrument used for measuring blood pressure in the arteries.

spinal drape Covering for the spine during surgery or spinal anesthesia.

spinal puncture The removal of cerebrospinal fluid (CSF) for diagnostic purposes.

spinal tap tray A collection of instruments and supplies for use in puncture of the spine to obtain spinal fluid for analysis and to determine the pressure within the cerebrospinal cavities.

spirochete A slender, spiral microorganism.

spirometer Device used for intermittent positive pressure exercises.

splint An appliance designed for immobilization of fractures or ligamentous injuries.

sponge, gauze Material used to absorb blood and other fluids.

spore A microorganism that has adapted to withstand unfavorable conditions.

sporicidal Describing an agent's ability to kill spores.

sputum Expectorate; discharge of bronchial fluids or substances.

standard The level of requirement established as a measure or model; an item dealing with, for example, quantity, weight, extent, value, quality, or time.

standard precautions An approach to infection control. All human blood and body fluids are to be treated as if highly infectious with bloodborne pathogens, such as HIV, HBV.

stapedectomy Surgical removal of the stapes in the ear.

stat Abbreviation for Latin term "statim," meaning immediately or at once.

static Word element meaning inhibition of bacterial growth or reproduction.

steam sterilizer Device used for complete destruction of microorganisms by subjecting them to saturated steam under pressure at a particular temperature for a specified period.

STEL Short-term exposure limit; the maximum concentration to which workers can be exposed for a 15-minute period only 4 times throughout an 8-hour day, with at least 1 hour between exposures (not enforceable by OSHA).

sterile Free from living organisms.

sterile technique Practices designed to prevent microbial contamination.

sterility maintenance cover See *dust cover.*

sterilization Destruction of all living microorganisms by exposure to physical or chemical agents.

sterilizer A device used in destroying all living microorganisms.

sternal Pertaining to the sternum.

sternal puncture Procedure used to obtain a sample of bone marrow from the sternum.

sternoid Resembling the sternum.

sternotomy Incision through the sternum to expose tissue.

sternum A long, flat bone or cartilage at the center front of the chest connecting the ribs on the two sides.

stethoscope An instrument used to detect and study sounds produced in the body.

stockless A distribution method that involves the manufacturer or vendor delivering items as they are needed; very little inventory kept in the facility.

stoma Artificially created opening.

stomatitis Inflammation of the mouth.

stomatogastric Pertaining to the stomach and the mouth.

stopcock Instrument used to regulate the flow of fluid through a tube or pipe.

strabismus A weakness of the muscle of the eye.

stretcher A narrow, bed-like device with wheels used for transporting a person from one point to another.

subdural tray A collection of instruments and supplies used to relieve intracranial pressure.

sublingual Pertaining to under the tongue.

suction Sucking up by reduction of air pressure over the surface of a substance.

suction catheter Device used for removal of liquids or secretions such as those of the respiratory tract.

suction pump Device that provides suction by alternating the expansion and contraction of air within a cylinder at regular intervals.

suffix Modifying word or syllable placed at the end of a word.

supine Lying on the back.

surfactant A substance that facilitates the spreading of another substance.

surgery A room or department where surgeons perform operative procedures.

surgical gloves Gloves designed for natural fit, sensitivity, and comfort necessary for complicated procedures.

surgical prep Preparation of the operative site for surgery.

surveillance Process of monitoring closely.

suture A strand or fiber used for securing parts of the living body together.

suture removal set A collection of instruments and supplies used to remove stitches.

suturing The process of securing skin edges together.

swab A wad of absorbent material wound around a small stick.

synthesis The combining of elements to produce a compound.

syringe A device in various sizes used to inject or withdraw fluids.

T

technique A method of accomplishing a desired aim.

terminology Specific terms used in any specialized field.

test A means of analysis or diagnosis.

therapy A remedial treatment of a bodily disorder.

thermocouple Two lengths of wire, each made of a different homogeneous metal; used to measure temperature changes.

thermometer An instrument used to determine temperature.

thoracentesis The surgical puncture and drainage of the chest cavity for diagnosis of lung disease or removal of fluid from the thorax.

thoracic Pertaining to the chest.

thoracotomy The surgical incision of the chest wall.

thorax The cavity in which the heart and lungs lie.

thumb forceps Instrument used for grasping tissue or other objects.

tincture A chemical dissolved in alcohol.

tissue forceps Instrument that is serrated or has teeth; used for grasping tissue.

tongue depressor Instrument used to depress the tongue for examination of the mouth and throat.

tourniquet A band used to constrict the blood flow in the veins.

toxic Caused by a poison.

toxin Poisonous substance produced by certain bacteria.

TPN Total parenteral nutrition; parenteral hyperalimentation (intravenous administration of total nutrient requirements via a central venous catheter).

trachea Tube through which air passes to and from the lungs.

tracheotomy The act of cutting into the trachea through the neck, usually for insertion of a tube to provide an artificial airway.

tracheotomy catheter A device used for tracheal aspirations.

tracheotomy mask A covering used for providing oxygen and moisture through a tracheostomy.

tracheotomy tube A device used to provide a continuous artificial airway.

traction A pulling force exerted on a skeletal structure by a special device.

transfusion The process of injecting the blood or fluid of one person into the blood vessels of another person.

transurethral resection (TUR) Removal of a portion of the prostate through the urethra.

triage The sorting and allocation of initial treatment to patients.

trocar A device used to insert a cannula into a body cavity to create a drainage outlet.

tube feeding A method or procedure used to feed liquids into the stomach.

TWA time-weighted average; the amount of a hazardous substance beyond which a person should not be exposed in an 8-hour period.

U

ulcer A sore of the skin or mucous membrane.

ultrasonic cleaner A device that uses ultrasound waves in water to clean instruments by means of cavitation.

ultrasound An imaging modality that provides a method for visualizing internal body structure with sound waves.

underpads A soft, absorbent material placed under incontinent patients for protection of the skin.

ureteral catheter A sterile tube which is passed through the urethra, the bladder, and into the ureter to remove urine from the kidney.

ureter A tube that connects the kidney with the urinary bladder.

urethra A tube that connects the urinary bladder with the outside of the body and carries off the urine from the bladder.

urimeter A device used to collect urine and measure small amounts of output.

urinal A vessel for receiving urine.

urinalysis Chemical analysis of urine.

urinary bag A receptacle designed to collect urine when a catheter is in place in the bladder.

urination Passage of urine from the body, also called micturition.

urine Waste material that is secreted by the kidneys.

urinometer A small hydrometer used to measure the specific gravity of urine.

urologist A physician who specializes in the urinary or urogenital tract.

urology The branch of medicine that deals with the diagnosis and treatment of diseases of the urinary tract and of the male reproductive organs.

utility room Space used for the storage either of clean or of soiled materials and equipment.

V

vaccination To inoculate a person with a vaccine so as to produce immunity to a particular disease.

vagina A canal in a female that leads from the uterus to the external orifice of the genital canal.

vaginal packing Dressing material inserted into the vagina to medicate or stop vaginal bleeding.

vaginal speculum An instrument used for expanding the vagina to allow for visual examination of the vagina and cervix.

vaginal tampon A device to arrest hemorrhage or absorb secretions.

vasectomy Excision of the vas deferens or a portion of the vas deferens to produce sterility in the male.

vector An agent that carries pathogens from one host to another.

vein A blood vessel that carries deoxygenated blood to the heart.

venipuncture Entry into a vein by means of a needle.

venous pressure Measure of the pressure of the blood within the peripheral veins.

virucidal Describing an agent's ability to kill viruses.

virus One of a group of minute infectious agents composed of proteinaceous and genetic material that are capable of growth and reproduction only in living cells.

VRE Vancomycin-resistant enterococcus; a microorganism that is resistant to antibiotics.

W

washer/decontaminator A mechanical device used to wash bedpans, glassware, instruments, basins, decontaminator and trays, etc.; commonly used in the decontamination process.

washer/sterilizer A mechanical device designed to wash, disinfect, and sterilize instruments and metalware; most commonly used in the decontamination process.

wound An injury to the body.

Appendix B
Medical Terminology for Central Service Department Employees

An understanding of basic medical terminology is necessary for the employees of sterile processing and distribution. Many of the operations and procedures performed in the hospital or clinic and some of the supplies and instrumentation are described by medical terms that are derived from Greek or Latin. Medical terms are composed of a root word, which is sometimes combined with a prefix or suffix or both. Properly, Greek words should only be used with Greek prefixes and suffixes, and Latin words with Latin prefixes and suffixes. Sometimes a vowel, usually a, i, or o, is added between root words and prefixes or suffixes for euphony (the arrangement of sounds so as to be pleasing to the ear). Following is a list of the most common root words, prefixes, and suffixes used to form medical terms, and their definitions. "G" indicates those derived from Greek, and "L" indicates those derived from Latin.

Root Words

Acr- (G) pertaining to extremity

Aden- (G) pertaining to a gland

Andr- (L) pertaining to male, masculine

Angi- (L) pertaining to vessel, channel

Arterio- (L) pertaining to artery

Arthro- (L) pertaining to joint

Bio- (G) pertaining to life

Bleph- (G) pertaining to eyelids

Cardi- (G) pertaining to heart

Cephal- (G) pertaining to head

Cheil- (G) pertaining to lip

Cheir- (G) pertaining to hand

Chole- (G) pertaining to bile

Chondr- (G) pertaining to cartilage

Cleid- (G) pertaining to clavicle

Col-, colo- (L) pertaining to large intestine

Colp- (G) pertaining to vagina

Cost- (G) pertaining to rib

Crani- (L) pertaining to skull

Crypt- (G) pertaining to anything hidden

Cyan- (L) blue

Cyst- (G) pertaining to any fluid-containing sac, bladder

Cyt- (G) pertaining to a cell

Dacry- (G) pertaining to lachrymal glands

Dent- (L) pertaining to the teeth

Derm-, dermat- (G) pertaining to skin

Encephal- (G) pertaining to brain

Enter- (G) pertaining to intestine

Fibr- (L) pertaining to fiber, connective tissue

Galact- (G) pertaining to milk

Gastr- (G) pertaining to stomach

Gloss- (L) pertaining to tongue

Gynec- (G) pertaining to woman

Hem-, hemat- (G) pertaining to blood

Hepato- (L) pertaining to liver

Hyster- (G) pertaining to uterus

Iie-, Ilo- (L) pertaining to hip bone

Kerat- (G) pertaining to horn, cornea

Kopr-, copr- (G) pertaining to feces

Leuk-, leuc- (G) pertaining to anything white

Lymph- (L) pertaining to lymphs

Masto- (L) pertaining to breast

Mer- (G) part

Metr- (G) pertaining to uterus

My- (G) pertaining to muscle

Myc- (G) pertaining to fungi

Myel- (L) pertaining to bone marrow

Myel- (G) pertaining to spinal cord

Naso- (L) pertaining to nose

Neo- (G) new

Neph- (G) pertaining to kidney

Neuro- (L) pertaining to nerves

Ocul- (L) pertaining to eye

Odont- (G) pertaining to tooth

Omo- (G) pertaining to shoulder

Oo- (G) pertaining to egg

Oophor- (G) pertaining to ovary

Ophthalm- (G) pertaining to eye

Orchi- (L) pertaining to testis

Oss- (L) pertaining to bone

Oste- (G) pertaining to bone

Ot- (G) pertaining to ear

Ovar- (G) pertaining to ovary

Path- (G) pertaining to disease

Ped- (G) pertaining to children

Ped- (L) pertaining to feet

Pharyng- (L) pertaining to pharynx

Phleb- (L) pertaining to vein

Pneum-, pneumon- (G) pertaining to lung (pneum-air)

Polio- (G) gray

Proct- (G) pertaining to anus or rectum

Psych- (G) pertaining to soul or mind

Py- (G) pertaining to pus

Pyel- (G) pertaining to pelvis of the kidney

Rach- (G) pertaining to spine

Renal- (L) pertaining to kidneys

Rhin- (G) pertaining to nose

Sacr- (L) pertaining to tailbone

Salping- (G) pertaining to a tube

Sapr- (G) pertaining to pus or decomposition

Septic- (G and L) pertaining to poison

Spir- (L) pertaining to breath or breathing

Stomat- (L) pertaining to mouth or opening

Synovi- (L) pertaining to joint fluid

Teno- (L) pertaining to tendons

Thorac- (L) pertaining to chest

Thyro- (L) pertaining to thyroid

Tox-, toxic- (G) pertaining to poison

Trache- (G) pertaining to trachea

Trich- (G) pertaining to hair

Ureter- (L) pertaining to ureters
Uro- (L) pertaining to urine

Vas- (L) pertaining to vessel, duct

Zoo- (G) pertaining to animal

Prefixes

A-, ab- (L) away, lack of
A-, an- (G) from, without
Ad- (L) to, toward, near
Aer- (L) pertaining to air, gas
Ambi- (L) both
Ante- (L) before
Anti- (G) against
Auto- (G) self

Bi-, bin- (L) two
Brady- (G) slow

Circum- (L) around
Contra- (L) against, opposed
Counter- (L) against

Di- (L) two
Dis- (L) apart
Dys- (G) pain or difficulty

Ecto- (G) outside
Em-, en- (G) in
End- (G) within

Epi- (G) above or upon

Erythro- (G) red

Eu- (G) well

Ex-, e- (L) out

Exo- (G) outside

Extra- (G) outside

Glyco- (G) sugar

Hemi- (G) half

Hetero- (G) other (opposite of homo)

Homo- (G) same

Hyper- (G) above, excess of

Hypo- (G) under, deficiency of

Im-, in- (L) not

Infra- (L) below

Inter- (L) between

Intra- (L) within

Macro- (G) large

Meg-, megal- (G) great

Mesa- (G) middle

Meta- (G) beyond, over, change

Micro- (G) small

Mycet- (G) fungus

Olig- (G) little

Para- (G) wrong, irregular, in the neighborhood of, around

Per- (L) through, excessively

Peri- (G) around, immediately around (in contradistinction to para)

Poly- (G) many

Post- (L) after

Pre- (L) before

Pro- (G and L) before

Pseud- (G) false

Retro- (L) backward

Semi- (L) half

Sub- (L) under

Super- (L) above, excessively

Supra- (L) above, upon

Sym-, syn- (G) with, together

Tachy- (G) fast

Trans- (L) across

Tri- (G and L) three

Uni- (L) one

Suffixes

-algia (G) pain

-asis, -osis (G) affected with

-asthenia (G) weakness

-blast (G) germ

-cele (G) tumor, hernia

-clysis (G) injection

-coccus (G) round bacterium

-cyte (G) cell

-ectasis (G) dilation, stretching

-ectomy (G) excision

-emia (G) blood

-esthesia (G) (noun) relating to sensation

-genic (G) producing

-gram or -graph (L) picture, diagram of

-iatrics (G) pertaining to a physician or the practice of healing or medicine

-itis (G) inflammation

-logy (G) science of

-lysis (G) losing, flowing, dissolution

-malacia (G) softening

-oma (G) tumor

-osis (-asis) (G) being affected with

-(o)stomy (G) creation of an opening

-(o)tomy (G) cutting into

-pathy (G) disease

-penia (G) lack of

-pexy (G) to fix

-phagia (G) eating

-phasia (G) speech

-phobia (G) fear

-plasty (G) molding, reforming

-pnea (G) air or breathing

-poiesis (G) making, forming

-ptosis (G) falling

-rhythmia (G) rhythm

-rrhagia (G) flowing or bursting forth

-rrhaphy (G) suture of

-rrhea (G) discharge

-rrhexis (G) rupture

-scope (L) device used to view an object

-sthen [**-ia**] [**-ic**] (G) pertaining to strength

-taxia, -taxis (G) order, arrangement of

-trophia, -trophy (G) nourishment

-ulation (G) act of

-uria (G) referring to urine

An understanding of these various root words, prefixes, and suffixes will enable CSD employees to understand what other medical personnel are talking about when they use these words. It will also enable them to understand what supplies and instrumentation are being requested when these are described to them or asked for by an unfamiliar name.

To help employees to understand these terms, an explanation of various words follows. These terms and their definitions are presented according to the different body systems to which they refer, plus a miscellaneous category.

Skeletal System

achondroplasia Birth defect that results in abnormal development of the cartilage and bone, commonly called dwarfism.

arthritis Inflammation of the joint arthroplasty; molding or reforming of a joint.

arthroscope A device used to view a joint.

chondroma A slowly developing tumor growing from tissue or cartilage.

osteitis Inflammation of the bone.

osteoarthritis Inflammation of the bone and joint.

osteomyelitis Inflammation of the bone and bone marrow.

patellectomy Excision or removal of the patella (knee cap).

synovitis Inflammation of the synovial fluid.

Muscular System

fibrositis An inflammation of the connective tissue mingled throughout a muscle.

myelography A diagnostic test that shows a picture or chart of the spinal subarachnoid space.

myocardial pacing electrode A pacing electrode that is attached to the muscular layer of the heart.

myocardium A muscular layer of the heart.

myoma Tumor made of muscular tissue.

tendonectomy Excision of a tendon.

tenotomy scissors (Stevens, Westcott) Scissors used for cutting into tendons.

Nervous System

ataxia Lack of order or coordination of the muscles caused by a nervous system disorder.

encephalitis An inflammation of the brain.

encephalogram A chart or picture of the electrical activity of the brain.

intracranial pressure monitor A device used to measure the pressure of the spinal fluid in the cranial cavity.

meningitis An inflammation of the meninges, the membranes that encase both the brain and spinal cord.

neuralgia Pain in a nerve.

neuritis Inflammation of a nerve.

neurology The science of the nerves.

neurosis Being affected with a neurologic disorder, usually emotional in nature.

poliomyelitis An inflammation of the gray matter of the spinal cord.

Circulatory System

arteriogram A diagnostic test that maps the arteries and notes any abnormalities.

cardiology The science of the heart.

endarteritis Inflammation of the inner wall of an artery.

endocarditis Inflammation of the lining of the heart.

erythrocyte A red blood cell.

hemodialysis Dialysis (removal of impurities) of the blood.

hemorrhage A bursting forth of blood.

hypoglycemia Deficiency of sugar in the blood.

intravenous catheter A catheter placed inside a vein.

leukocyte A white blood cell.

phlebitis Inflammation of a vein.

septicemia Poisoned condition of blood.

tachycardia Rapid heart beat.

toxemia Poisoned condition of blood.

Respiratory System

anesthesia Without sensation; a partial or total loss of sensation.

bronchitis Inflammation of the bronchi.

bronchoscope Device used to view the bronchi in the lungs.

incentive spirometer Device used to measure breathing.

laryngectomy Excision, removal of the larynx.

nasal airway Airway inserted into the nasal passages.

pharyngitis Inflammation of the pharynx.

pneumatic powered instruments Instruments powered with air.

pneumonectomy Excision of the lung.

pneumonia Disease of the lungs.

thoracotomy Cutting into the chest.

tracheotomy Cutting into the trachea.

Digestive System

cholecystectomy Excision of the gallbladder.

colitis Inflammation of the colon.

colostomy Creation of an opening into the large intestine.

enteroptosis Falling of the intestine.

enterorrhaphy Act of sewing up a gap in the intestine.

gastritis An inflammation of the stomach.

gastroenteritis An inflammation of the stomach and intestines

gastroenterology Science of the stomach and intestines.

hepatitis Inflammation of the liver.

nasogastric tube A tube inserted through the nose into the stomach.

proctopexy Fixation of the rectum by suture.

proctoscope Device used to view the inside of the rectum.

Urinary System

cystitis Inflammation of the bladder.

cystoscope A device used to view the urinary bladder.

dysuria Difficulty urinating.

glycosuria Sugar in the urine.

hematuria Blood in the urine.

nephrectomy Excision of the kidney.

nephritis Inflammation of the kidney.

pyelitis Inflammation of the pelvis of the kidney.

polyuria Excessive secretion of urine.

suprarenal Above or on the kidney.

urethritis Inflammation of the urethra.

urology Science of the urinary system.

Reproductive System

colporrhaphy Act of sewing up a gap in the vagina.

galactose Milk sugar.

gynecology Science of diseases affecting women.

gynecomastia A condition in which males develop large breasts like females.

hysterectomy Excision of the uterus.

metritis Inflammation of the uterus.

oophorectomy Removal of an ovary.

orchiopexy Fixation of a testicle.

ovariorrhexis Rupture of an ovary.

prostatectomy Removal of the prostate gland.

spermatocele An intracoastal mass usually caused by an obstruction of the tubular system that conveys the sperm.

vasectomy Excision of a section of the vas deferens

Endocrine System

adenitis Inflammation of a gland.

adenoma Tumor of a gland.

adenopathy Disease affecting a gland.

adrenal gland A gland located near the kidneys.

hyperthyroidism Overactive thyroid.

hypothyroidism Underactive thyroid.

pancreatectomy Excision, removal of the pancreas.

pancreatitis Inflammation of the pancreas.

thyroidectomy Removal of the thyroid gland.

Sensory System

binocular Pertaining to both eyes.

blepharoplasty Molding or reforming of an eyelid.

dermatitis Inflammation of the skin.

dermatoid Skinlike.

ectoretina Outermost layer of the retina.

keratitis Inflammation of the cornea.

otorrhea Discharge from the ear.

otoscope A device used to view the internal structures of the ear.

ophthalmometer An instrument for measuring the eye.

ophthalmoscope Device used to view the internal structure of the eye.

percutaneous Through the skin.

rhinoplasty Molding or reforming of the nose.

Miscellaneous

ambidextrous Referring to both hands.

antiseptic Against or preventing sepsis.

aphasia Loss of ability to speak.

asepsis Without infection.

auscultation Listening for sound in the body.

autointoxication Poisoning by toxin generated in the body.

cytometer A device for measuring and counting cells.

endocrine Excreting inwardly.

exocrine Excreting outwardly.

hydrophobia Fear of water.

hyperthermia Over or above the normal body temperatures.

hypothermia Under or below the normal body temperature.

metastasis Change in site of a disease.

pathology Science of disease.

pediatrics Science of medicine for children.

pedograph Imprint of foot.

prognosis Forecast as to result of disease.

pyogenic Producing pus.

pyorrhea Discharge of pus.

transplant Transfer of tissue from one place to another.

Summary

As you can see, many medical terms have become a part of our everyday language. However, others are used only in discussions relating to health care. It is important for CSD employees to have a basic understanding of these terms to help them better perform their jobs by knowing how the various medical equipment and supplies are used in the treatment and diagnosis of diseases and injury.

Appendix C
Symbols Used by Device Manufacturers

Device manufacturers are using symbols in an attempt to reduce the need for multiple translations of information printed on packaging, to simplify labeling wherever possible, and to prevent separate development of different symbols to convey the same information.

The following symbols are currently being used by many manufacturers. These symbols are being reviewed by the International Standards Organization (ISO), which is a worldwide federation of national standards bodies. The European Standards Committee (CEN) has also reviewed these standards, and they are currently being used in Europe.

Note that the relative size and location of these symbols on the packaging materials varies. Also, be aware that some manufacturers have come up with their own symbols: you may need to consult these manufacturers directly to learn the meanings.

LOT	Batch code
	Biological risk
REF	Catalogue number
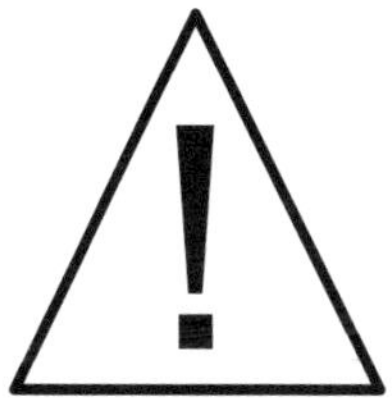	Caution. Consult accompanying documents

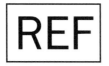

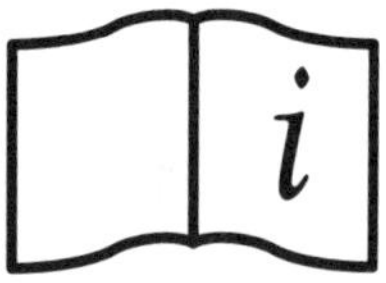

Consult instructions for use

CONTROL

Control

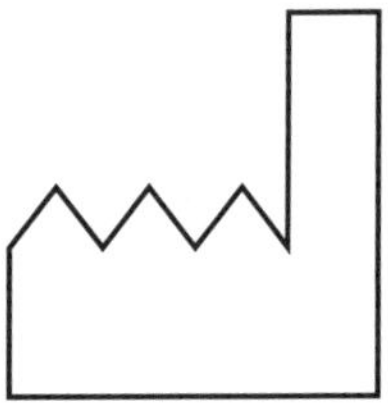

Date of manufacture

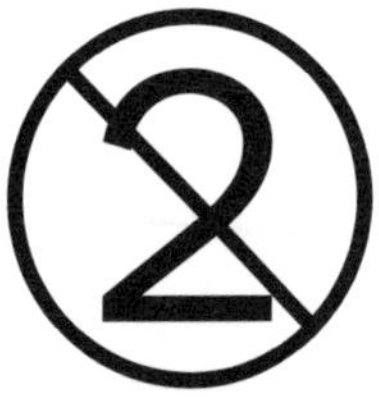

Do not reuse

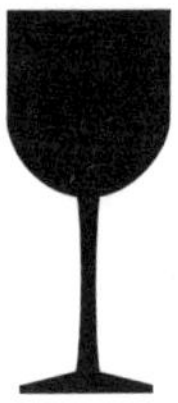

Fragile. Handle with care

Keep away from heat

Keep dry

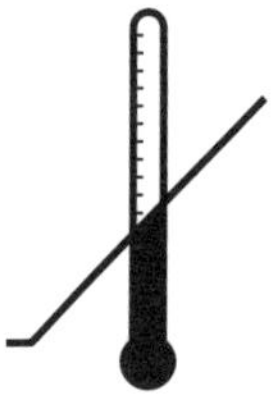

Lower limit of temperature

CONTROL –	Negative control
CONTROL +	Positive control
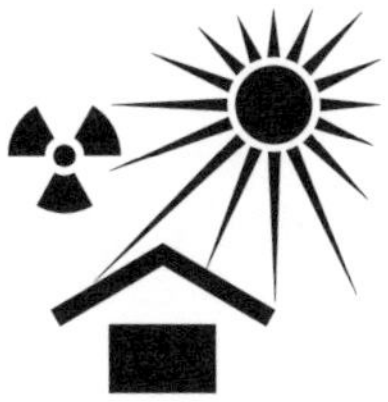	Protect from heat and radioactive sources
SN	Serial number
STERILE	Sterile
STERILE A	Sterilized using aseptic processing techniques
STERILE EO	Sterilized using ethylene oxide
STERILE R	Sterilized using irradiation
STERILE ǀǀ	Sterilized using steam or dry heat
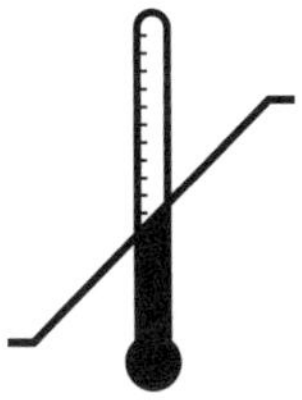	Temperature limitation

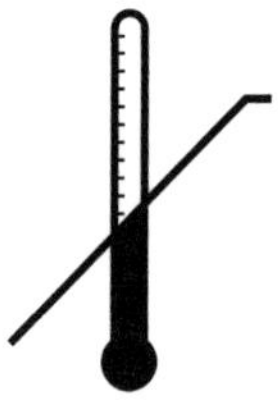

Upper limit of temperature

Use by

Bibliography

General

American Society for Healthcare Central Service Professionals. *Recommended Practices for Central Service: Continuous Quality Management.* Chicago: American Hospital Association, 1993.

Association for the Advancement of Medical Instrumentation. *Recommended Practices, Sterilization, Part I: Sterilization in Health Care Facilities.* Arlington, Va: Author, 2001.

Block, S. S. *Disinfection, Sterilization, and Preservation,* 4th ed. Philadelphia: Lea and Febiger, 1991.

Cokendolpher, J., and Haukos, J. *The Practical Application of Disinfection and Sterilization in Health Care Facilities.* Chicago: American Hospital Association, 1996.

Joint Commission on Accreditation of Healthcare Organizations. *Accreditation Manual for Hospitals.* Chicago: Author, 1996.

Perkins, J. J. *Principles and Methods of Sterilization in Health Sciences,* 2nd ed. Springfield, Ill.: Charles C. Thomas, 1983.

Reichert, M., and Young, J. H. *Sterilization Technology for the Health Care Facility.* Gaithersburg, Md.: Aspen, 1997.

Chapter One: Introduction to Central Service

American Society for Healthcare Central Service Professionals. *Recommended Practice for Central Service: Potential Injury Creating Events.* Chicago: American Hospital Association, 1996.

Friedman, B. B. "The Four C's of a Successful Central Sterile Supply–Operating Room Relationship." *Hospital Materials Management Quarterly,* Nov. 1990, *12*(2), 26–31.

Kennard, B. "A Realistic View of the Changing Role of Central Supply." *Hospital Materials Management Quarterly,* Aug. 1989, *11*(1), 32–35.

Marieb, E. N. *Essentials of Human Anatomy & Physiology.* Redwood City, Calif.: Benjamin Cummings, 1993.

Miller, J. K. "Microsurgical Instrument Systems Promote Handling with Care." *Materials Management Health Care,* June 1993, *2*(6), 27, 30.

Montague, J. "Breaking Away from On-the-Job Stress." *Materials Management Health Care,* June 1993, *2*(6), 18–21.

Murphy, Laurie J. *Techniques of Effective Telephone Communication.* Kansas City, Mo: *National Press Publications,* 1989.

O'Shaughnessy, K. L. "Steam Sterilization Costs: A Guide for the Central Service Manager. *Journal of Healthcare Materials Management,* July 1993, *11*(6), *40*, 42–45.

Sherwood, L. *Human Physiology: From Cells to Systems.* St. Paul: West Publishing Co., 1989.

Soltesz, S., Smith, S., Love, G., and Davis, P. E. *Quick Medical Terminology: A Self-Teaching Guide,* 3rd ed. New York: John Wiley & Sons, 1992.

Chapter Two: Human Anatomy and Physiology

Anderson, J. E. *Grant's Atlas of Anatomy.* Baltimore: Williams & Wilkins, 1978.

Gray, H. (T. P. Pick and R. Howden, eds.) *Gray's Anatomy.* New York: Bounty Books, 1977.

Kapit, W., and Elson, L. M. *The Anatomy Coloring Book,* 2nd ed. New York: HarperCollins, 1993.

Memmler, R. L., Cohen, B. I., and Wood, D. L. *The Human Body in Health and Disease.* Philadelphia: J. B. Lippincott, 1992.

Netter, E. H. *The CIBA Collection of Medical Illustrations.* (7 vols.). West Caldwell, N.J.: CIBA Pharmaceutical, 1953–1985.

Sherwood, L. *Human Physiology: From Cells to Systems.* St. Paul: West Publishing Co., 1989.

Smith, D. *Quick Medical Terminology: A Self-Teaching Guide,* 2nd ed. New York: John Wigeson, 1984.

Swan, R. *The Human Body on File.* New York: Facts on File, 1983.

Chapter Three: Microbiology and Infection Control

Association for Practitioners of Infection Control. "Guidelines for Handwashing and Hand Antiseptics in Health Care Settings." *American Journal of Infection Control,* Aug. 1995.

Association for Professionals in Infection Control and Epidemiology. *APIC Text of Infection Control and Epidemiology.* Washington, D.C.: Author, 2000.

Birnbaum, D. "Microbiology for Central Supply Workers." *Journal of Healthcare Materials Management,* Apr. 1992, *10*(3), 74–78.

Burton, G. *Microbiology for the Health Sciences,* 4th ed. Philadelphia: J. B. Lippincott, 1992.

Centers for Disease Control and Prevention. "Public Health: Surveillance, Prevention, and Control of Nosocomial Infections. *Journal of American Medical Association,* Dec. 2, 1992, *268*(21), 11–14.

Centers for Disease Control and Prevention. "Guidelines for Isolation Precautions in Hospitals." *American Journal of Infection Control,* 1996, *24,* 24–52.

Centers for Disease Control and Prevention. *Guideline for Prevention of Nosocomial Pneumonia.* Atlanta: Author, 1994.

Crow, S., and King, J. "Health Care Personnel's Perception of Infection Control." *Canada Journal of Infections Control.* Spring 1991, *6*(1), 16–19.

Gardner, I. E., and Peel, M. M. *Introduction to Sterilization, Disinfection, and Infection Control,* 2nd ed. New York: Livingstone, 1991.

Meers, P. D., Jacobsen, W., and McPherson, M. *Hospital Infection Control for Nurses.* San Diego: Singular Publishing Group, 1992.

Miller, C. H. "Cleaning, Sterilization and Disinfection: Basics of Microbial Killing for Infection Control." *Journal of American Dental Association,* Jan. 1993, *124*(1), 48–56.

Chapter Four: Decontamination

American Society for Healthcare Central Service Professionals. *Recommended Practices for Central Service: Decontamination.* Chicago: American Hospital Association, 1999.

Association for the Advancement of Medical Instrumentation. *Recommended Practice, Safe Use and Handling of Glutaraldehyde-Based Products in Health Care Facilities.* Arlington, Va.: Author, 1996.

Association of Operating Room Nurses. *Recommended Practices for: 1. Cleaning and Processing Anesthesia Equipment; 2. Chemical Disinfection; 3. Care of Instruments, Scopes and Powered Surgical Instruments.* Author, 1996.

Bonds, D. "Understanding Decontamination." *Journal of Healthcare Materials Management,* Oct. 1991, *9*(9), 78–79.

Fluke, C. "Cart Cleaning." *Journal of Healthcare Materials Management,* July 1991, *9*(6), 68–69.

Gurevich, I. "Efficacy of Chemical Sterilants/Disinfectants: Is There a Light at the End of the Tunnel?" *Infections Control Hospital Epidemiology,* May 1993, *14*(5), 276–278.

Gurevich, I., Yanneffi, B., and Cunha, B. A. "The Disinfectant Dilemma Revisited." *Infection Control Hospital Epidemiology.* Feb. 1990, *11*(2), 96–100.

Harrison, S. K., Evans, W. J., Jr., LeBlanc, D. A., and Bush, L. W. "Cleaning and Decontaminating Medical Instruments." *Journal of Healthcare Materials Management,* Jan. 1990, *8*(1), 36–42.

Russell, A. D. "Glutaraldehyde: Current Status and Uses." *Infection Control and Hospital Epidemiology,* Nov. 1994, *15*(11), 724–733.

Sierocinski, D. M., and Gore, R. J. "OSHA and the Decontamination Area." *Journal of Healthcare Materials Management,* June 1993, *11*(5), 62–65.

Souhrada, L. "OSHA Standard Prompts Questions from CS." *Materials Management Health Care,* May 1992, *1*(3), 30–32.

Weisman, E. "PPE (Personal Protective Equipment) Selection: Don't Ignore Employees' Concerns." *Health Facility Management,* Mar. 1993, *6*(3), 56, 58–60, 62–63.

Chapter Five: Instrumentation

Association of Operating Room Nurses. *Standards and Recommended Practices: Care of Instruments, Scopes, and Powered Surgical Instruments.* Author, Mar. 1992.

Becker, G. E. "Surgical Instruments: The Unmanaged Asset." *Journal of Healthcare Materials Management,* Apr. 1990, *8*(3), 40, 42, 44–46.

Great Plains Society for Hospital Central Service Personnel. *Instrument Manual.* Author: 1980.

Miller, J. K. "Microsurgical Instrument Systems Promote Handling with Care." *Materials Management Health Care,* June 1993, *2*(6), 27, 30.

Murphy, E. K. "Counts, Documentation Revisited." *Association of Operating Room Nurses Journal,* Oct. 1991, *54*(4), 875–878.

Reichert, M., and Young, J. H. *Sterilization Technology for the Health Care Facility.* Gaithersburg, Md.: Aspen, 1997, Chapter Four.

Ryan, P., and Romey, S. "Instrument 'Milk': The Controversy Continues: Survey on Instrument Lubrication." *Journal of Healthcare Materials Management,* Aug.-Sept. 1989, *7*(6), 26–36.

Smith, M. F., and Stelm, J. L. *Basic Surgical Instrumentation.* Philadelphia: W. B. Saunders, 1993.

Chapter Six: Preparation and Packaging for Sterilization

American Society for Hospital Central Service Professionals. *Recommended Practice for Central Service: Sterile Storage Inventory Management and Distribution.* Chicago: American Hospital Association, 1986.

Association for the Advancement of Medical Instrumentation. *Guidelines for the Selection and Use of Reusable Rigid Container Systems for Ethylene Oxide Sterilization and Steam Sterilization in Health Care Facilities.* ANSI/AAMI ST33–1996. Arlington, Va: Author, 1996.

Association of Operating Room Nurses. *Standards and Recommended Practices: Selection and Use of Packaging Systems.* Author, May 1996.

Fluke, C. "CSR Wrapping and Packaging." *Journal of Healthcare Materials Management,* Aug.-Sept. 1989, *7*(6), 77–80.

Mathias, J. M. "Why Use Double-Barrier Sterile Packaging?" *OR Manager,* Nov. 1991, *7*(11), 5, 9.

Taylor, W. "Anatomy of an Instrument Tray from Central Sterile Supply to the Operating Room." *Hospital Materials Management Quarterly,* Nov. 1990, *12*(2), 1–8.

Wells, M. P., and Bradley, M. *Surgical Instruments: A Pocket Guide.* Philadelphia: W. B. Saunders Co., 1993.

Chapter Seven: Sterilization

Alfa, M. "Plasma-Based Sterilization." *Infection Control and Sterilization Technology,* Mar. 1996, 19.

American Society for Healthcare Central Service Professionals. *Recommended Practice for Central Service Personnel Sterilization.* Chicago: American Hospital Association, 1994.

American Society for Healthcare Central Service Professionals. *Ethylene Oxide Use in Hospitals: A Manual for Health Care Personnel.* (3rd ed.). Chicago: American Hospital Association, 1998.

American Society for Healthcare Central Service Professionals. *Steam and Its Use in Sterilization: Resolving Observed Problems with the Purity of Steam.* Chicago: Author, 1985.

Association for the Advancement of Medical Instrumentation. *Good Hospital Practice: Performance Evaluation of Ethylene Oxide Sterilizers—Ethylene Oxide Test Packs.* AAMI EOTP-2/85. Arlington, Va.: Author, 1985.

Association for the Advancement of Medical Instrumentation. *Good Hospital Practice: Ethylene Oxide Gas—Ventilation Recommendations and Safe Use.* AAMI EOVRSU-3/81. Arlington, Va.: Author, 1987.

Association for the Advancement of Medical Instrumentation. *Good Hospital Practice: Steam Sterilization and Sterility Assurance.* AAMI ST46–2002. Arlington, Va.: Author, 2001.

Association for the Advancement of Medical Instrumentation. *Hospital Steam Sterilizers.* ANSI/AAMI ST8–1994. Arlington, Va.: Author, 2001.

Association of Operating Room Nurses. "Recommended Practices: Steam and Ethylene Oxide (EO) Sterilization." *Association of Operating Room Nurses Journal,* Oct. 1992, *56*(4), 721–730.

Association of Operating Room Nurses. "Recommended Practices for Sterilization in the Practice Setting." *1996 Standards and Recommended Practices.* Denver: Author, 1996, 271.

Emergency Care Research Institute. "EtO Monitors." *Journal of Healthcare Materials Management,* Apr. 1992, *10*(3), 60–67.

Emergency Care Research Institute. "Washer/Sterilizers." *Journal of Healthcare Materials Management,* Oct. 1991, *9*(9), 62–67.

Emergency Care Research Institute. "Sterilization Containers." *Journal of Healthcare Materials Management,* July 1990, *8*(5), 50, 52, 54–61.

Ferdinand, M. "Current Low Temperature Sterilization in the CS Department: Case Studies and Recommendations." *Infection Control and Sterilization Technology,* May 1996, 47–53.

Green, V. W. "Surgery, Sterilization and Sterility." *Journal of Healthcare Materials Management,* Mar. 1993, *11*(2), 46, 48–52.

Gschwandtner, G. "Aeration of Respiratory Therapy Items: Are You Really Aerating?" *Journal of Healthcare Materials Management,* Feb.-Mar. 1990, *8*(2), 48–49, 51.

Harris, M. H. "Flash Sterilization: Is It Safe for Routine Use?" *Association of Operating Room Nurses Journal,* June 1992, *55*(6), 1547–1551.

Hunstiger, C. *Maintaining Sterile Integrity in Hospital Sterilized Devices.* Chicago: American Society for Healthcare Central Service Professionals of the American Hospital Association, 1987.

Kaczmarek, R. G., and others. "Multistate Investigation of the Actual Disinfection/Sterilization of Endoscopes in Health Care Facilities." *American Journal of Medicine,* Mar. 1992, *92*(3), 257–261.

LaMontagne, A. D., and others. "A Participatory Workplace Health and Safety Training Program for Ethylene Oxide." *American Journal of Indiana Medicine,* 1992, *22*(5), 651–664.

Lind, N. "Just-in-Time Sterilization." *Infection Control Sterilization Technology,* Apr. 1995, 36.

Lind, N. "Sterilization Quality Control." *Journal of Healthcare Materials Management,* Feb. 1994, *12*(2), 62.

Lind, N. "Steam Sterilization." *Journal of Healthcare Materials Management,* Nov. 1994, *12*(11), 56.

Notarianni, G. "OSHA's Eye-Wash Standards." *Infection Control and Sterilization Technology,* May 1995, *1*(5).

OSHA. "Occupational Exposure to Ethylene Oxide, Final Standard." *Federal Register 49*(122), 25734–25809, June 22, 1984; *Code of Federal Regulations,* Title 29, Part 1910. Washington, D.C.: Occupational Safety and Health Administration, 1984.

O'Shaughnessy, R. "Steam Sterilization Costs: A Guide for Central Services Managers." *Journal of Healthcare Medical Management,* July 1993, *2*(6), 62.

Patterson, P. "Recommendations for Flash Sterilizing Implants Differ." *OR Manager.* Mar. 1992, *8*(3), 1, 12.

Reichert, M., and Young, J. H. (eds.). *Sterilization Technology for the Health Care Facility.* Gaithersburg, Md.: Aspen, 1997.

Reichert, M., and Young, J. H. "Part III: Sterilization and Disinfection." *Sterilization Technology for the Healthcare Faculty.* Gaithersburg, Md.: Aspen, 1997.

Steelman, V. M. "Ethylene Oxide: The Importance of Aeration." *Association of Operating Room Nurses Journal,* Mar. 1992, *55*(3), 773–775, 778–779, 782–783.

Stout, E. W., and Lado, E. A. "Practical Approach to Sterilization." *Today's FDA,* July 1990, *2*(7), 1C, 6C.

U.S. Dept. of Health and Human Services. *Ethylene Oxide Sterilizers in Health Care Facilities: Engineering Controls and Work Practices.* Cincinnati, Ohio: U.S. Dept. of Health and Human Services, Public Health Service, Centers for Disease Control, National Institute for Occupational Safety and Health, Division of Standards Development and Technology Transfer, 1989.

Widmer, A. E., Houston, A., Bollinger, E., and Wenzel, R. P. "A New Standard for Sterility Testing for Autoclaved Surgical Trays." *Journal of Hospital Infections,* Mar.-Apr. 1992, *14*(2), 20–25, 28–29.

World Health Organization. *Guidelines on Sterilization and High-Level Disinfection Methods Effective Against Human Immunodeficiency Virus (HIV).* Geneva: World Health Organization; Albany, N.Y.: WHO Publications Center USA, 1988.

Young, M. "Rapid Readout Biological Monitoring System." *Journal of Healthcare Materials Management,* July 1992, *10*(6), 74–75.

Chapter Eight: Sterile Storage

Brooks, L., and McDonald, S. "Do Receiving and Sterile Storage Mix? Only with Great Care, Say CS Experts." *Materials Management Health Care,* Apr. 1993, *2*(4), 36.

Fluke, C. "Handling Dropped Packaged Items." *Journal of Healthcare Materials Management,* June 1992, *10*(5), 74–76.

Mathias, J. M. "Sterility Assurance Replaces Expiration Dating." *OR Manager,* Mar. 1992, *8*(3), 1, 20–22.

Moss, M. T. "OR Supply Storage Takes on a New Look." *Association of Operating Room Nurses Journal,* Oct. 1991, *54*(4), 868–869, 872–874.

Chapter Nine: Distribution

American Society for Heathcare Central Service Professionals. *Recommended Practice for Central Service: Administration and Organization.* Chicago: American Hospital Association, 1989.

Becker, G. E. "Case Carts: Myths and Realities." *Journal of Healthcare Materials Management,* July 1991, *9*(6), 43–47.

Emergency Care Research Institute. "Surgical Case Carts." *Journal of Health Care Materials Management,* July 1991, *9*(6), 52–63.

Mathias, J. M. "What Makes a Case Cart System Work?" *OR Manager,* June 1992, *8*(6), 16–18.

Sommers, R. W., Chapelle, W. A., and Wooster, J. "Successful Implementation of a Par-Level Supply Distribution System: It's Everybody's Business." *Hospital Materials Management Quarterly,* May 1991, *12*(4), 44–52.

Wilson, J. W., Cunningham, W. A., and Westbrook, K. W. "Stockless Inventory Systems for the Health Care Provider: Three Successful Applications." *Journal of Health Care Marketing,* June 1992, *12*(2), 39–45.

Chapter Ten: Inventory Control

Bennett-Woods, R., and Wilver, M. "Is Stockless JIT Right for Your Organization? It Wasn't for Ours." *Journal of Healthcare Materials Management,* Mar. 1991, *9*(2), 24, 26–28.

Ferdinand, M. "Custom Case Carts: One Hospital's Approach to Controlling OR Inventory." *Journal of Healthcare Materials Management,* Nov.-Dec. 1989, *7*(8), 40–42.

Kerr, M. I. "Stockless/Just-in-Time: The Next Step in Inventory Management." *Journal of Healthcare Materials Management,* Mar. 1991, *9*(2), 14, 16, 20–22.

Russ, A. M. "Planning and Implementation of a Computerized Inventory System in Central Service." *Hospital Materials Management Quarterly,* May 1993, *14*(4), 55–59.